A CLINICAL GUIDE FOR CONTRACEPTION

SECOND EDITION

A CLINICAL GUIDE FOR CONTRACEPTION

SECOND EDITION

Leon Speroff, M.D.

Professor of Obstetrics and Gynecology
Oregon Health Sciences University
Portland, Oregon

Philip D. Darney, M.D., M.Sc.

Professor in Residence
Obstetrics, Gynecology and Reproductive Sciences
University of California, San Francisco
San Francisco, California

Illustration and Page Design
by Lisa Million, Portland, Oregon

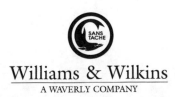

Williams & Wilkins
A WAVERLY COMPANY

BALTIMORE • PHILADELPHIA • LONDON • PARIS • BANGKOK
BUENOS AIRES • HONG KONG • MUNICH • SYDNEY • TOKYO • WROCLAW

Editor: Charles W. Mitchell
Managing Editor: Marjorie Kidd Keating
Illustration and Page Design: Lisa Million
Production Coordinator: Marette Magargle-Smith
Printer: Victor Graphics, Inc.
Binder: Victor Graphics, Inc.

351 West Camden Street
Baltimore, Maryland 21201-2436 USA

Rose Tree Corporate Center
1400 North Providence Road
Building II, Suite 5025
Media, Pennsylvania 19063-2043 USA

Accurate indications, adverse reactions and dosage schedules for drugs are provided in this book, but it is possible that they may change. The reader is urged to review the package information data of the manufacturers of the medications mentioned.

Printed in the United States of America

First Edition 1992

ISBN 0-683-18035-5

96 97 98 99
1 2 3 4 5 6 7 8 9 10

Dedication

This book is dedicated to our children, one son and seven daughters.
As Sherlock Holmes said: "You know my methods, use them!"

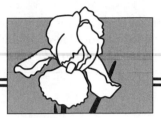

Preface

CONTRACEPTION, socially recognized and accepted only in the last 20 years, is both an essential and a complicated part of modern life. Contraception has separated sex from procreation, and has provided couples greater control and enjoyment of their lives. It is a critical element in limiting population, thus preserving our planet's resources and maintaining quality of life for ourselves and our children. Contraception is both a personal and a social responsibility.

The above accomplishments could not be achieved by the simple contraceptive methods employed before the late 20th century. Greater effectiveness and ease of use required more complicated methods, associated with greater consequences to our health. Intensive study of these issues has yielded an enormous wealth of information, making an informed choice possible but not easy.

In this book, we have distilled and formulated the information essential for the intelligent use of contraception. The current state of knowledge and variety of contraceptive options allow clinicians and patients to select methods best suited to an individual's personal, social, and medical characteristics and requirements. But even now science is still sometimes inadequate, and medical judgments must be made without the comfort of scientific support. In these situations we have expressed our opinion, reflecting our knowledge and our clinical experience.

In addition to our children, we dedicate this book to all health care professionals who have assumed the social responsibility of assisting couples to use safe, effective contraception. We hope our text will help you and your patients.

Leon Speroff, M.D.
Portland, Oregon

Philip D. Darney, M.D.
San Francisco, California

Contents

1

Contraception in the U.S.A.

A S SOCIETIES become more affluent, fertility decreases. This decrease is in response to the use of contraception and abortion. During her reproductive lifespan, the average !Kung woman, a member of an African tribe of hunter-gathers, experienced 15 years of lactational amenorrhea, 4 years of pregnancy, and only 48 menstrual cycles.[1] In contrast, a modern urban woman will experience 420 menstrual cycles. Contemporary women undergo earlier menarche and start having sexual intercourse earlier in their lives than in the past. Even though breastfeeding has increased in recent years, its duration is relatively brief, and its contribution to contraception in the developed world is trivial. Therefore, it is more difficult today to limit the size of a family unless some method of contraception is utilized.

More young women (under age 25) in America become pregnant than do their contemporaries in other Western countries.[2] The teenage pregnancy rates in 5 northern European countries and Canada range from 13 to 53% of the U.S. rate. The differences disappear almost completely after age 25. This is largely because American men and women after age 25 utilize surgical sterilization at a great rate.

It is obviously not true that young American women wish to have these higher pregnancy rates. American teenagers abort about half of their pregnancies, and this proportion is only slightly higher than that

2

seen in other countries. However, from ages 20–34, American women have the highest proportion of pregnancies aborted compared to other countries, indicating an unappreciated, but real problem, of unintended pregnancy existing beyond the teenage years. About half of all pregnancies in the U.S. are estimated to be unplanned and more than half of these are aborted.[3]

Another possible contribution to the problem of unintended pregnancy is the delay of marriage. Delaying marriage prolongs the period in which women are exposed to the risk of unintended pregnancy. This, however, cannot be documented as a major reason for the large differential between young adults in Europe and the U.S. The evidence available also indicates that a difference in sexual activity is not an important explanation. The major difference between American women and European women is that American women under age 25 are less likely to use any form of contraception.[2] Significantly the use of oral contraceptives (the main choice of younger women) is lower in the U.S. than in other countries.

Why are Americans different? The cultures in countries such as Canada and Britain are certainly very similar. A major difference must be attributed to the availability of contraception. In the rest of the world, contraceptive services can be obtained in more accessible resources and relatively inexpensively. In the rest of the world, contraception can be advertised on television. A further problem is the enormous diversity of people as well as the unequal distribution of income in the U.S. These factors influence the ability of our society to effectively provide education regarding sex and contraception, and to effectively make contraception services available.

The era of modern contraception dates from 1960 when oral contraception was first approved by the U.S. Food and Drug Administration, and intrauterine devices were re-introduced. For the first time, contraception did not have to be a part of the act of coitus. However, national family planning services and research were not funded by the U.S. Congress until 1970, and the last U.S. law prohibiting contraception was not reversed until 1973.

In 1966, a report from NASA placed our technological achievements into historical perspective.[4] Eight hundred lifespans can bridge more than 50,000 years. But of those 800 people:

- 650 spent their lives in caves,
- only the last 70 had a truly effective means of communication,
- only the last 6 saw the printed word,
- only the last 4 could measure time with precision,
- only the last 2 used an electric motor,
- and the majority of items which make up our current world were developed within the lifespan of the 800th person.

Contraception is not new; but its widespread development and application are new. It is in the latest tick of the Earth's timeclock, that safe control of fertility is now possible. This book is dedicated to that end. *This chapter will present an overview of the efficacy of contraceptive methods, a summary of contraceptive use in the U.S. and the world, and a brief look at the future.*

Efficacy of Contraception

A clinician's anecdotal experience is truly insufficient to provide the accurate information necessary for patient counseling. The clinician must be aware of the definitions and measurements used in assessing contraceptive efficacy, and must draw upon the talents of appropriate experts in this area to summarize the accurate and comparative failure rates for the various methods of contraception. A most helpful publication accomplishes these purposes and is highly recommended.[5]

Definition and Measurement

Contraceptive efficacy is generally assessed by measuring the number of unplanned pregnancies that occur during a specified period of exposure and use of a contraceptive method. The two methods which have been used to measure contraceptive efficacy are the Pearl index and life table analysis.

The Pearl Index. The Pearl index is defined as the number of failures per 100 woman-years of exposure. The denominator is the total months or cycles of exposure from the onset of a method until completion of the study, or an unintended pregnancy, or discontinuation of the method. The quotient is multiplied by 1200 if the denominator consists of months or by 1300 if the denominator consists of cycles.

4

With most methods of contraception, failure rates decline with duration of use. The Pearl index is usually based on a lengthy exposure (usually about a year) and therefore fails to accurately compare methods at various durations of exposure. This limitation is overcome by using the method of life table analysis.

Life Table Analysis. Life table analysis calculates a failure rate for each month of use. A cumulative failure rate can then compare methods for any specific length of exposure. Women who leave a study for any reason other than unintended pregnancy are removed from the analysis, contributing their exposure until the time of the exit.

Contraceptive failures do occur, and for many reasons. Thus "method effectiveness" and "use effectiveness" have been used to designate efficacy with correct and incorrect use of a method. It is less confusing to simply compare the very best performance (the lowest expected failure rate) with the usual experience (typical failure rates) as noted in the table of failure rates during the first year of use. The lowest expected failure rates are determined in clinical trials, where the combination of highly motivated subjects and frequent support from the study personnel yields the best results.

Failure Rates During the First Year of Use, United States [6]

5

Method	Percent of Women with Pregnancy	
	Lowest Expected	Typical
No method	85.0%	85.0%
Combination Pill	0.1	3.0
Progestin only	0.5	3.0
IUDs		3.0
Progesterone IUD	2.0	<2.0
Copper T 380A	0.8	<1.0
Norplant	0.2	0.2
Female sterilization	0.2	0.4
Male sterilization	0.1	0.15
Depo-Provera	0.3	0.3
Spermicides	3.0	21.0
Periodic abstinence		20.0
Calendar	9.0	
Ovulation method	3.0	
Symptothermal	2.0	
Post-ovulation	1.0	
Withdrawal	4.0	18.0
Cervical cap	6.0	18.0
Sponge		
Parous women	9.0	28.0
Nulliparous women	6.0	18.0
Diaphragm and spermicides	6.0	18.0
Condom	2.0	12.0

Contraceptive Use in the U.S.

The National Survey of Family Growth is conducted every 5–6 years by the National Center for Health Statistics. Data are available from 1972, 1976, 1982, and 1988.[7,8] The sample is very large, and therefore, the estimates are very accurate.

Contraceptive Status and Method in Women 15–44 in 1988 [7,8]

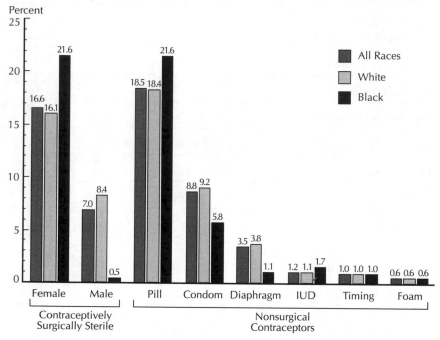

Contraceptive Use by Age in 1988 [7,8]

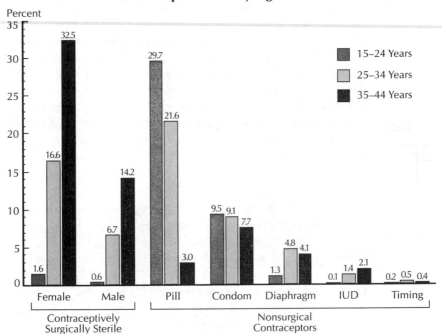

Percent

- 15–24 Years
- 25–34 Years
- 35–44 Years

Female: 1.6, 16.6, 32.5
Male: 0.6, 6.7, 14.2
Pill: 29.7, 21.6, 3.0
Condom: 9.5, 9.1, 7.7
Diaphragm: 1.3, 4.8, 4.1
IUD: 0.1, 1.4, 2.1
Timing: 0.2, 0.5, 0.4

Contraceptively
Surgically Sterile

Nonsurgical
Contraceptors

Changes in Contraceptive Use by Married Couples [7,8]

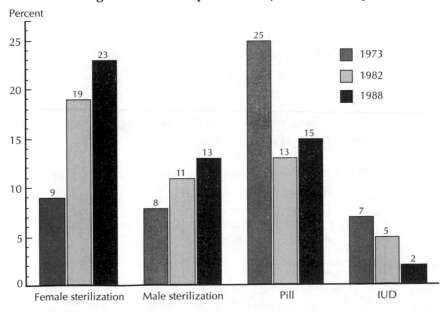

Percent

- 1973
- 1982
- 1988

Female sterilization: 9, 19, 23
Male sterilization: 8, 11, 13
Pill: 25, 13, 15
IUD: 7, 5, 2

8

The percent of married couples using sterilization as a method of contraception more than doubled from 1972 to 1988. In contrast, the percent of married couples using oral contraception declined sharply between 1973 and 1982. Recently, however, the use of oral contraception has increased, reaching new highs in the 1990s. About 10.7 million American women used oral contraceptives in 1988. Among never married women, oral contraception has been the leading method of birth control, and oral contraception is the favorite method for women who plan to have children in the future. Although condom use has not changed significantly among married couples, it did increase among never married women and is the second leading method.

In 1988, 60% of women, 15–44 years of age, were using contraception. Contraceptive sterilization was utilized by 24% of these women (the next leading method was oral contraception, 18.5%) The number of couples using the IUD decreased by two-thirds from 1981 to 1988, from 2.2 million to 0.7 million (7.1% to 2%). IUD use is concentrated in married women over age 35. A total of 35 million of the 57.9 million women of reproductive age were using some method of contraception in 1988, and this number has been relatively stable for the last several years.[9]

Of the 40% not using contraception, 7% were at risk of having an unintended pregnancy. Of the other 33%:

- 5% — sterilized for medical reasons,
- 1% — nonsurgically sterilized,
- 5% — pregnant,
- 4% — trying to get pregnant,
- 18% — not sexually active.

Thus, of those who are at risk of getting pregnant, 90% are using some method of contraception.

About 20 million women have one or more visits for contraceptive services per year in the U.S.

- 64% from a private doctor, group of doctors, or HMO,
- 36% from a public clinic.

A difference by race in contraceptive visits (greater among blacks) is present only until age 20. By ages 35–44, over half of women or their husbands are surgically sterile, either for contraceptive or medical reasons.

The Ortho Pharmaceutical Corporation performs an annual birth control study involving thousands of women.[9] According to this study, the current use of oral contraception by U.S. women aged 15–44 increased from 21% in 1984 to 25% in 1993, followed by a slight decline to 24% in 1994. Women are using oral contraception for longer durations (the average length of time in the 1994 Ortho Study was 5.8 years), and more older women are using oral contraception. Oral contraceptive use quadrupled from 1990 to 1993 in women aged 40–45. These changes undoubtedly reflect clinician and patient awareness of the greater safety in low-dose formulations. Besides the 24% of reproductive age women who are current users of oral contraception, 54% are former users; thus, 78% of women can be expected to be exposed to oral contraception at some point in their lifetimes. IUD use decreased from 4% of reproductive age women in 1984 to 1% in 1989, and this percentage has remained stable since then. Most IUD users (73%) are in the age group 35–50. The percentage of women using condoms has increased from 8% in 1979 to 19% in 1994, and most (74%) are under age 34. According to the Ortho Study, 45% of women use condoms only for contraception; 41% for both contraception and protection against STDs, and 14% only because of a fear of STDs.

10

1994 Ortho Annual Study — Method of Contraception [9]

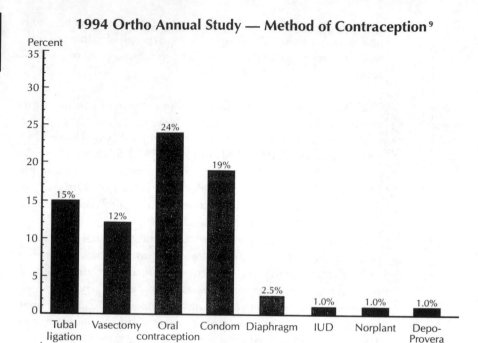

Percent

- Tubal ligation: 15%
- Vasectomy: 12%
- Oral contraception: 24%
- Condom: 19%
- Diaphragm: 2.5%
- IUD: 1.0%
- Norplant: 1.0%
- Depo-Provera: 1.0%

Sterilization
(27% of women age 15–50)

For added insight, it is useful to compare the choices of American women with Swedish women.[10,11] Swedish women mostly use oral contraception, condoms or the IUD; 95% of those exposed to risk of pregnancy practice contraception. Older Swedish women are more likely to rely on the IUD or barrier methods.

Contraceptive Choices in Sweden and the U.S. [10,11]

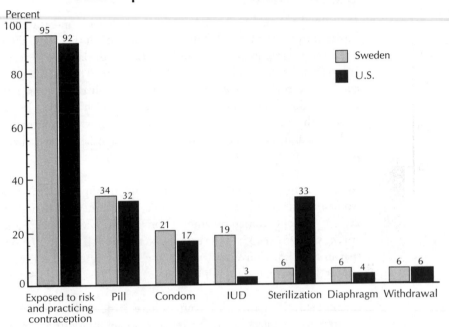

Abortion in the U.S.A.

The number of abortions performed in the United States has been decreasing in recent years, totaling 1.5 million in 1992.[12] About one-third of pregnancies not ending in miscarriage or stillbirth are terminated by abortion. The proportion of abortions performed in hospitals has steadily declined, reaching 7% in 1992. The proportion handled by specialized abortion clinics has increased, while the percentage of abortions performed by physicians in their own offices has remained low, about 3–5% of all abortions. More than 50% of abortions are obtained by women younger than 25, with the rate peaking at ages 18–19, and about 80% are unmarried.[12,13]

U.S. Characteristics

Malcolm Potts reviewed the history, development, and future of birth control in the United States.[14] He pointed out that while there was rapid progress in the 1960s and 1970s, over the last 10–15 years, "everything began to fall apart." Today U.S. women have fewer birth control choices than women in other industrialized nations, and contraception is more expensive. He concluded that these are the reasons that American women have higher rates of unintended childbirth and abortion compared to women in other industrialized nations.

Another contrast is oral contraceptive use among older married women. In the Netherlands, for example, it is nearly twice as high in 20–29 year old women as among comparable U.S. women, and among women over 35, the level in the Netherlands is nearly 10 times that in the U.S. Conversely, the total abortion rate in the U.S. is almost 3 times that of Dutch women.

It is not surprising that U.S. couples have made up for the lack of contraceptive choices by greater reliance on voluntary sterilization. With the current trend, it wouldn't be long before 3 out of 4 American couples choose sterilization within 15 to 20 years of their last wanted birth. During the years of maximal fertility, oral contraceptives are the most common method peaking at age 20–24. Most IUD users are concentrated between ages 35 and 50, and even here there are differences: four times as many French women over 40 use IUDs compared to American women.

Among 30–44 year olds, therefore, sterilization is the most utilized method of family planning. Between 1973 and 1982, oral contraception and sterilization changed places as the most popular contraceptive method among married women over the age of 25. The rate of sterilization among American women over 35 is about the same compared to Great Britain and the Netherlands, but under the age of 30 it is 50% higher in American women.

In the United States, there are no major differences in expected family size among the various religious groups, an exception being the higher level of family size desired by Mormons.[15] Religion does influence choice of contraceptive method; however, with Protestant levels of female sterilization higher than that of Catholics and

Catholic utilization of oral contraception and condoms higher than that of Protestants.[15]

In young women, the frequency of sexual intercourse is associated with the choice of contraceptive.[16] Young people who are very active sexually prefer oral contraception because it is perceived as very effective and allows sex to be worry free. As concern with AIDS grew, a more favorable attitude towards the condom emerged.

Another problem in the U.S. is the prevalence of misconceptions. More than half of women, even well-educated women, are not accurately aware of the efficacy or the benefits and side effects associated with contraception.[17,18] Unfortunately, a significant percentage of women still do not know that there are many health benefits with the use of oral contraception. Misconceptions regarding contraception have, in many instances, achieved the stature of myths. Myths are an obstacle to good utilization and can only be dispelled by accurate and effective educational efforts.

Worldwide Use of Contraception

The world population is expected to stabilize at between 10 and 11 billion by the year 2100.[19] Approximately 95% of the growth will occur in developing countries, so that by 2100, 13% of the population will live in developed countries, a decrease from the current 25%.

World Population

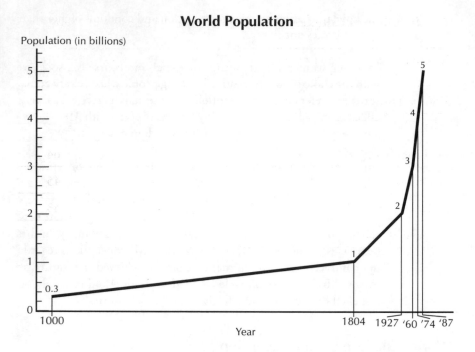

Throughout the world, 45% of married women of reproductive age practice contraception. However, there is significant variation from area to area; for example, 69% in East Asia, but only 11% in Africa. Female sterilization and the IUD are most popular in developing countries, while oral contraceptives and condoms are post popular in developed countries. Of the 400 million women of reproductive age, less than 60 million (15%) are using oral contraceptives, and more than half live in the U.S., Brazil, France, and Germany.

Number of Couples Using Birth Control Methods in 1986 [20]

Method	China	Rest of Developing World	Developed World	Total World
Female sterilization	53 mill.	45 mill.	15 mill.	113 mill.
IUDs	59	13	11	83
Oral contraceptives	9	28	27	64
Condoms	5	12	28	45
Male sterilization	17	18	8	43
Other methods	3	8	13	24

The 76% of the world's population living in developing countries accounts for:

- 85% of all births,
- 95% of all infant and childhood deaths,
- 99% of all maternal deaths.

The problem in the developing world is self-evident. The ability to regulate fertility has a significant impact on infant, child, and maternal mortality and morbidity. A pregnant woman has a 200 times greater chance of dying living in a developing country rather than in a developed country.[19] The health risks associated with pregnancy and childbirth in the developing world are far greater than risks secondary to the use of modern contraception.[21]

In recent years, there has been an appropriate shift from a narrow focus on contraception to a broader view that encompasses the impact of poverty, emphasizes overall well-being and the rights of individuals, endorses gender equality, and examines the interactions among these issues.[22] It is not enough to simply limit fertility. Contraception is only one component of reproductive health.

The Impact of Use and Non-Use

Inadequate access to contraception is associated with a high abortion rate. Effective contraceptive use largely, although not totally, replaces the resort to abortion.[23] The combination of restrictive abortion laws and the lack of safe abortion services continues to make unsafe abortion a major cause of morbidity and mortality throughout the world. Both safe and unsafe abortions can be minimized by maximizing contraceptive services. However, the need for safe abortion services will persist. Contraceptive failures account for about half of the 1.5 million annual induced abortions in the U.S.

In the U.S. in the late 1980s, $1 spent on public funding for family planning saved an average of $4.40 spent on medical, welfare, and nutritional services.[24] The investment in family planning leads to short-term reductions in expenditures on maternal and child health services, and after 5 years, a reduction in costs for education budgets. Contraception is cost-effective; preventing unintended pregnancies saves money.[25]

Cutting back on publicly funded family planning services impacts largely on poor women, increasing the number of unintended births and abortions. In California, in the 1980s, there was an average of $7.70 saved for every $1 spent to provide contraceptive services.[26] This estimate is higher than the national estimate because the income ceiling for eligibility is higher in California.

There is a gap between the low levels of unintentional pregnancy that can be achieved and the actual levels being obtained, most of which is in couples using reversible contraception. A major thrust, in addition to providing services, must include education and counseling of couples in effective contraception.

STDs and Contraception

The interaction between clinician and patient for the purpose of contraception provides an opportunity to control sexually transmitted diseseases (STDs). The World Health Organization estimates that by the year 2000, over 13 million women will have been affected with the human immunodeficiency virus (HIV).[27] The modification of unsafe sexual practices reduces the risk of unplanned pregnancy and the risk of infections of the reproductive tract. A patient visit for contraception is an excellent time for STD screening; if an infection is symptomatic, it should be diagnosed and treated during the same visit in which contraception is requested. A positive history for STDs should trigger both screening for asymptomatic infections and counseling for safer sexual practices. Attention should be given to the contraceptive methods which have the greatest influence on the risk of STDs. Unfortunately, according to the Ortho Annual Study, only 43% of the women who reported in 1994 that their contraceptive advice was received from a physician also experienced a discussion about STDs.[9]

Contraception and Litigation

Clinicians are concerned about the prospect of bad outcomes associated with contraceptive use leading to litigation. Multimillion dollar verdicts and settlements in favor of plantiffs who have used products as innocent as spermicides capture national attention. Actually, these events are very unusual compared to the widespread use of contraception.

The best way to avoid litigation is good patient communication. Patients who sue usually claim there were contraindications or risks that were not conveyed by the clinician. The best way to influence litigation is to keep good records. Good clinician's records are the most formidable weapon for the defense. Documentation is vital, but it is useless without thorough history taking. Good records and good history taking put the responsibility on the patient's honesty in response to the clinician.

> *Document that the risks and benefits of all methods were discussed.*
> *Document a plan for follow-up.*
> *Document all interactions with the patient, including phone calls.*

The Future

From 1970 to 1986, the number of births in women over age 30 quadrupled; however, since 1990, the fertility rate among women over 30 has remained relatively stable.[28] As more and more couples have defered pregnancy until later in life, the use of sterilization under age 35 should decline, and the need for reversible contraception will increase. In 1988, 75% of pill users were under age 30. Only 5% of women 35–44 used oral contraception, compared to 38% under age

25. These numbers will change as clinicians and patients understand and accept that low-dose oral contraception is safe for healthy, nonsmoking older women.

The percent of married couples using sterilization as a method of contraception more than doubled from 1972 to 1988. In contrast, the percent of married couples using oral contraception declined sharply between 1973 and 1982.[8] Nevertheless, the need for reversible contraception in women over the age of 30 is growing, not diminishing.

The highest ever number of births in the U.S. occurred between 1947 and 1965 — the post World War II baby boom. Women born in this period won't be through reaching their 45th birthday until around 2010. For approximately a 20-year period, therefore, there will be an unprecedented number of women in the later child-bearing years. It is estimated that the number of women ages 35–49 will increase 61% between 1982 and 1995. The proportion of births accounted for by this group of women will increase by about 72%, from 5% in 1982 to 8.6% in 2000.[29] This group of women is not only increasing in number, but it is changing its fertility pattern.

The deferment of marriage is a significant change in our society. In 1960, 28% of women 20–24 were single; in 1985, 58.5%. In 1960, 10% of women 25–29 were single; in 1985, 26%. But only 16% of the decline in the total fertility rate is accounted for by the increase in the average age at first marriage. Eighty-three percent of the decline in total fertility rate is accounted for by changes in marital fertility rates. In other words postponement of pregnancy in marriage is the more significant change.[30] This combination of increasing numbers, deferment of marriage, and postponement of pregnancy in marriage is responsible for the fact that we will be seeing more and more older women who will need reversible contraception.

In short, there will be longer duration of use in younger women and greater use in older women. Indeed, this pattern of use was being observed by 1990.

Change in Female Demographics 1985–2000 [31]

Age	1985	1990	1995	2000	% Change 1985–2000
15–24	19.5 mill.	17.4 mill.	16.7 mill.	17.7 mill.	-9.2%
25–29	10.9	10.6	9.3	8.6	-21.1
30–34	10.0	11.0	10.8	9.4	-6.0
35–44	16.2	19.1	21.1	21.9	+35.2
Total 15–44	56.6	58.1	57.9	57.6	+1.8

One solution to the problem of a restricted number of choices for American women is to develop new methods. However, experts are pessimistic when it comes to looking forward to new methods. There are many obstacles to the development of new methods, including the attitudes of the American public (Besides America's traditionally conservative, religion-oriented views towards sex and family, polarization is produced by responses evoked by specific issues such as sterilization and abortion.), the funding available for research, the time and cost required to meet federal regulations, and the problems of product liability.[32]

Fortunately clinicians and patients have recognized that low dose oral contraception is very safe for healthy, nonsmoking older women. However, as the above statistics indicate, their use is still not sufficient to meet the need. Besides fulfilling a need, this population of women has a series of benefits to be derived from oral contraception that tilt the risk/benefit ratio to the positive side. The following benefits are especially pertinent for older women:

> **Effective contraception**
> > • **less need for therapeutic abortion**
> > • **less need for surgical sterilization**
> **Less endometrial cancer**
> **Less ovarian cancer**
> **Fewer ovarian cysts**
> **Fewer ectopic pregnancies**

More regular menses
- less flow
- less dysmenorrhea
- less anemia

Less salpingitis

Less rheumatoid arthritis

Increased bone density

Probably less endometriosis

Possibly protection against atherosclerosis

Possibly less benign breast disease

Possibly fewer uterine fibroids

The growing need for reversible contraception would also be served by increased utilization of the IUD. After several years of use, efficacy with the IUD is similar to that of oral contraceptives. The decline in IUD use in the U.S. is in direct contrast to the experience in the rest of the world, a complicated response to publicity and litigation. An increased risk of pelvic infection with contemporary IUDs in use is limited to the act of insertion and the transportation of pathogens to the upper genital tract. This risk is effectively minimized by careful screening with pre-insertion cultures and the use of good technique. A return to IUD use by American couples is both warranted and desirable.

Contraceptive advice is a component of good preventive health care. The approach is a key. This is an era of informed choice by the patient. Patients deserve to know the facts and need help in dealing with the state of the art and the uncertainty. But there is no doubt that patients, especially young patients, are influenced in their choice by their clinician's advice and attitude. While the role of a clinician is to provide the education necessary for the patient to make proper choices, one should not lose sight of the powerful influence exerted by the clinician in the choices ultimately made.

If one attempts to sum up the impact of the benefits of contraception on public health, as some have done with models focusing on hospital admissions, there is no doubt that the benefits outweigh the risks. The impact can be measured in terms of both morbidity and mortality. But the impact on public health is of little concern during the private clinician-patient interchange in the medical office. Here personal risk is paramount, and compliance with effective contraception requires accurate information.

In our view, the attitude of the clinician is a crucial influence on the ultimate patient take home message. In the 70s we approached the patient with great emphasis on risk. In the 90s the approach should be different, highlighting the benefits and the greater safety of appropriate contraception.

The challenge for the next 20 years is to do as Sherlock Holmes said: "You know my methods, use them."[33] A stable global population of about 8–10 billion is possible. Without better contraceptive education and services, global population could reach 15 billion before stabilization.

22

References

1. **Djerassi C,** *The Politics of Contraception, Vol I. The Present,* Stanford Alumni Association, Stanford, California, 1979.

2. **Westoff CF,** Unintended pregnancy in America and abroad, Fam Plann Perspect 20:254, 1988.

3. **Harlap S, Kost K, Forrest JD,** *Preventing pregnancy, protecting health: a new look at birth control choices in the United States,* The Alan Guttmacher Institute, New York, 1991.

4. **Lesher RL, Howick GJ,** Assessing technology transfer, NASA Report SP-50671, 1966.

5. **Trussell J, Hatcher RA, Cates W Jr, Stewart FH, Kost K,** A guide to interpreting contraceptive efficacy studies, Obstet Gynecol 76:558, 1990.

6. **Trussell J, Hatcher RA, Cates W Jr, Stewart FH, Kost K,** Contraceptive failure in the United States: an update, Stud Fam Plann 21:51, 1990.

7. **Mosher WD, Pratt WF,** Contraceptive use in the United States, 1973–88, Advance data from vital and health statistics; No. 182, National Center for Health Statistics, Hyattsville, Maryland, 1990.

8. **Mosher WD,** Use of family planning services in the United States: 1982 and 1988, Advance data from vital and health statistics, No. 184, National Center for Health Statistics, Hyattsville, Maryland, 1990.

9. **Ortho Pharmaceutical Corporation,** Annual birth control study, 1994.

10. **Forrest JD, Fordyce RR,** U.S. women's contraceptive attitudes and practice: How have they changed in the 1980s? Fam Plann Perspect 20:112, 1988.

11. **Riphagen FE, von Schoultz B,** Contraception in Sweden, Contraception 39:633, 1989.

12. **Henshaw SK, Van Vort J,** Abortion services in the United States, 1991 and 1992, Fam Plann Perspect 26:100, 1994.

13. **Henshaw SK,** Induced abortion: a world review, 1990, Fam Plann Perspect 22:76, 1990.

14. **Potts M,** Birth control methods in the United States, Fam Plann Perspect 20:288, 1988.

15. **Goldscheider C, Mosher WD,** Patterns of contraceptive use in the United States: the importance of religious factors, Studies Fam Plann 22:102, 1991.

16. **Glor JE, Severy LJ,** Frequency of intercourse and contraceptive choice, J Biosoc Sci 22:231, 1990.

17. **Peipert JF, Gutmann J,** Oral contraceptive risk assessment: a survey of 247 educated women, Obstet Gynecol 82:112, 1993.

18. Murphy P, Kirkman A, Hale RW, A national survey of women's attitudes toward oral contraception and other forms of birth control, Women's Health Issues 5:94, 1995

19. Diczfalusy E, The worldwide use of steroidal contraception, Int J Fertil 34 (Supplement):56, 1989.

20. Population Crisis Committee, Access to birth control: a world assessment, Population Briefing Paper No. 19, Washington, DC, 1986.

21. DaVanzo J, Parnell AM, Foege WH, Health consequences of contraceptive use and reproductive patterns: summary of a report from the US National Research Council, JAMA 265:2692, 1991.

22. Garcia-Moreno C, Türmen T, International perspectives on women's reproductive health, Science 269:790, 1995.

23. Potts M, Rosenfield A, The fifth freedom revisited: I. Background and existing programs, Lancet 336:1227, 1990.

24. Forrest JD, Singh S, Public-sector savings resulting from expenditures for contraceptive services, Fam Plann Perspect 22:6, 1990.

25. Forrest JD, Singh S, The impact of public-sector expenditures for contraceptive services in California, Fam Plann Perspect 22:161, 1990.

26. Trussell J, Leveque JA, Koenig JD, London R, Borden S, Henneberry J, LaGuardia KD, Stewart F, Wilson TG, Wysocki S, Strauss M, The economic value of contraception: a comparison of 15 methods, Am J Public Health 85:494, 1995.

27. World Health Organization, *Women's Health,* Geneva, 1994.

28. Ventura SJ, et al, Advance report of final natality statistics, 1992, *Monthly Vital Statistics Report,* Vol. 43, No. 5, Supplement, 1994.

29. Spencer G, Projections of the population of the United States, by age, sex, and race: 1983–2080. Current Population Reports — Population Estimates and Projections, US Department of Commerce, Series P-25, No. 952, 1984.

30. Westoff CF, Fertility in the United States, Science 234:554, 1986.

31. Spencer G, Projections of the population of the United States by age, sex and race: 1988–2080, Current Population Reports 1989, Series P-25, No. 1018, GPO, Washington, DC, 1989.

32. Mastroianni L Jr, Donaldson PJ, Kane TT, editors, *Developing New Contraceptives: Obstacles and Opportunities,* National Academy Press, Washington, DC, 1990.

33. Doyle AC, *The Sign of Four.*

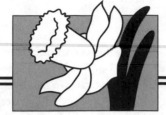

2

Oral Contraception

CONTRACEPTION is commonly viewed as a modern event, a recent development in human history. On the contrary, efforts to limit reproduction predate our ability to write about it. It is only oral contraception with synthetic sex steroids that is recent.

History[1,2]

It wasn't until the early 1900s, that inhibition of ovulation was observed to be linked to pregnancy and the corpus luteum. Ludwig Haberlandt, professor of physiology at the University of Innsbruck, Austria, was the first to demonstrate that ovarian extracts given orally could prevent fertility (in mice). In the 1920s, Haberlandt and a Viennese gynecologist, Otfried Otto Fellner, were administering steroid extracts to a variety of animals and reporting the inhibition of fertility. By 1931, Haberlandt was proposing the administration of hormones for birth control. An extract was produced, named Infecundin, ready to be used, but Haberlandt's early death in 1932, at age 47, brought an end to this effort. Fellner disappeared after the annexation of Austria to Hitler's Germany.

The concept was annunciated by Haberlandt, but steroid chemistry wasn't ready. The extraction and isolation of a few milligrams of the sex steroids required starting points measured in gallons of urine, or thousands of pounds of organs. Edward Doisy processed 80,000 sow ovaries to produce 12 mg of estradiol.

25

Russell Marker

The supply problem was solved by an eccentric chemist, Russell E. Marker, who completed his thesis, but not his course work, for his Ph.D. Marker, born in 1902 near Hagerstown, Maryland, received his Bachelor's degree in organic chemistry and his Master's degree in colloidal chemistry from the University of Maryland. After leaving the University of Maryland, Marker worked with the Ethyl Gasoline Corporation, and in 1926, developed the process of octane rating, based on the discovery that knocking in gasoline was due to hydrocarbons with an uneven number of carbons.

From 1927 to 1935, Marker worked at the Rockefeller Institute, publishing a total of 32 papers on configuration and optical rotation as a method of identifying compounds. He became interested in solving the problem of producing abundant and cheap amounts of progesterone, but he was told to continue with his work in optical technology. In 1935, he moved to Pennsylvania State University at a reduced salary, but with the freedom to pursue any field of research. At that time it required the ovaries from 2,500 pregnant pigs to produce 1 mg of progesterone. In 1939, Marker devised the method (called the Marker degradation) to covert a sapogenin molecule into a progestin. Marker became convinced that the solution to the problem of obtaining large quantities of steroid hormones was to find plants (in the family that includes the lily, the agave, and the yam) that contained sufficient amounts of diosgenin, a plant steroid (a sapogenin) which could be used as a starting point for steroid hormone production. This conviction was strengthened with his discovery that a species of *Trillium,* known locally as Beth's root, was collected in North Carolina and used in the preparation of Lydia Pinkham's Compound, popular at the time to relieve menstrual troubles. The active ingredient in Beth's root was diosgenin, but the rhizome was too small to provide sufficient amounts for commercial production. Marker's search for an appropriate plant took him to California, Arizona, and Texas.

On a visit to Texas A & M University, Marker found a picture of a large dioscorea (*Dioscorea mexicana)* in a book that he just happened to pick up and browse through while spending the night at the home of a retired botanist. After returning to Pennsylvania, he decided to go to Veracruz, Mexico, (it took 3 days by train) to search for this dioscorea. He made several attempts in 1941 and early 1942, but was frustrated first by the lack of a plant-collecting permit from the

Mexican government and then by his failure to find the plant. He remembered that the book with the picture reported that this dioscorea was known locally as "cabeza de negro," black tubers that grew near Orizaba and Cordoba. Marker took a bus to Cordoba, and near Orizaba, an Indian who owned a small store brought him two plants. Each tuber was 9–12 inches high and consisted of a white material like a turnip, used by local Mexicans as a poison to catch fish.

Marker managed to get one bag of tubers back to Penn State and isolated diosgenin. Unable to obtain support from the pharmaceutical industry, Marker used his life savings and in 1942, he returned to Veracruz, collected the roots of the Mexican yam, and prepared a syrup from the roots. Back in Pennsylvania with his 5-gallon cans of syrup, Marker worked out the degradation of diosgenin to progesterone. One 5-gallon can yielded 3 kg of progesterone. United States pharmaceutical companies refused to back Marker, and even the University refused, despite Marker's urging, to patent the process.

In 1943, Marker resigned from Pennsylvania State University and went to Mexico where he collected the roots of *Dioscorea mexicana,* ten tons worth! Looking through the yellow pages in a Mexico City telephone directory, Marker found a company called Laboratorios Hormona, owned by a lawyer, Emeric Somlo, and a physician, Frederick Lehman. Marker arranged a meeting, and the three agreed to form a Mexican company to produce hormones. In an old pottery shed in Mexico City (the laboratories of Laboratorios Hormona), in two months, he prepared several pounds of progesterone (worth $300,000) with the help of four young women who had little education and spoke no English (Marker did not speak Spanish). The two partners and Marker formed a company in 1944 which they called Syntex (from *synthesis* and *Mexico*). In 1944, Marker produced over 30 kg of progesterone. The price of progesterone fell from $200 to $50 a gram.

During this time, Marker received expenses, but he was not given his share of the profits or the 40% share of stock due to him. Failing to reach a settlement, Marker left Syntex after only one year and started a new company in Texcoco, called Botanica-Mex. He changed to *Dioscorea barbasco,* which gave a greater yield of diosgenin, and the price of progesterone dropped to $10 a gram, and later to $5. This company was allegedly harassed (legally and physically) by Syntex, and in 1946, sold, eventually reaching ownership by Organon of Holland, which still uses it.

In 1949, Marker retired to Pennsylvania to devote the rest of his life to making replicas of antique works in silver, a successful business that allowed him, in the 1980s, to endow scientific lectureships at both Pennsylvania State University and the University of Maryland. However, he took his knowhow with him. Fortunately for Syntex, he had published a scientific description of his process, and there still was no patent on his discoveries. Syntex recruited George Rosenkranz, a Hungarian immigrant living in Cuba, to reinstitute the commercial manufacture of progesterone (and testosterone) from Mexican yams, a task which took him (with the help of the women left behind by Marker) 2 years.

In 1970, the Mexican government recognized Marker and awarded him the Order of the Aztec Eagle; he declined. In 1984, Pennsylvania State University established the annual Marker Lectures in Science, and in 1987, the Russell and Mildred Marker Professorship of Natural Product Chemistry. In 1987, Marker was granted an honorary Doctorate in Science from the University of Maryland, the degree he failed to receive in 1926. At the age of 92, Russell Earl Marker died in Wernersville, Pennsylvania, in 1995, from complications after a broken hip.

Carl Djerassi[3]

The Djerassi family lived in Bulgaria for hundreds of years after escaping Spain during the Inquisition. Carl Djerassi, the son of a Bulgarian physician, was born in Vienna (as was his physician mother). Djerassi, at the age of 16, and his mother emigrated to the United States in 1939. A Jewish refugee aid organization placed Djerassi with a family in Newark, New Jersey. With a scholarship to Tarkio College in Tarkio, Missouri, he was exposed to middle America, where he earned his way giving talks to church groups about Bulgaria and Europe. His education was further supported by another scholarship from Kenyon College in Ohio, where he pursued chemistry. After a year working for CIBA, Djerassi received his graduate degree from the University of Wisconsin. Returning to CIBA and being somewhat unhappy, he responded to an invitation to visit Syntex. Rosenkranz proposed that Djerassi head a research group to concentrate on the synthesis of cortisone.

In 1949, it was discovered that cortisone relieved arthritis, and the race was on to develop an easy and cheap method to synthesize cortisone. Carl Djerassi, at age 26, joined Syntex to work on this synthesis using the Mexican yam plant steroid diosgenin as the starting point. This was quickly achieved (in 1951), but soon after, an even better method of cortisone production was discovered at Upjohn, using microbiologic fermentation. This latter method used progesterone as the starting point, and therefore, Syntex found itself as the key supplier to other companies for this important process, at the rate of 10 tons of progesterone per year and a price of 48 cents per gram.

Djerassi and other Syntex chemists then turned their attention to the sex steroids. They discovered that the removal of the 19 carbon from yam-derived progesterone increased the progestational activity of the molecule. Ethisterone had been available for a dozen years, and the Syntex chemists reasoned that removal of the 19 carbon would increase the progestational potency of this orally active compound. In 1951, norethindrone was synthesized; the patent for this drug is the first patent for a drug listed in the National Inventor's Hall of Fame in Akron, Ohio. A closely related compound, norethynodrel, was actually the first orally active progestational agent to receive a patent, assigned to Frank Colton, a chemist at G.D. Searle & Company.

Gregory Pincus

Gregory Goodwin (Goody) Pincus was born in 1903 in New Jersey, the son of Russian Jewish immigrants who lived on a farm colony founded by a German-Jewish philanthropic organization. Pincus was the oldest of 6 children and grew up in a home of intellectual curiosity and energy, but even his family regarded him as a genius.

Pincus graduated from Cornell and went to Harvard to study genetics, joining Hudson Hoagland and B.F. Skinner as graduate students of W.J. Crozier in physiology, receiving degrees in 1927. Crozier's hero was Jacques Loeb who discovered artificial partheno-genesis working with sea urchin eggs. Most importantly, Loeb was a strong believer in applying science to improve human life. Thus Crozier, influenced by Loeb, taught Pincus, Hoagland, and Skinner (respectively, in reproductive biology, neurophysiology, and psychology) to apply science to human problems. This was to be the cornerstone of Pincus's own philosophy.

Hoagland, after a short stay at Harvard, spent a year in Cambridge, England, then moved to Clark University in Worcester, Massachusetts, to be the chair of biology at the age of 31. Pincus went to England and Germany, and returned to Harvard as an assistant professor of physiology.

Pincus performed pioneering studies of meiotic maturation in mammalian oocytes, in both rabbit and human oocytes. In 1934, Pincus reported the achievement of in vitro fertilization of rabbit eggs, earning him a headline in the New York Times that alluded to Haldane and Huxley. An article in Colliers depicted him as an evil scientist. By 1936, Harvard had cited Pincus's work as one of the university's outstanding scientific achievements of all time, but Harvard denied him tenure in 1937.

At Clark University, Hudson Hoagiand was in constant conflict with the president of the university, Wallace W. Atwood, the senior author of a widely used textbook on geography. In 1931, the Department of Biology consisted of one faculty member and his graduate student, and their chair, Hudson Hoagland. Hoagland, upset and angry over Harvard's refusal to grant tenure to his friend (suspecting that this was because of anti-Semitism), invited Pincus to join him.

Hoagland secured funds for Pincus from philanthropists in New York City, enough for a laboratory and an assistant. This success impressed the two men, especially Hoagland, planting the idea that it would be possible to support research with private money.

Min-Chueh Chang received his Ph.D. degree from Harvard on an infamous day, December 7, 1941, and thus he was forced to remain in this country. He was drawn to Pincus because of Pincus's book, *The Eggs of Mammals,* published in 1936, a book that had a major impact on biologists at that time. The successful recruitment of M-C Chang by Hoagland and Pincus was to pay great dividends.

Soon Hoagland had put together a group of outstanding scientists, but because of his on-going antagonism with President Atwood, the group was denied faculty status. Working in a converted barn, they were totally supported by private funds. By 1943, 12 of Clark's 60 faculty were in the department of biology.

Frustrated by the politics of academia, Hoagland and Pincus (who both enjoyed stepping outside of convention) had a vision of a private research center devoted to their philosophy of applied science.

Indeed, the establishment of the Worcester Foundation for Experimental Biology in 1944 can be attributed directly to Hoagland and Pincus, their friendship for each other, their confidence, enthusiasm, ambition and drive. It was their spirit that turned many members of Worcester society into financial supporters of biologic science. Hoagland and Pincus accomplished what they set out to do. They created and sustained a vibrant, productive scientific institution where it was a pleasure to work.

Although named the Worcester Foundation for Experimental Biology, the Foundation was located in the summer of 1945 across Lake Quinsigamond in a house on an estate in Shrewsbury. The Board of Trustees was chaired by Harlow Shapley, a distinguished astronomer, vice-chaired by Rabbi Levi Olan, and included 3 Nobel laureates and a group of Worcester businessmen.

From 1945 to the death of Pincus in 1967, the staff grew from 12 to 350 (scientists and support people), 36 of whom were independently funded and 45 were postdoctoral fellows. The annual budget grew from $100,000 to $4.5 million. One hundred acres of adjoining land were acquired and the campus grew to 11 buildings. In its first 25 years, approximately 3,000 scientific papers were published.

But in those early years, Pincus was the animal keeper, Mrs. Hoagland the bookkeeper, M-C Chang was the night watchman, and Hoagland mowed the lawn. During the years of World War II, Pincus and Hoagland combined their interests in hormones and neurophysiology to focus on stress and fatigue in industry and the military.

The initial discoveries that led to an oral contraceptive can be attributed to M-C Chang (also the first to describe the capacitation process of sperm). In 1951, he confirmed the work of Makepeace (in 1937) demonstrating that progesterone could inhibit ovulation in rabbits. When norethindrone and norethynodrel became available, Chang found them to be virtually 100% effective in inhibiting ovulation when administered orally to rabbits.

Katherine Dexter McCormick was a very rich woman; in 1904, she married Stanley McCormick, the son of Cyrus McCormick, the founder of International Harvester. She was also intelligent, the second woman to graduate from the Massachusetts Institute of Technology, socially conscious, and a generous contributor to family planning efforts. McCormick's husband suffered from schizophrenia, and she established the Neuroendocrine Research Foundation at Harvard to study schizophrenia. This brought her together with Hoagland who told her of the work being done by Chang and Pincus.

Pincus attributed his interest in contraception to his growing appreciation for the world's population problem, and to a 1951 visit with Margaret Sanger, at that time president of the Planned Parenthood Federation of America. At that visit Sanger expressed hope that a method of contraception could be derived from the laboratory work being done by Pincus and Chang.

In 1952, Margaret Sanger brought Pincus and Katherine McCormick together. During this meeting, Pincus formulated his thoughts derived from his mammalian research. He envisioned a progestational agent in pill form as a contraceptive, acting like progesterone in pregnancy. Sanger and McCormick provided a research grant for further animal research. By the time of her death, McCormick had contributed more than $2 million to the Worcester Foundation, and left another $1 million in her will. In his book, *The Control of Fertility*, published in 1965, Pincus wrote: "This book is dedicated to Mrs. Stanley McCormick because of her steadfast faith in scientific inquiry and her unswerving encouragement of human dignity."[4]

It was Pincus who made the decision to involve a physician because he knew human experiments would be necessary. John Rock, chief of gynecology at Harvard, met Pincus at a scientific conference and discovered their mutual interest in reproductive physiology. Rock and his colleagues pursued Pincus's work. Using oocytes from oophorectomies, they reported in vitro fertilization in 1944, probably the first demonstration of fertilization of human oocytes in vitro. Rock was interested in the work with progestational agents, not for contraception, however, but because he hoped the female sex steroids could be used to overcome infertility.

Sanger and McCormick needed some convincing that Rock's Catholicism would not be a handicap, but they were eventually won over because of his stature. Rock was a physician who literally transformed his personal values in response to his recognition of the problems secondary to uncontrolled reproduction. With the help of Luigi Mastroianni, the first administration of synthetic progestins to women was to Rock's patients in 1954. Of the first 50 patients to receive 10–40 mg of synthetic progestin for 20 days each month, all failed to ovulate during treatment (causing Pincus to begin referring to the medication as "the pill") and 7 of the 50 became pregnant after discontinuing the medication (pleasing Rock who all along was motivated to treat infertility).

Pincus and Chang decided to announce their findings at the International Planned Parenthood meeting in Tokyo, in the fall of 1955. Rock refused to join in this effort, believing that Pincus and Chang were moving too fast. Despite this disagreement (which apparently was spirited and strong), it was done, and the Tokyo presentation generated world-wide publicity.

In 1956, with Celso-Ramon Garcia and Edris Rice-Wray, working in Puerto Rico, the first human trial was performed. The initial progestin products were contaminated with about 1% mestranol. In the amounts being used, this added up to 50–500 μg of mestranol, a sufficient amount of estrogen to inhibit ovulation by itself. When efforts to lower the estrogen content yielded breakthrough bleeding, it was decided to retain the estrogen for cycle control; thus establishing the principle of the combined estrogen-progestin oral contraceptive. Early clinical trials were conducted by J.W. Goldzieher in San Antonio and E.T. Tyler in Los Angeles.

Pincus, a long-time consultant to Searle, picked the Searle compound for extended use, and with great effort, convinced Searle that the commercial potential of an oral contraceptive warranted the risk of possible negative public reaction. Pincus also convinced Rock, and together they pushed the U.S. Food and Drug Administration for acceptance of oral contraception. In 1957, Enovid was approved for the treatment of miscarriages and menstrual disorders, and in 1960, for contraception. Neither Pincus nor the Worcester Foundation got rich on the pill; alas there was no royalty agreement.

The Pill did bring Pincus fame and travel. There is no doubt that he was very much aware of the accomplishment and its implications. As he traveled and lectured in 1957, he said: "How a few precious facts obscurely come to in the laboratory may resonate into the lives of men everywhere, bring order to disorder, hope to the hopeless, life to the dying. That this is the magic and mystery of our time is sometimes grasped and often missed, but to expound it is inevitable."[4]

Pincus was the perfect person to bring oral contraception into the public world, at a time when contraception was a private, suppressed subject. Difficult projects require people like Pincus. A scientific entrepreneur, he could plow through distractions. He could be hard and aggressive with his staff. He could remain focused. He hated to lose, even in meaningless games with his children. Yet he combined a gracious, charming manner with his competitive hardness. He was filled with the kind of self-confidence that permits an individual to forge ahead, to translate vision into reality. Pincus died in 1967 (as did Katherine McCormick at the age of 92), of aplastic anemia that some have argued was caused by his long-term exposure to solvents and chemicals. Rock died in 1984, at the age of 94, and Chang, in 1991, was buried at the age of 82, in Shrewsbury, near his laboratory and close to the grave of Pincus.

Pincus wrote his book, *The Control of Fertility*, in 1964–65, only because "a break came in the apparent dam to publication on reproductive physiology and particularly its subdivisions concerned with reproductive behavior, conception, and contraception."[4]

> "We have conferred and lectured in many countries of the world, seen at first hand the research needs and possibilities in almost every European, Asiatic, Central, and South American country. We have faced the hard fact of over-population in country after country, learned of the bleak demographic future, assessed the prospects for the practice of efficient fertility control. This has been a saddening and a heartening experience; saddening because of the sight of continuing poverty and misery, heartening because of the dedicated colleagues and workers seeking to overcome the handicap of excess fertility and to promote healthy repro-ductive function. Among these we have made many friends, found devoted students."[4]

Syntex, a wholesale drug supplier, was without marketing experience or organization. By the time Syntex had secured arrangements with Ortho for a sales outlet, Searle marketed Enovid in 1960 (150 µg mestranol and 9.85 mg norethynodrel). Ortho-Novum, using norethindrone from Syntex, appeared in 1962. Wyeth Laboratories introduced norgestrel in 1968, the same year in which the first reliable prospective studies were initiated. It was not until the late 1970s that a dose-response relationship between problems and the amount of steroids in the pill was appreciated. As a result, health care providers and patients, over the years, have been confronted by a bewildering array of different products and formulations. The solution to this clinical dilemma is relatively straightforward: use the lowest doses that provide effective contraception.

Pharmacology of Steroid Contraception

The Estrogen Component of Combination Oral Contraceptives

Estradiol is the most potent natural estrogen and is the major estrogen secreted by the ovaries. The major obstacle to the use of sex steroids for contraception was inactivity of the compounds when given orally. A major breakthrough occurred in 1938 when it was discovered that the addition of an ethinyl group at the 17 position made estradiol orally active. Ethinyl estradiol is a very potent oral estrogen and is one of the two forms of estrogen in every oral contraceptive. The other estrogen is the 3-methyl ether of ethinyl estradiol, mestranol.

Ethinyl estradiol   Mestranol

Mestranol and ethinyl estradiol are different from natural estradiol and must be regarded as pharmacologic drugs. Animal studies have suggested that mestranol is weaker than ethinyl estradiol, because mestranol must first be converted to ethinyl estradiol in the body. Indeed, mestranol will not bind to the cellular estrogen receptor. Therefore, unconjugated ethinyl estradiol is the active estrogen in the blood for both mestranol and ethinyl estradiol. In the human body, differences in potency between ethinyl estradiol and mestranol do not appear to be significant, certainly not as great as indicated by assays in rodents. This is now a minor point since all of the low-dose oral contraceptives contain ethinyl estradiol.

The metabolism of ethinyl estradiol (particularly as reflected in blood levels) varies significantly from individual to individual, and from one population to another.[5] There is even a range of variability at different sampling times within the same individual. Therefore, it is not surprising that the same dose can cause side effects in one individual and none in another.

The estrogen content (dosage) of the pill is of major clinical importance. Thrombosis is one of the most serious side effects of the pill, playing a key role in the increased risk of death from a variety of circulatory problems. This side effect is related to estrogen, and it is dose related. Therefore, the dose of estrogen is a critical issue in selecting an oral contraceptive.

The Progestin Component of Combination Oral Contraceptives

The discovery of ethinyl substitution and oral potency led (at the end of the 1930s) to the preparation of ethisterone, an orally active derivative of testosterone. In 1951, it was demonstrated that removal of the 19 carbon from ethisterone to form norethindrone did not destroy the oral activity, and most importantly, it changed the major hormonal effect from that of an androgen to that of a progestational agent. Accordingly, the progestational derivatives of testosterone were designated as 19-nortestosterones (denoting the missing 19 carbon). The androgenic properties of these compounds, however, were not totally eliminated and minimal anabolic and androgenic potential remains within the structure.

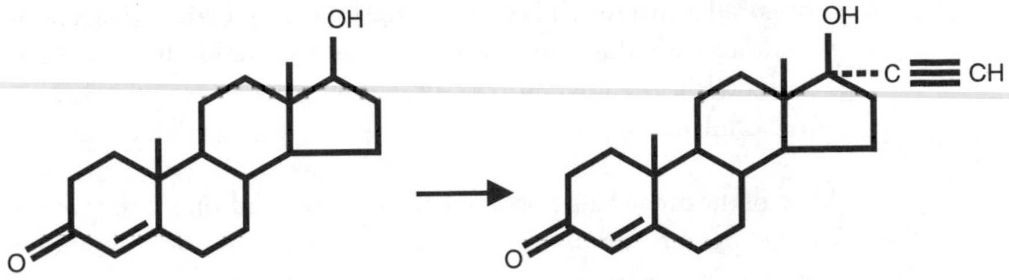

Testosterone

Ethisterone

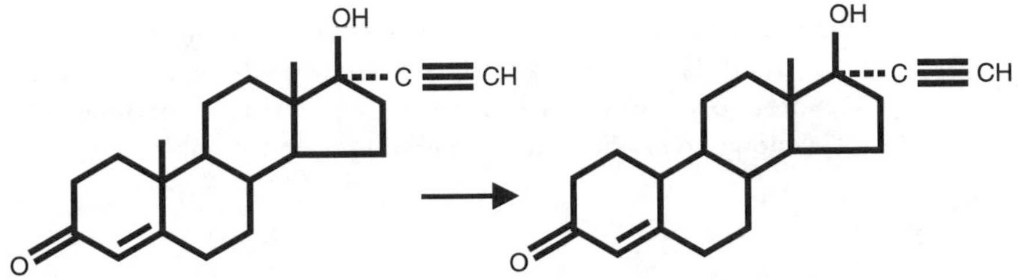

Ethisterone

Norethindrone

The "impurity" of 19-nortestosterone, i.e. androgenic as well as progestational effects, was further complicated in the past by a belief that they were metabolized within the body to estrogenic compounds. This question was restudied, and it was argued that the previous evidence for metabolism to estrogenic compounds was due to an artifact in the laboratory analysis. More recent studies indicate that norethindrone can be converted to ethinyl estradiol, however the rate of this conversion is so low that insignificant amounts of ethinyl estradiol can be found in the circulation or urine following the administration of the commonly used doses of norethindrone.[6] Any estrogenic activity, therefore, would have to be due to a direct effect. In animal and human studies, however, only norethindrone, norethynodrel, and ethynodiol diacetate have estrogen activity, and it is very slight due to weak binding to the estrogen receptor.[7] Clinically, androgenic and estrogenic activities of the progestin component are, therefore, insignificant due to the low dosage in the current oral contraceptives. As with the estrogen component, serious side effects have been related to the high-doses of progestins used in old formulations, not the particular progestin, and routine use of oral contraceptives should now be limited to the low-dose products.

The norethindrone family contains the following 19-nortestosterone progestins: norethindrone, norethynodrel, norethindrone acetate, ethynodiol diacetate, lynestrenol, norgestrel, norgestimate, desogestrel, and gestodene.

Most of the progestins closely related to norethindrone are converted to the parent compound. Thus the activity of norethynodrel, norethindrone acetate, ethynodiol diacetate, and lynestrenol is due to rapid conversion to norethindrone.

Norgestrel is a racemic equal mixture of the dextrorotatory enantiomer and the levorotatory enantiomer. These enantiomers are mirror images of each other and rotate the plane of polarized light in opposite directions. The dextrorotatory form is known as d-norgestrel, and the levorotatory form is l-norgestrel (known as levonorgestrel). Levonorgestrel is the active isomer of norgestrel.

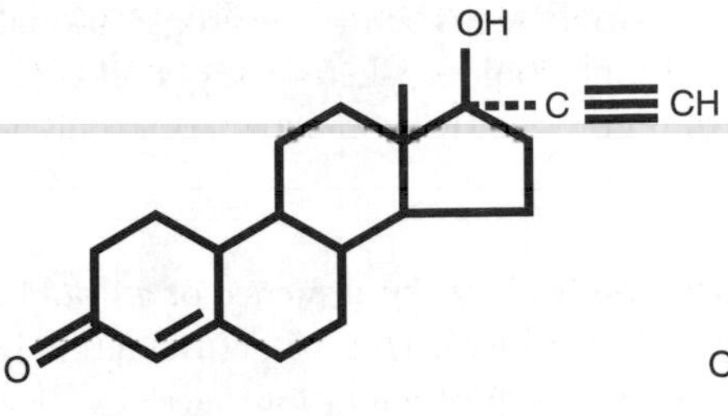

Norethindrone

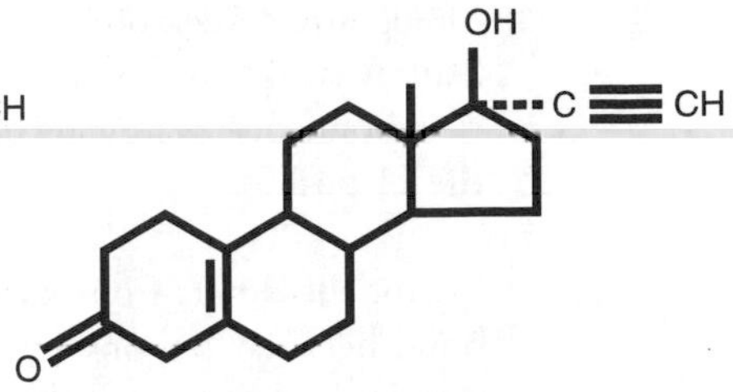

Norethynodrel

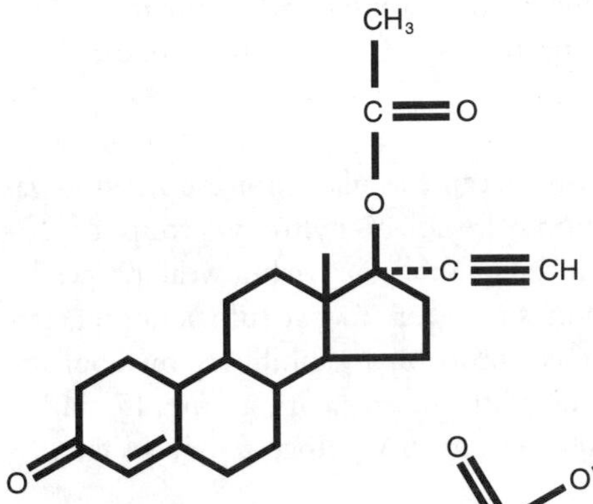

Norethindrone acetate

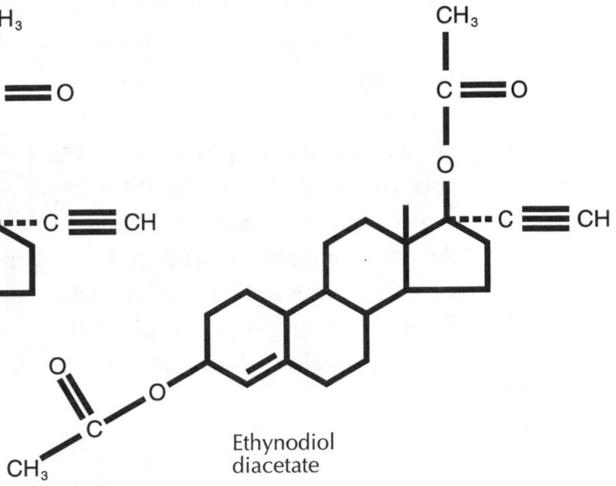

Ethynodiol diacetate

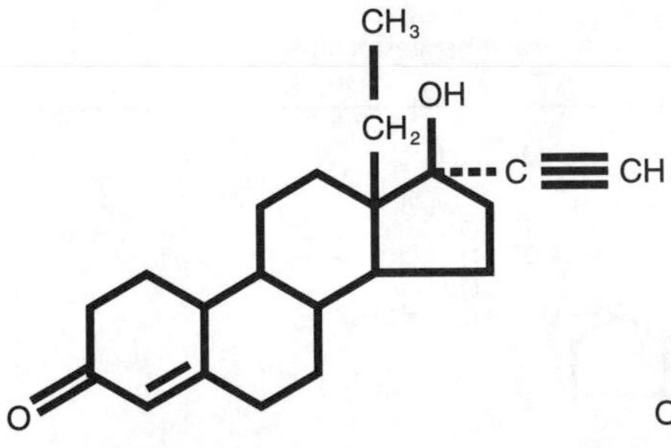

Levonorgestrel

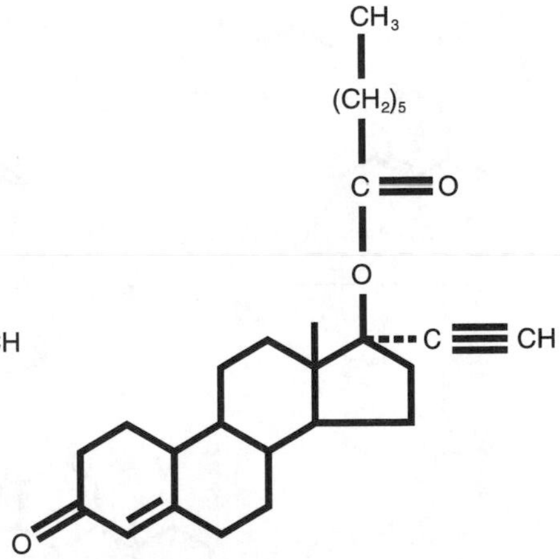

Norethindrone enanthate

Desogestrel undergoes two metabolic steps before the progestational activity is expressed in its active metabolite, 3-keto-desogestrel. This metabolite differs from levonorgestrel only by a methylene group in the 11 position.

Gestodene differs from levonorgestrel by the presence of a double bond between carbons 15 and 16, thus it is Δ-15 gestodene. It is metabolized into many derivatives with progestational activity, but not levonorgestrel.

Several metabolites contribute to the activity of norgestimate, including 17-deacetylated norgestimate, 3-keto norgestimate, and levonorgestrel.

A second group of progestins became available for use when it was discovered that acetylation of the 17-hydroxy group of 17-hydroxyprogesterone produced an orally active but weak progestin. An addition at the 6 position is necessary to give sufficient progestational strength for human use, probably by inhibiting metabolism. Derivatives of progesterone with substituents at the 17 and 6 positions include the widely used medroxyprogesterone acetate.

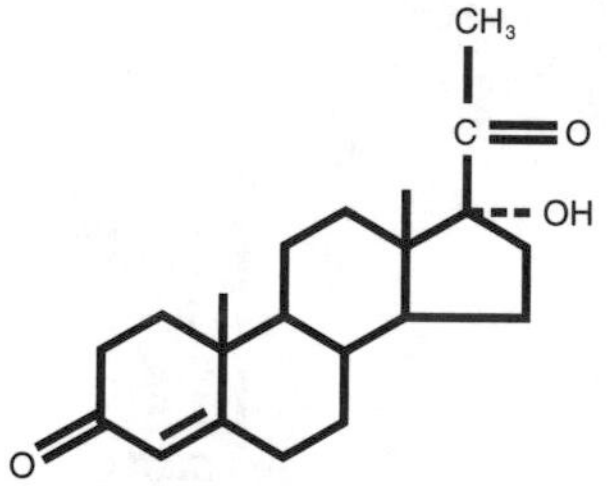

17α-Hydroxyprogesterone

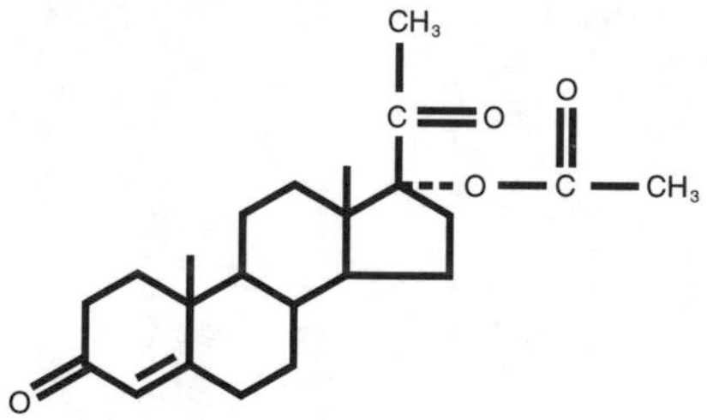

17-Acetoxy progesterone

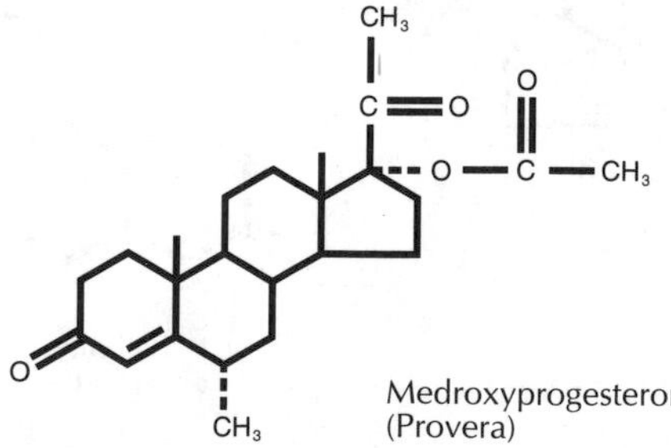

Medroxyprogesterone acetate
(Provera)

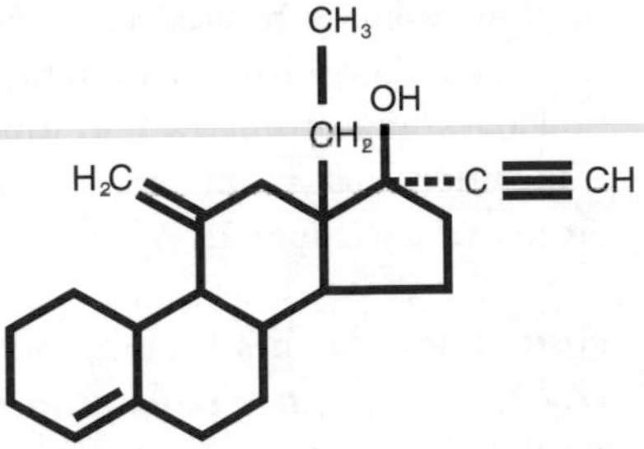

Desogestrel

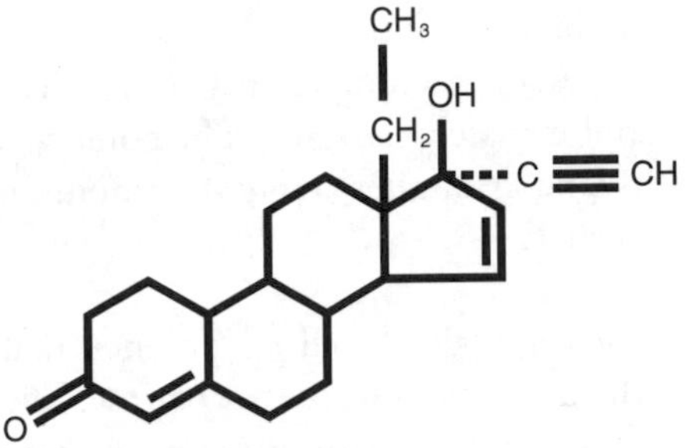

Gestodene

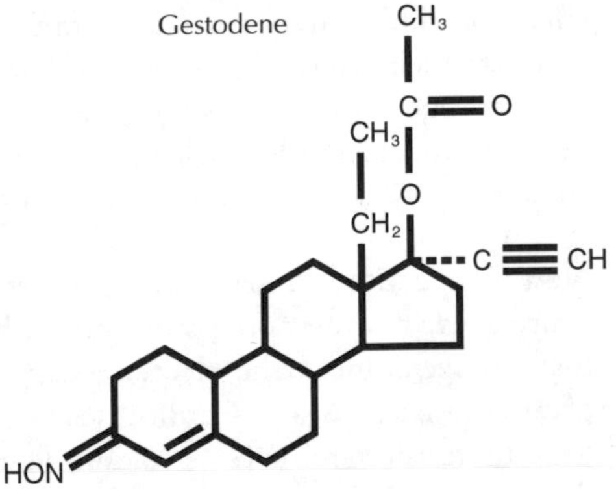

Norgestimate

Potency. For many years, clinicians, scientists, medical writers, and even the pharmaceutical industry have attempted to assign potency values to the various progestational components of oral contraceptives. An accurate assessment, however, has been difficult to achieve for many reasons. Progestins act on numerous target organs (e.g., the uterus, the mammary glands, and the liver), and potency varies depending upon the target organ and endpoint being studied. In the past, animal assays, such as the Clauberg test and the rat ventral prostate assay, were used to determine progestin potency. While these were considered acceptable methods at the time, a better understanding of steroid hormone action and metabolism, and a recognition that animal and human responses differ, have led to greater reliance upon data collected from human studies.

Historically, this has been a confusing issue as publications and experts used potency ranking to provide clinical advice. There is absolutely no need for confusion. Oral contraceptive progestin potency is no longer a consideration when it comes to prescribing oral contraception, because the potency of the various progestins has been accounted for by appropriate adjustments of dose. In other words, the biologic effect (in this case the clinical effect) of the various progestational components in current low-dose oral contraceptives is approximately the same. The potency of a drug does not determine its efficacy or safety, only the amount of a drug required to achieve an effect.

Clinical advice based on potency ranking is an artificial exercise which has not stood the test of time. There is no clinical evidence that a particular progestin is better or worse in terms of particular side effects or clinical responses. Thus oral contraceptives should be judged by their clinical characteristics: efficacy, side effects, risks, and benefits. Our progress in lowering the doses of the steroids contained in oral contraceptives has yielded products with little serious differences. Potency is no longer an important clinical issue.

New Progestins. Probably the greatest influence on the effort which yielded the new progestins was the belief throughout the 80s that androgenic metabolic effects were important, especially in terms of cardiovascular disease. (Cardiovascular side effects are now known to be due to a dose-related stimulation of thrombosis by estrogen). In the search to find compounds which minimize androgenic effects, however, the pharmaceutical companies succeeded.

The new progestins include desogestrel, gestodene, and norgestimate.[8] With the combined products containing the new progestins, the changes in the coagulation system are very similar to those with the current low-dose formulations. A slight prothrombotic effect is characterized by increased levels of fibrinopeptide A which is balanced by antithrombin III and protein C. Thus any coagulation tendency is counteracted. The protime and the activated partial thromboplastin time measure the overall activity of the coagulation pathways — there is no significant increase in these measurements with the new formulations.

In regard to cycle control (breakthrough bleeding and amenorrhea), the new formulations are comparable to existing low-dose products. All progestins derived from 19-nortestosterone have the potential to decrease glucose tolerance and increase insulin resistance. The impact of the current low-dose formulations is very minimal, and the impact of the new progestins is negligible. Most changes are not statistically significant, and when they are, they are so subtle as to be of no clinical significance. For example, there are no changes in hemoglobin A1c. In a controversial issue, it was argued that gestodene affects the pharmacokinetics of ethinyl estradiol differently, causing higher circulating levels of the estrogen component.[9] Intense evaluation of this issue, however, failed to reveal any effects unique to gestodene.[10,11]

The decreased androgenicity of the progestins in the new products is reflected in increased sex hormone binding globulin and decreased free testosterone concentrations to a greater degree than the older established oral contraceptives. This difference may be of greater clinical value in the treatment of acne and hirsutism, but whether a better clinical response is possible is yet to be documented in clinical studies.

The new progestins, because of their reduced androgenicity, predictably do not adversely affect the cholesterol-lipoprotein profile. Indeed, the estrogen-progestin balance of combined oral contraceptives containing one of the new progestins may even promote favorable lipid changes. Thus, the new formulations have the potential to offer protection against cardiovascular disease, an important consideration as we enter an era of women using oral contraceptives for longer durations and later in life. But one must be cautious regarding the clinical significance of subtle changes, and it will be a long time before epidemiologic data on this issue are available.

New Formulations

The multiphasic preparation alters the dosage of both the estrogen and progestin components periodically throughout the pill-taking schedule. The future will bring even more products and different formulations. The aim of these new formulations is to alter steroid levels in an effort to achieve lesser metabolic effects and minimize the occurrence of breakthrough bleeding and amenorrhea, while maintaining efficacy. We are probably at or very near the lowest dose levels which can be achieved without sacrificing efficacy. Metabolic studies with the multiphasic preparations indicate no differences or slight improvements over the metabolic effects of low-dose monophasic products. Clinicians and patients are urged to choose a new multiphasic preparation or to use the low-dose (less than 50 µg estrogen) monophasic pills. The use of higher dose pills should be discontinued, and all women on higher dose pills should be changed to low-dose preparations. Stepping down the dose can be safely accomplished with absolutely no decrease in efficacy. The therapeutic principle remains: utilize the pills which give effective contraception and the greatest margin of safety.

Mechanism of Action

The combination pill, consisting of estrogen and progestin components, is given daily for 3 out of every 4 weeks. The combination pill prevents ovulation by inhibiting gonadotropin secretion via an effect on both pituitary and hypothalamic centers. The progestational agent in the pill primarily suppresses luteinizing hormone (LH) secretion (and thus prevents ovulation), while the estrogenic agent suppresses follicle-stimulating hormone (FSH) secretion (and thus prevents the selection and emergence of a dominant follicle). Therefore, the estrogenic component significantly contributes to the contraceptive efficacy. However, even if follicular growth and development were not sufficiently inhibited, the progestational component would prevent the surge-like release of LH necessary for ovulation.

The estrogen in the pill serves two other purposes. It provides stability to the endometrium so that irregular shedding and unwanted breakthrough bleeding can be minimized; and the presence of estrogen is required to potentiate the action of the progestational agents. The latter function of estrogen has allowed reduction of the progestational dose in the pill. The mechanism for this action is probably estrogen's effect in increasing the concentration of intracellular progestational receptors. Therefore, a minimal pharmacologic level of estrogen is necessary to maintain the efficacy of the combination pill.

Since the effect of a progestational agent will always take precedence over estrogen (unless the dose of estrogen is increased many, many fold), the endometrium, cervical mucus, and perhaps tubal function reflect progestational stimulation. The progestin in the combination pill produces an endometrium which is not receptive to ovum implantation, a decidualized bed with exhausted and atrophied glands. The cervical mucus becomes thick and impervious to sperm transport. It is possible that progestational influences on secretion and peristalsis within the Fallopian tubes provide additional contraceptive effects.

Efficacy

In view of the multiple actions of oral contraceptives, it is hard to understand how the omission of a pill or two can result in a pregnancy. Indeed, careful review of failures suggests that pregnancies usually occur because initiation of the next cycle is delayed allowing escape from ovarian suppression. Strict adherence to 7 pill-free days is critical in order to obtain reliable, effective contraception. For this reason, the 28-day pill package, incorporating 7 pills which do not contain steroids, is a very useful aid to assure adherence to the necessary schedule.

The contraceptive effectiveness of the new progestin and multiphasic formulations are unequivocally comparable to low-dose (less than 50 µg estrogen) and higher dose monophasic combination birth control pills. While carefully monitored studies with motivated subjects achieve an annual failure rate of 0.1%, typical usage is associated with a 3.0% failure rate during the first year of use.[12] Efficacy decreases significantly when the estrogen component is removed, and only a small dose of the progestin is administered (the progestin-only minipills).

46

Failure Rates During the First Year of Use, United States [12]

Method	Percent of Women with Pregnancy Lowest Expected	Typical
No method	85.0%	85.0%
Combination Pill	0.1	3.0
Progestin only	0.5	3.0
IUDs		3.0
Progesterone IUD	2.0	<2.0
Copper T 380A	0.8	<1.0
Norplant	0.2	0.2
Female sterilization	0.2	0.4
Male sterilization	0.1	0.15
Depo-Provera	0.3	0.3
Spermicides	3.0	21.0
Periodic abstinence		20.0
Calendar	9.0	
Ovulation method	3.0	
Symptothermal	2.0	
Post-ovulation	1.0	
Withdrawal	4.0	18.0
Cervical cap	6.0	18.0
Sponge		
Parous women	9.0	28.0
Nulliparous women	6.0	18.0
Diaphragm and spermicides	6.0	18.0
Condom	2.0	12.0

Metabolic Effects of Oral Contraception

Cardiovascular Disease

A major problem for clinicians is that we and our patients live in the present but we must use data from the past. Nowhere is this more true than in the area of oral contraception where the data are derived from older pills of higher dosage while current clinical practice utilizes lower-dose pills and new formulations.

In the 1970s, data emerged from two major British prospective cohort studies (the Royal College of General Practitioners [RCGP] study and the Oxford/Family Planning Association [OFPA] study) derived from experience with high-dose oral contraceptives (greater than 50 µg estrogen).[13-20] These reports indicated increased risks for venous thrombosis, myocardial infarction, and stroke. In response to these reports, lower-dose formulations (less than 50 µg estrogen) came to dominate the market, and clinicians become more careful in their screening of patients and prescribing of oral contraception. Two forces, therefore, were at work simultaneously to bring greater safety to women utilizing oral contraception: the use of lower dose formulations and the avoidance of oral contraception by high risk patients. For these reasons, the Walnut Creek study and the Puget Sound study in the United States did not find an increased risk of myocardial infarction with the use of oral contraceptives.[21,22]

In the older studies, the risk of myocardial infarction was noted to be increased in women over age 35, and consideration of other risk factors (hypertension, hypercholesterolemia, cigarette smoking, obesity, and diabetes mellitus) indicated that oral contraceptives acted synergistically with them, rather than additively.[23-26] In the 1983 RCGP report, only older (over age 35) smokers currently using oral contraceptives had a statistically significant increased risk of ischemic heart disease compared to controls.[17] The British data also indicated a relationship between progestin doses and the risk of cardiovascular disease, *but it is important to note that the British studies found an increased risk only with progestin doses no longer utilized.*[27,28] Because older high-dose pills were used by older women in these studies, the results were further confounded by their inclusion of women at higher risk because of age. Thus, it was not until the early 1980s that it became apparent that the major mortality risk was in smokers over the age of 35, and nonsmokers without risk factors for vascular disease could expect the benefits of oral contraception to outweigh the risks.

Mortality data using the current low-dose pills support this favorable outlook.[22,29]

Epidemiologic evaluations of oral contraceptives and vascular disease indicate that venous thrombosis is a dose-related effect of estrogen, limited to current users, with a disappearance of the risk by 3 months after discontinuation. Women who use 50 µg estrogen pills have an increased incidence of venous thrombosis.[30] A review of the massive Medicaid data in the state of Michigan confirmed the fact that the risk of venous thrombosis is increased at the 50 µg dose.[31]

A case-control study of all 794 women in Denmark who suffered a cerebral thromboembolic attack during 1985–1989 concluded that there was an almost two-fold increased relative risk associated with oral contraceptives containing 30–40 µg estrogen, and the risk was significantly influenced by both smoking and the dose of estrogen in additive (not synergistic) fashion.[32] Whether the conclusion of this retrospective case-control study (which relied upon questionnaires) is real or not must be verified by the ongoing cohort studies. Even if real, however, the modest increase in relative risk with low-dose oral contraceptives would yield only a very small number of cases since this is such a rare event. A case-control analysis of data collected by the Royal College of General Practitioners' Oral Contraception Study concluded that current users were at increased risk of stroke (with a persisting effect in former users); however, this outcome was limited mainly to smokers and to formulations with 50 µg or more of estrogen.[33] There is no evidence that varicose veins have any influence on thrombosis associated with oral contraceptive use.[15]

Embolism must be a very rare consequence of thrombosis secondary to oral contraception. An analysis of fatal venous thromboembolism in England and Wales between 1986 and 1988 failed to find a statistically significant increase in relative risk for current users of oral contraceptives.[34] Thromboembolic disease, therefore, is a consequence of pharmacologic administration of estrogen, and the level of risk is related to the estrogen dose. *It is likely that a slight increase of nonfatal venous thromboembolism is still present at estrogen doses less than 50 µg, but the actual incidence is low (about 15 per 100,000 woman-years), lower than that associated with pregnancy (about 60 per 100,000 woman-years).*[31,32,35,36]

Estimated Annual Mortality Rates Associated with Oral Contraceptive Use and Smoking Compared to Pregnancy

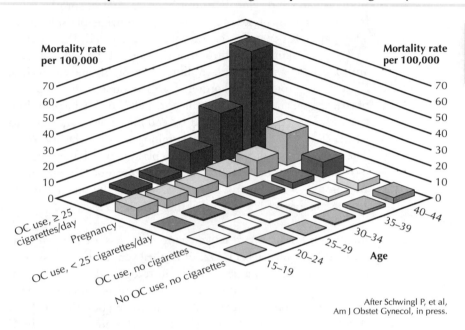

After Schwingl P, et al,
Am J Obstet Gynecol, in press.

Smoking. Smoking continues to be a difficult problem, not only for patient management, but for analysis of data as well. In large national surveys in 1982 and 1988, the decline in the prevalence of smoking was similar in users and nonusers of oral contraception; however, 24.3% of 35 to 45-year old women who used oral contraceptives were smokers![37] In this group of smoking, oral contraceptive-using women, 85.3% smoked 15 or more cigarettes per day (heavy smoking). Despite the widespread teaching and publicity that smoking is a contraindication to oral contraceptive use over the age of 35, more older women who use oral contraceptives smoke and smoke heavily, compared to young women. This strongly implies that older smokers are less than honest with clinicians when requesting oral contraception, and this further raises serious concern over how well this confounding variable can be controlled in case-control and cohort studies. *A former smoker must have stopped smoking for at least 12 consecutive months to be regarded as a nonsmoker. Women who have nicotine in their bloodstream obtained from patches or gum should be regarded as smokers.*

The Coagulation System and Oral Contraception. The goal of the clotting mechanism is to produce thrombin, which converts fibrinogen to a fibrin clot. Thrombin is generated from prothrombin by factor Xa in the presence of factor V, calcium, and phospholipids. The vitamin K-dependent factors include factors VII, IX, and X, as well as prothrombin. Antithrombin III is one of the body's natural anticoagulants, an irreversible inhibitor of thrombin and factors IXa, Xa, and XIa. Protein C and protein S are two other major inhibitors of coagulation and are also vitamin K-dependent. Tissue plasminogen activator (t-PA) is produced by endothelial cells and released when a clot forms. Both t-PA and plasminogen bind to the fibrin clot. The t-PA converts the plasminogen to plasmin which lyses the clot by degrading the fibrin. Deficiencies of antithrombin III, protein C, and protein S are inherited in an autosomal dominant pattern, accounting for 5–10% of familial thrombosis.

An inherited resistance to activated protein C has been identified as the basis for about 50% of cases of familial venous thrombosis, due in almost all cases to a gene alteration recognized as the factor V Leiden mutation.[38,39] Oral contraceptives and pregnancy increase the risk of thrombosis in protein C deficient women (less than 0.5% of all women), but probably only in those who are also protein C resistant.[40] Heterozygotes for the factor V Leiden mutation have an 8-fold increased risk of venous thrombosis, and homozygotes, an 80-fold increased risk, and this risk appears to be further enhanced by oral contraceptive use. The highest prevalence (3–4% of the general population) of factor V Leiden is found in Europeans, and its occurrence outside Europe is very rare, perhaps explaining the low frequency of thromboembolic disease in Africa, Asia, and in Native Americans.[41]

Some studies of the blood coagulation system have concluded that both monophasic and multiphasic low-dose oral contraceptives have no significant clinical impact on the coagulation system. Slight increases in thrombin formation are offset by increased fibrinolytic activity.[42,43] On the other hand, recent studies of formulations containing 30 and 35 µg of ethinyl estradiol indicate an increase in clotting factors associated with an increase in platelet activity.[44] Smoking produces a shift to hypercoagulability, and these adverse changes are dose-related to the amount of estrogen in the oral contraceptive.[45] Indeed, a 20 µg estrogen formulation has no effect on clotting parameters, even in smokers.[45,46]

Today, the rare woman on oral contraception who has a thrombotic episode probably represents someone with an underlying clotting problem, an individual who shows an extreme response to oral contraceptives, or an individual with an unknown lesion of a vessel wall or an unknown local disturbance of circulation. The minimal risk of thrombosis associated with oral contraceptive use does not justify the cost of routine screening for deficiencies in the coagulation system. **If a patient has a family history of idiopathic thrombosis or develops a thrombotic complication while taking oral contraceptives, an evaluation to search for an underlying abnormality in the coagulation system is warranted (measurement of antithrombin III, protein C, activated protein C resistance, protein S, activated partial thromboplastin time, fibrinogen, and plasminogen).**[47] Other risk factors for thromboembolism that should be considered by clinicians include an acquired predisposition such as the presence of lupus anticoagulant or malignancy, and immobility or trauma. Varicose veins are not a risk factor unless they are very extensive.

Combination oral contraception is contraindicated in women who have a history of idiopathic venous thromboembolism, and also in women who have a family history of idiopathic venous thromboembolism. These women will have a higher incidence of congenital deficiencies in important clotting measurements, especially antithrombin II, protein C, protein S, and resistance to activated protein C.[48]

There is no evidence of an increase in risk of cardiovascular disease among past users of oral contraception.[49-51] In the Nurses' Health Study, long-term past use of oral contraceptives was not associated with an increase in overall mortality.[52] Part of the concern for a possible lingering effect of oral contraceptive use was based upon a presumed adverse impact on the atherosclerotic process which would then be added to the effect of aging and thus would be manifested later in life. Instead, the findings are consistent with the contention that cardiovascular disease due to oral contraception is secondary to acute effects, specifically estrogen-induced thrombosis, a dose-related event.

The Desogestrel-Gestodene Controversy. In October, 1995, the United Kingdom Committee on Safety of Medicines recommended that women should use oral contraceptives containing desogestrel or gestodene only if prepared to accept an increased risk of thromboembolism. This action was based on observational studies that indicated a 2–3-fold increase in the risk of thromboembolism when desogestrel and gestodene-containing contraceptives were compared to products with levonorgestrel.[53-56] The risk of idiopathic venous thromboembolism associated with formulations containing less than 50 µg ethinyl estradiol was increased 3–4-fold compared to nonusers, suggesting that low-dose formulations still carry a risk of venous thrombosis. The number of cases and controls using 20 µg estrogen products and formulations with other progestins were too few to allow precise analysis. Using data derived from the General Practice Research Database (a computerized system involving the general practitioners in the U.K.), it is important to note that no increase could be detected in the death rate from pulmonary embolism, stroke, and myocardial infarction in the users of low-dose oral contraceptives.[54]

The fact that these studies point in the same direction is concerning, but it is possible that these observational studies, somewhat similar in design, are influenced by the same unrecognized biases. Furthermore, the case numbers are relatively small (20–40 cases), and, for example, preferential prescribing to women at greater risk could affect the results. It is difficult to reconcile the conclusions with the strong belief supported by good evidence that thrombosis is an estrogen dose-related complication, and that progestational agents have no impact on clotting parameters. Even if the results of these observational studies are accurate; however, the overall real risk is small. Remember, there is no evidence of increased mortality with low-dose oral contraceptives. Indeed, pregnancy is associated with greater risk. In our view, these equivocal reports are not of sufficient strength to escape biases and to change our prescribing of oral contraceptives.

Lipoproteins and Oral Contraception. The balance of estrogen and progestin potency in a given oral contraceptive formulation can potentially influence cardiovascular risk by its overall effect on lipoprotein levels. Oral contraceptives with relatively high-doses of progestins (doses not used in today's low-dose formulations) do produce unfavorable lipoprotein changes.[57] The levonorgestrel triphasic exerts no significant changes on HDL-cholesterol, LDL-cholesterol, apoprotein B, and no change or an increase in apoprotein A, while the levonorgestrel monophasic combination (with a higher dose of levonorgestrel) has a tendency to increase LDL-cholesterol and apoprotein B, and to decrease HDL-cholesterol and apoprotein A.[58-61] The monophasic desogestrel and desogestrel pills have a favorable effect on the lipoprotein profile, while the triphasic norgestimate and gestodene pills produce beneficial alterations in the LDL/HDL and apoprotein B/apoprotein A ratios.[58–61] Like the triphasic levonorgestrel pills, norethindrone multiphasic pills have no significant impact on the lipoprotein profile over 6–12 months.[62] *In summary, studies of low-dose formulations indicate that the adverse effects of progestins are limited to the fixed dose combination with levonorgestrel, a dose of levonorgestrel that exceeds that in the multiphasic formulation.*

In the past decade we have been subjected to considerable marketing hype about the importance of the impact of oral contraceptives on the cholesterol-lipoprotein profile. If indeed certain oral contraceptives had a negative impact on the lipoprotein profile, one would expect to find evidence of atherosclerosis as a cause of an increase in subsequent cardiovascular disease. There is no such evidence. Thus the mechanism of the cardiovascular complications is undoubtedly a short-term acute mechanism—thrombosis (an estrogen-related effect).

This conclusion is reinforced by angiographic and autopsy studies. Young women with myocardial infarctions who have used oral contraceptives have less diffuse atherosclerosis than non-users.[63,64] Indeed, a case-control study indicated that the risk of myocardial infarction in patients taking older, high-dose levonorgestrel-containing formulations is the same as that experienced with pills containing other progestins.[65]

An important study in monkeys indicated a protective action of estrogen against atherosclerosis, but by a mechanism independent of the cholesterol-lipoprotein profile. Oral administration of a combination of estrogen and progestin to monkeys fed a high cholesterol, atherogenic diet decreased the extent of coronary atherosclerosis despite a reduction in HDL-cholesterol levels.[66–68] In somewhat similar experiments, estrogen treatment markedly prevented arterial lesion development in rabbits.[69–71] In considering the impact of progestational agents, lowering of HDL is not necessarily atherogenic if accompanied by a significant estrogen impact. These animal studies help explain why older, higher-dose combinations which had an adverse impact on the lipoprotein profile did not increase subsequent cardiovascular disease.[49–52] The estrogen component provided protection through a direct effect on vessel walls, especially favorably influencing vasomotor and platelet factors such as nitric oxide and prostacyclin. Perhaps the low-dose combinations will eventually be associated with a favorable impact on the risk of cardiovascular disease.

Epidemiologic data on this issue derived from low-dose oral contraception come from Finland and England. Preliminary analysis of cardiovascular deaths among women under 40 years of age in Finland indicated a statistically significant reduction in low-dose oral contraceptive users in the relative risk of myocardial infarction and stroke.[72] In England, studies from the RCGP and OFPA report no increased risk in *current* users, as previously indicated in studies of higher-dose pills.[73] A case-control study of fatal strokes in England and Wales found no statistically significant increase in risk of stroke with low-dose oral contraceptives; however, the statistical power was limited because of the relatively small number of stroke cases under the age of 40.[74] In the large WHO case-control study and in the analysis of the General Practice Research Database in the United Kingdom, no increase in mortality due to stroke or myocardial infarction could be detected in oral contraceptive users.[36,53,54] There truly is greater safety associated with lower doses and better screening.

Conclusion. These considerations have significant bearing on the choice of a contraceptive. It certainly is a good pharmacologic principle to utilize a medication with the least impact on normal physiology. However, if this impact is so subtle that it is clinically insignificant, then this issue is of relatively little importance when it comes to selecting an oral contraceptive. Current evidence suggests there is no advantage or disadvantage associated with any of the current low-dose formulations in regards to cardiovascular disease. *Furthermore, it should be recognized that the clinical relevance of lipid modifications remains to be substantiated by epidemiologic data. It is appropriate to question the clinical and biological significance of the reported changes because the great majority of the changes have still been within the physiologic ranges for age and sex.* However, it seems prudent to avoid the higher doses of progestins such as 150–250 μg levonorgestrel. The low-doses of levonorgestrel (such as in the multiphasic formulations) do not have an adverse impact on the lipid profile.

Epidemiologic and laboratory data convincingly indicate that there is a dose-response relationship between the risk of arterial and venous thrombosis and the amount of estrogen in the combination oral contraceptive. Smoking and estrogen dose are additive factors, not synergistic, except in the now unused very high-dose estrogen preparations and in very heavy smokers. It is not known whether there is any risk of thrombosis at the 20 μg dose of estrogen; however, it is worth noting that the 20 μg formulations have no effect on clotting parameters, even in smokers.[45,46] Therefore, we can provide the following conclusions and recommendations.

The relative risk of cardiovascular events (arterial thrombosis) is increased for women of all ages who smoke and use oral contraceptives. However, because the actual incidence of cardiovascular events is so low at a young age, the real risk is very, very low for young women, although it increases with age. Given the lack of impact on clotting parameters of 20 μg estrogen,[45,46] a 20 μg formulation may benefit smoking women, regardless of age. This also applies to all women using nicotine-containing products as an aid to stop smoking. We further recommend this same consideration for women who have other cardiovascular risk factors, such as diabetes mellitus, migraine headaches, and obesity. Ex-smokers (for at least one year) should be regarded as nonsmokers. However, keep in mind that the theoretical greater safety of 20 μg estrogen has not been confirmed by epidemiologic data.

Smokers over age 35 should continue to be advised that combined oral contraceptives are not a good choice, regardless of the number of cigarettes smoked. In view of the unreported high rate of smoking in older women who use oral contraceptives,[37] clinicians should consider using 20 μg estrogen products for women over age 35.

The newest oral contraceptive formulations contain the new progestins: desogestrel, gestodene, and norgestimate. The metabolic effects of these new products are minimal to negligible. It is even possible that the estrogen balance of combined oral contraceptives with the new progestins can promote favorable lipid changes and protect against cardiovascular disease.[8] It will be a long time, however, before epidemiologic data will reveal the clinical impact, if any, of subtle metabolic changes.

Hypertension

Oral contraceptive-induced hypertension was observed in approximately 5% of users of higher-dose pills. More recent evidence indicates that small increases in blood pressure can be observed even with 30 μg estrogen, monophasic pills, including those containing the new progestins. However, an increased incidence of clinically significant hypertension has not been reported.[75–78] No significant clinical changes in blood pressure have been noted with any of the multiphasic formulations. It is possible for an occasional patient to experience an idiosyncratic reaction and develop hypertension; therefore, an annual assessment of blood pressure is still an important element of clinical surveillance, even when low-dose oral contraceptives are used. Variables such as previous toxemia of pregnancy or previous renal disease do not predict whether a woman will develop hypertension on oral contraception.[79] Likewise, women who have developed hypertension on oral contraception are not more predisposed to develop toxemia of pregnancy.

The mechanism for an effect on blood pressure is thought to involve the renin-angiotensin system. The most consistent finding is a marked increase in plasma angiotensinogen, the renin substrate, up to 8 times normal values (on higher dose pills). In nearly all women, excessive vasoconstriction is prevented by a compensatory decrease in plasma renin concentration. If hypertension does develop, the renin-angiotensinogen changes take 3–6 months to disappear after stopping combined oral contraception.

One must also consider the effects of oral contraceptives in patients with pre-existing hypertension or cardiac disease. Data from the RCGP continue to indicate that the presence of hypertension in oral contraceptive users increases the risk of myocardial infarction.[51] It is still unknown whether this risk is present with low-dose pills. In our view, with medical control of the blood pressure and close follow-up (at least every 3 months), the patient and her clinician may choose low-dose oral contraception. Close follow-up is also indicated in women with a history of pre-existing renal disease or a strong family history of hypertension or cardiovascular disease. It seems prudent to suggest that patients with marginal cardiac reserve should utilize other means of contraception. Significant increases in cardiac output and plasma volume have been recorded with oral contraceptive use (higher-dose pills), probably a result of fluid retention.

Carbohydrate Metabolism

With the older high-dose oral contraceptives, an impaired glucose tolerance test was present in many women. In these women, plasma levels of insulin as well as the blood sugar were elevated. Generally the effect of oral contraception is to produce an increase in peripheral resistance to insulin action. Most women can meet this challenge by increasing insulin secretion, and there is no change in the glucose tolerance test, although 1-hour values may be slightly elevated.

57

Carbohydrate metabolism is affected mainly by the progestin component of the pill. The derangement of carbohydrate metabolism may also be affected by estrogen influences on lipid metabolism, hepatic enzymes, and elevation of unbound cortisol. The glucose intolerance is dose-related, and once again effects are less with the low-dose formulations. *Insulin and glucose changes with low-dose monophasic and multiphasic oral contraceptives are so minimal, that it is now believed that they are of no clinical significance.*[78–82] This includes long-term evaluation with hemoglobin A1c. The one exception is the claim that the levonorgestrel monophasic has an excessively negative impact.

The observed changes in studies of oral contraception and carbohydrate metabolism are in the nondiabetic range. In order to measure differences, investigators have resorted to analysis by measuring the area under the curve for glucose and insulin responses during glucose tolerance tests. A highly regarded cross-sectional study utilizing this technique reported that even lower-dose formulations have detectable effects on insulin resistance.[83] The reason this is important is that it is now recognized that hyperinsulinemia due to insulin resistance is a contributor to cardiovascular disease. However, there are several critical questions that remain unanswered. Can the results from a cross-sectional study be duplicated in a study of sufficient size with patients serving as their own controls? Is a statistically significant hyperinsulinemia detected in a study clinically meaningful?

Because long-term, follow-up studies of large populations have failed to detect any increase in the incidence of diabetes mellitus or impaired glucose tolerance (even in past and current users of high-dose pills),[84,85] the concern now appropriately focuses on the slight impairment as a potential risk for cardiovascular disease. If slight hyperinsulinemia were meaningful, wouldn't you expect to see evidence of an increase in cardiovascular disease in past users who took oral contraceptives when doses were higher? As we have emphasized before, there is no such evidence. The data strongly indicate that the changes in lipids and carbohydrate metabolism that have been measured are not clinically meaningful.

It can be stated definitively that oral contraceptive use does not produce an increase in diabetes mellitus.[84,85] The hyperglycemia associated with oral contraception is not deleterious and is completely reversible. Even women who have risk factors for diabetes in their history are not affected. In a large study of women with recent gestational diabetes, no significant impact could be demonstrated over 6–13 months comparing a low-dose monophasic and a multiphasic to a control group.[86] A high percentage of women with previous gestational diabetes develop overt diabetes and associated vascular complications. Until overt diabetes develops, it is appropriate for these patients to use low-dose oral contraception.

In clinical practice, it may, at times, be necessary to prescribe oral contraception for the overt diabetic. The effect on insulin requirement is neither consistent nor predictable, but one would expect little, if any, change with low-dose pills. According to the older epidemiologic data, the use of oral contraceptives increases the risk of thrombosis in women with insulin-dependent diabetes mellitus; therefore, women with diabetes have been encouraged to use other forms of contraception. However this effect in women under age 35 who are otherwise healthy is probably very minimal with low-dose oral contraception, and reliable protection against pregnancy is a benefit for these patients that outweighs the small risk. A case-control study could find no evidence that oral contraceptive use by young women with insulin-dependent diabetes mellitus increased the development of retinopathy and nephropathy.[87] In a one-year study of women with insulin-dependent diabetes mellitus who were using a low-dose oral contraceptive, no deterioration could be documented in lipoprotein or hemostatic biochemical markers for cardiovascular risk.[88]

The Liver

The liver is affected in more ways and with more regularity and intensity by the sex steroids than any other extragenital organ. Estrogen influences the synthesis of hepatic DNA and RNA, hepatic cell enzymes, serum enzymes formed in the liver, and plasma proteins. Estrogenic hormones also affect hepatic lipid and lipoprotein formation, the intermediary metabolism of carbohydrates, and intracellular enzyme activity.

The active transport of biliary components is impaired by estrogens as well as some progestins. The mechanism is unclear, but cholestatic jaundice and pruritus were occasional complications of higher-dose oral contraception, and are similar to the recurrent jaundice of pregnancy, i.e., benign and reversible. The incidence with lower-dose oral contraception is uknown, but it must be a rre occurrence.

The only absolute hepatic contraindication to oral contraceptive use is acute or chronic cholestatic liver disease. Cirrhosis and previous hepatitis are not aggravated. Once recovered from the acute phase of liver disease, a woman can use oral contraception.

Data from the RCGP prospective study indicated that an increase in the incidence of gallstones occurred in the first years of oral contraceptive use, apparently due to an acceleration of gallbladder disease in women already susceptible.[89] In other words, the overall risk of gallbladder disease was not increased, but the first years of use disease was activated or accelerated in women who were vulnerable because of asymptomatic disease or a tendency toward gallbladder disease. The mechanism appears to be induced alterations in the composition of gallbladder bile, specifically a rise in cholesterol saturation that is presumably an estrogen effect.[90] The Nurses' Health Study reported no significant increase in the risk of symptomatic gallstones among ever-users, but slightly elevated risks among current and long-term users.[91] Although oral contraceptive use has been linked to an increased risk of gallbladder disease, the epidemiologic evidence has been inconsistent. Indeed an Italian case-control study and a current report from the Oxford Family Planning Association cohort find no increase in the risk of gallbladder disease in association with oral contraceptive use and no interaction with increasing age or body weight.[92,93] Keep in mind that even though some studies found a statistically significant modest increase in the relative risk of gallbladder disease, even if the effect were real, it is of little clinical importance because the actual incidence of this problem is very low.

Other Metabolic Effects

Nausea, breast discomfort, and weight gain continue to be disturbing effects, but their incidence is significantly less with low-dose oral contraception. Fortunately, these effects are most intense in the first few months of use and, in most cases, gradually disappear. Weight gain usually responds to dietary restriction, but for some patients, the weight gain is an anabolic response to the sex steroids, and discontinuation of oral contraception is the only way that weight loss can be achieved. This must be rare with low-dose oral contraception because data in published studies fail to indicate a difference in body weight between users and nonusers. There is no association between oral contraception and peptic ulcer disease or inflammatory bowel disease.[94,95] Oral contraception is not recommended for patients with problems of gastrointestinal malabsorption because of the possibility of contraceptive failure.

Chloasma, a patchy increase in facial pigment, was, at one time, found to occur in approximately 5% of oral contraceptive users. It is now a rare problem due to the decrease in estrogen dose. Unfortunately, once chloasma appears, it des only gradually following discontinuation of the pill and may never disappear completely. Skin blanching medications may be useful.

Hematologic effects include an increased sedimentation rate due to increased levels of fibrinogen, increased total iron binding capacity due to the increase in globulins, and a decrease in prothrombin time. The continuous use of oral contraceptives may prevent the appearance of symptoms in porphyria precipitated by menses. Changes in vitamin metabolism have been noted: a small nonharmful increase in vitamin A and decreases in blood levels of pyridoxine (B_6) and the other B vitamins, folic acid, and ascorbic acid. Despite these changes, routine vitamin supplements havnot been shown to be of benefit for women eating adequate, normal diets.

Mental depression is very rarely associated with oral contraceptives. In studies with higher-dose oral contraceptives, the effect was due to estrogen interference with the synthesis of tryptophan that could be reversed with pyridoxine treatment. It seems wiser, however, to discontinue oral contraception if depression is encountered. Though infrequent, a reduction in libido is occasionally a problem and may be a cause for seeking an alternative method of contraception.

Because estrogen is known to stimulate prolactin secretion and to cause hypertrophy of the pituitary lactotrophs, it was appropriate to be concerned over a possible relationship between oral contraception and prolactin-secreting pituitary adenomas. Several case-control studies have uniformly concluded that no such relationship exists. Previous use of oral contraceptives is not related to the size of prolactinomas at presentation and diagnosis[6] Oral contraception can be prescribed to patients with pituitary microadenomas without fear of subsequent tumor growth.[97]

The Risk of Cancer

Endometrial Cancer

The use of oral contraception protects against endometrial cancer. Use for at least 12 months reduces the risk of developing endometrial cancer by *50%*, with the greatest protective effect gained by use for more than 3 years.[98–100] This protection persists for 15 or more years after discontinuation (the actual length of duration of protection is unknown) and is greatest in women at highest risk: nulliparous and low parity women. This protection is equally protective for all 3 major histologic subtypes of endometrial cancer: adenocarcinoma, adenoacanthoma, and adenosquamous cancers. Finally, protection is seen with all monophasic formulations of oral contraceptives, including pills with less than 50 μg estrogen. There are no data as yet with multiphasic preparations or the new progestin formulations, but since these products are still dominated by their progestational component, there is every reason to believe that they will be protective.

Ovarian Cancer

Protection against ovarian cancer, the most lethal of female reproductive tract cancers, is one of the most important benefits of oral contraception. Because this cancer is detected late and prognosis is poor, the impact of this protection is very significant. Indeed, a decline in mortality from ovarian cancer has been observed in several countries since the early 1970s, perhaps an effect of oral contraceptive use.[101] The risk of developing epithelial ovarian cancer in users of oral contraception is reduced by *40%* compared to that of nonusers.[100,102–104] This protective effect increases with duration of use and continues for at least 10–15 years after stopping the medication. This protection is seen in women who use oral contraception for as little as 3 to 6 months (although at least 3 years of use are required for a notable impact), reaches an 80% reduction in risk with more than 10 years of use, and is a benefit associated with all monophasic formulations, including the low-dose formulations.[105] Again, the multiphasic and new progestin products have not been in use long enough to yield any data on this issue, but because ovulation is effectively inhibited by these formulations, protection against ovarian cancer should be exerted.

Cancer of the Cervix

Studies have indicated that the risk for dysplasia and carcinoma-in-situ of the uterine cervix increases with the use of oral contraception for more than one year.[106–110] Invasive cervical cancer may be increased after 5 years of use, reaching a two-fold increase after 10 years. It is well recognized, however, that the number of partners a woman has had and age at first coitus are the most important risk factors fr cervical neoplasia. Other confounding factors include exposure to human papillomavirus, the use of barrier contraception (protective), and smoking. These are difficult factors to control, and therefore, the conclusions regarding cervical cancer are not definitive. An excellent study from the Centers for Disease Control and Prevention (CDC) concluded there is no increased risk of invasive cervical cancer in users of oral contraception, and an apparent increased risk of carcinoma-in-situ is due to enhanced detection of disease (because oral contraceptive users have more frequent Pap smears).[109] On the other hand, a case-control study of patients in Panama, Costa Rica, Colombia, and Mexico concluded that there is a minimal risk for invasive squamous cell carcinoma, but there is a significantly increased risk for invasive adenocarcinoma.[111] Similar results were obtained in a case-control study in Los Angeles. The relative risk of adenocarcinoma of the cervix increased from 2.1 with ever use to 4.4 with 12 or more years of oral contraceptive use.[112] Becausthe incidence of adenocarcinoma of the cervix has increased in young women over the last 20 years, there is concern that this increase reflects the use of oral contraception. Oral contraceptives increase cervical ectopia, but whether this increases the risk of cervical adenocarcinoma is unclear.

This concern obviously is an important reason for annual Pap smear surveillance. Fortunately, steroid contraception does not mask abnormal cervical changes, and the necessity for prescription renewals offers the opportunity for improved screening for cervical disease. It is reasonable to perorm Pap smears every 6 months in women using oral contraception for 5 or more years who are also at higher risk because of their sexual behavior (multiple partners, history of sexually transmitted diseases).

Liver Adenomas

Hepatocellular adenomas can be produced by steroids of both the estrogen and androgen families. Actually, there are two different lesions, peliosis and adenomas. Peliosis is characterized by dilated vascular spaces without endothelial lining, and may occur in the absence of adenomatous changes. The adenomas are not malignant; their significance lies in the potential for hemorrhage. The most common presentation is acute right upper quadrant or epigastric pain. The tumors may be asymptomatic, or they may present suddenly with hematoperitoneum. There is some evidence that the tumors regress when oral contraception is stopped. Epidemiologic data have not supported the contention that mestranol increased the risk more than ethinyl estradiol.

The risk appears to be related to duration of oral contraceptive use and to the steroid dose in the pills. This is reinforced by the rarity of the condition ever since low-dose oral contraception became available. The ongoing prospective studies have accumulated many woman-years of use and have not identified a single case of such a tumor. In our view it isn't even worth mentioning during the informed consent (choice) process.

No reliable screening test or procedure is currently available. Routine liver function tests are normal. Computed tomography (CT) scanning or magnetic resonance imaging (MRI) may be the best means of diagnosis; angiography and ultrasonography are not reliable. Palpation of the liver should be part of the periodic evaluation in oral contraceptive users. If an enlarged liver is found, oral contraception should be stopped, and regression should be evaluated and followed by imaging.

Liver Cancer

Oral contraception has been linked to the development of hepatocellular carcinoma.[113,114] However, the very small number of cases, and thus the limited statistical power, requires great caution in interpretation. The largest study on this question, the WHO Collaborative Study of Neoplasia and Steroid Contraceptives, found no association between oral contraception and liver cancer.[115] In the United States, the death rates from liver cancer have not changed over the last 3 decades despite introduction and widespread use of oral contraception.

Breast Cancer

Because of its prevalence and its long latent phase, concern over the relationship between oral contraception and breast cancer continues to be an issue in the minds of both patients and clinicians. Unfortunately, the iue is not resolved and probably will not be until another decade passes, allowing data to emerge from the modern era of lower-dose oral contraception.

Worth emphasizing is the protective effect of higher-dose oral contraception on benign breast disease, an effect that became apparent after 2 years of use.[116] After 2 years there was a progressive reduction (about 40%) in the incidence of fibrocystic disease of the breast. Women who used oral contraception were one-fourth as likely to develop benign breast disease as nonusers, but this protection was limited to current and recent users. It is still uncertain whether this same protection is provided by the lower-dose products. A French case-control study has indicated a reduction of non-proliferative benign breast disease associated with low-dose oral contraceptives used before a first full term pregnancy, but no effect on proliferative disease or with use after a pregnancy.[117]

The RCGP,[16] OFPA,[118,119] and Walnut Creek[21] cohort studies (and more recently, the Nurses' Health Study[120] indicated no significant differences in breast cancer rates between users and nonusers. However, patients were enrolled in these studies at a time when oral contraception was used primarily by married couples spacing out their children. By the 1980s, oral contraception was primarily being used by women early in life, for longer durations, and to delay an initial pregnancy (remember, a full-term pregnancy early in life protects against breast cancer).

Over the last decade, case-control studies have focused on the use of oral contraception early in life, for long duration, and to delay a first, full-term pregnancy. Because the cohort of women who have used oral contraception in this fashion is just now beginning to reach the ages of postmenopausal breast cancer, the studies had to examine the risk of breast cancer diagnosed before age 45 (only 13% of all breast cancer). The results of these studies have not been clear-cut. Some studies have indicated an overall increased relative risk of early, premenopausal breast cancer,[121-127] while others indicated no increase in overall risk.[128-130] The most impressive finding indicates a link in most studies[125,127-139] but not all,[140,141] of early breast cancer before age 40 in women who used oral contraception for long durations of time.

The Centers for Disease Control study is one of the largest case-control studies on the subject.[142–144] No overall increased risk of breast cancer was found in women using oral contraceptives before the age of 20 with a duration of use greater than 4 years, or before the age of 25 with a duration of use greater than 6 years, or with greater than 4 years use before a first pregnancy. In addition, no overall increased risk of breast cancer was found among any subgroups of users including women with benign breast disease or a family history of breast cancer.

In further analysis of the CDC study, there was no increased risk associated with any specific type of oral contraceptive, progestin only pills, or the use of 2 or more types. In addition, there was no increased risk associated with any specific progestin or estrogen component, and most importantly, it was demonstrated that long-term use (15 or more years) was not associated with an increased risk of breast cancer. The reliability of the CDC study is reinforced by the fact that the data confirmed the previously identified risk factors, such as nulliparity, late age at first birth, history of benign breast disease, and a family history of breast cancer. Thus far, the CDC study has found no evidence for a latent effect (increased risk many years later) on breast cancer risk through age 54.[145]

In view of the confusing and contradictory findings among the many case-control studies, the CDC reexamined their data to determine whether oral contraceptive use had different effects on the risk of breast cancer diagnosed at different ages.[146] The data indicated that oral contraceptive use increased slightly the risk of breast cancer diagnosed under the age of 35, had no effect on women diagnosed from age 35 to 44, and in women diagnosed from age 45 to 54, oral contraceptive use appeared to decrease the risk of breast cancer. However, these estimates did not achieve statistical significance. Nevertheless, the protection that oral contraceptive use appears to provide to older women is a more convincing argument because it was supported by several dose-response relationships (age with first use and time since first and last use). The elevated risk among the women with early breast cancer is a more tenuous conclusion, not strengthened by a supporting dose-response pattern. A large (1,991 patients with breast cancer) case-control study from Italy included 784 cases in the age group 55–64 years.[147] No association between oral contraceptives and the risk of breast cancer was found, including no link with duration of use. In contrast, a recent and large case control study in the U.S. concluded that there is an increased risk of eary premenopausal breast cancer associated with oral contraceptive use early in life for long durations.[139]

The crucial question is: as studies gain more statistical power, will they confirm a slightly increased risk for premenopausal breast cancer or will the present suggestion of an increased risk disappear? For example, an early report from New Zealand indicated an increased relative risk for premenopausal breast cancer, and as the study continued, this relative risk moved closer and closer to 1.0.[148] This excellent New Zealand study reports no increase in risk of breast cancer associated with long duration of use, use before a first full term pregnancy, or use at a young age.

Further comfort can be derived from the United States national cancer surveillance data.[149] **The increase in breast cancer in American women is in older women, those who did not have the opportunity to use oral contraception. In women under 56 years of age, there has been no change in the age-specific breast cancer rates from 1950 to 1985.**

Since oral contraceptive use decreases benign breast disease and benign breast disease increases a woman's risk of breast cancer, why doesn't oral contraception decrease the risk of breast cancer? It has been argued that the impact of oral contraception on benign breast disease must be limited to the type of tissue change that is not linked to breast cancer risk. It is also possible that oral contraception either accelerates the development of breast cancer that would have been diagnosed later, or leads to earlier diagnosis through greater involvement with a health care system, or perhaps both of these. Finally, the effect of oral contraception on benign breast disease may be limited to older high-dose formulations.

Conclusion. For some time to come, probably a decade or more, clinical advice will have to be based on the current conflicting findings. With considerable confidence, we believe that long-term use of oral contraception during the reproductive years is **NOT** associated with a significant increase in the risk of breast cancer after age 45. There is the possibility that a subgroup of young women who use contraception early and for a long time (greater than 4 years) has a slightly increased risk of breast cancer before the age of 45, a relative risk of less tha 1.5.[150] It is not cost effective to promote mammographic surveillance of this group of patients, but it should not be denied to any woman of this group who makes the request. Keep in mind that these conclusions depend upon data derived from use of higher-dose oral contraception. It is important to be aware that there has been consistent failure to demonstrate an increased risk with oral contraceptive use in women with positive family histories of breast cancer or in women with proven benign breast disease.[143,148,151]

Adding up the benefits of oral contraception, the possible slight increase in risk of breast cancer is far outweighed by positive effects on our public health. But the impact on public health is of little concern during the private clinician-patient interchange in the office. Here personal risk receives highest priority; fear of cancer is a motivating force, and compliance with effective contraception requires accurate information.

The clinician should not fail to take every opportunity to direct attention to all factors that affect breast cancer. Breastfeeding and control of alcohol intake are good examples, and are also components of preventive health care. Especially important is this added motivation to encourage breastfeeding. The protective effect of breastfeeding is greatest for premenopausal breast cancer, the cancer of concern to younger women using oral contraception.

Patients deserve to know the facts and need help in dealing with the state of the art and the uncertainty. But there is no doubt that patients, especially young patients, are influenced in their choice by their clinician's advice and attitude. We are concerned over the findings of the breast cancer reports, but the definitive answer awaits future studies. We believe the safety and benefits of low-dose oral contraception currently outweigh the potential risks.

Other Cancers

The Walnut Creek study suggested that melanoma was linked to oral contraception, however, the major risk factor for melanoma is exposure to sunlight. More recent and accurate evaluation utilizing both of the RCGP and OFPA prospective cohorts and accounting for exposure to suight, has not indicated a significant difference in the risk of melanoma comparing users to nonusers.[152,153] There is no evidence linking oral contraceptive use to kidney cancer, colon cancer, gallbladder cancer, or pituitary tumors.[154] Long-term oral contraceptive use may slightly increase the risk of molar pregnancy, but there is no convincing evidence of a cause and effect association.[15]

Endocrine Effects

Adrenal Gland

For some time it has been known that estrogen increases the cortisol-binding globulin (CBG). It had been thought that the increase in plasma cortisol while on oral contraception was due to increased binding by this globulin and not an increase in free active cortisol. Now it is apparent that free and active cortisol levels are also elevated. Estrogen decreases the ability of the liver to metabolize cortisol, and in addition, progesterone and related compounds can displace cortisol from transcortin, and thus contribute to the elevation of unbound cortisol. The effects of these elevated levels over prolonged periods of time are unknown, but no obvious impact has become apparent. To put this into perspective, the increase is not as great as that which occurs in pregnancy, and, in fact, it is within the normal range for nonpregnant women.

The adrenal gland responds to adrenocorticotropic hormone (ACTH) normally in women on oral contraceptives, therefore there is no suppression of the adrenal gland itself. Initial studies showed that the response to metyrapone (an 11β-hydroxylase blocker) was abnormal, suggesting that the pituitary was suppressed. However, estrogen accelerates the conjugation of metyrapone by the liver, and therefore the drug has less effect, thus explaining the subnormal responses initially reported. The pituitary-adrenal reaction to stress is normal in women on oral contraceptive pills.

Thyroid

As with CBG, estrogen increases thyroxine-binding globulin. Prior to the introduction of new methods for measuring free thyroxine levels, evaluation of thyroid function was a problem. Measurement of TSH (thyroid-stimulating hormo) and the free thyroxine level in a woman on oral contraception provides an accurate assessment of a patient's thyroid state. Oral contraception affects the total thyroxine level in the blood as well as the amount of binding globulin, but the free thyroxine level is unchanged.

Oral Contraception and Reproduction

The impact of oral contraceptives on the reproductive system is less than initially thought. Early studies which indicated adverse effects have not stood the test of time and the scrutiny of multiple, careful studies. There are two major areas which deserve review: (1) Inadvertent use of oral contraceptives during the cycle of conception and during early pregnancy, and (2) Reproduction after discontinuing oral contraception.

Inadvertent Use During the Cycle of Conception and During Early Pregnancy

One of the reasons, if not the major reason, why a lack of withdrawal bleeding while using oral contraceptives is such a problem is the anxiety produced in both patient and clinician. The patient is anxious because of the uncertainty regarding pregnancy, and the clinician is anxious because of the concerns stemming from the retrospective studies which indicated an increased risk of congenital malformations among the offspring of women who were pregnant and using oral contraception.

Organogenesis does not occur in the first 2 embryonic weeks (first 4 weeks since last menstrual period), however teratogenic effects are possible between the third and eighth embryonic weeks (5 to 10 weeks since LMP).

Initial positive reports linking the use of contraceptive steroids to congenital malformations have not been substantiated. Many suspect a strong component of recall bias in the few positive studies due to a tendency of patients with malformed infants to recall details better than those with normal children. Other confounding problems have included a failure to consider the reasons for the administration of hormones (e.g., bleeding in an already abnormal pregnancy), and a failure to delineate the exact timing of the treatment (e.g., treatment was sometimes confined to a period of time during which the heart could not have been affected).

An association with cardiac anomalies was first claimed in the 1970s.[156,157] This link received considerable support with a report from the U.S. Collaborative Perinatal Project; however, subsequent analysis of these data uncovered several methodologic shortcomings.[158] Simpson, in a very thorough and critical review in 1990, concluded that there is no reliable evidence implicating sex steroids as cardiac teratogens.[159] In fact, in his review, Simpson found no relationship between oral contraception and the following problems: hypospadias, limb reduction anomalies, neural tube defects, and mutagenic effects which would be responsible for chromosomally abnormal fetuses. Even virilization is not a practical consideration because the doses required (e.g., 20–40 mg norethindrone per day) are in excess of anything currently used. These conclusions reflect use of combined oral contraceptives as well as progestins alone.

In the past there was a concern regarding the VACTERL complex. VACTERL refers to a complex of vertebral, anal, cardiac, tracheoesophageal, renal, and limb anomalies. While case-control studies indicated a relationship with oral contraception, prospective studies have failed to obsere any connection between sex steroids and the VACTERL complex.[160,161] A meta-analysis of 26 prospective studies of the risk of birth defects with oral contraceptive ingestion during pregnancy concluded that there was no increase in risk for major malformations, congenital heart defects, or limb reduction defects.[162]

Women who become pregnant while taking oral contraceptives or women who inadvertently take birth control pills early in pregnancy should be advised that the risk of a significant congenital anomaly is no greater than the general rate of 2–3%. This recommendation can be extended to those pregnant woman who have been exposed to a progestational agent such as medroxyprogesterone acetate or 17-hydroxyprogesterone caproate.[163,164]

Reproduction after Discontinuing Oral Contraception

Fertility. The early reports from the English prospective studies indicated that former users of oral contraception had a delay in achieving pregnancy. In the OFPA study, former use had an effect on fertility for up to 42 months in nulliavida women and for up to 30 months in multigravida women.[165] Presumably the delay is due to lingering suppression of the hypothalamic-pituitary reproductive system.

A later analysis of the Oxford data indicated that the delay is concentrated in women age 30–34 who have never given birth.[166] At 48 months 82% of these women had given birth compared to 89% of users of other contraceptive methods. No effect was observed in women younger than 30 or in women who had previously given birth. Childless women age 25–29 experienced some delay in return to fertility, but by 48 months, 91% had given birth compared to 92% in users of other methods. It should be noted that after 72 months the proportions of women who remained undelivered were the same in both groups of women.

This delay has been observed in the United States as well. In the Boston area, the interval from cessation of contraception to conception was 13 months or greater for 24.8% of prior oral contraceptive users compared to 10.6% for former users of all other methods (12.4% for IUD users, 8.5% for diaphragm uses, and 11.9% for other methods).[167] Oral contraceptive users had a lower monthly percentage of conceptions for the first 3 months, and somewhat lower percentage from 4 to 10 months. It took 24 months for 90% of previous oral contraceptive users to become pregnant, 14 months for IUD users, and 10 months for diaphragm users. Similar findings in Connecticut indicate that this delay lasts at least a year, and the effect is greater with higher-dose preparations.[168] Despite this delay, there is no evidence that infertility is increased by the use of oral contraception. In fact, in young women, oral contraceptive use is associated with a lower risk of primary infertility.[169]

Spontaneous Abortion. There is no increase in the incidence of spontaneous abortion in pregnancies after the cessation of oral contraception.[170] Indeed, the rate of spontaneous abortion and stillbirths is slightly less in former pill users, about 1% less for spontaneous abortions and 0.3% less for stillbirths.

Pregnancy Outcome. There is no evidence that oral contraceptives cause changes in individual germ cells that would yield an abnormal child at a later time.[159] There is no increase in the number of abnormal children born to former oral contraceptive users, and there is no change in the sex ratio (a sign of sex-linked recessive mutations).[170,171] These observations are not altered when analyzed for duration of use. Initial observations that women who had previously used oral contraception had an increase in chromosomally abnormal fetuses have not been confirmed. Furthermore, as noted above, there is no increase in the abortion rate after discontinuation, something one would expect if oral contraceptives induce chromosomal abnormalities since these are the principal cause of spontaneous abortion.

In a 3-year follow-up of children whose mothers used oral contraceptives prior to conception, no differences could be detected in weight, anemia, intelligence, or development.[172] Former pills users have no increased risks for the following: perinatal morbidity or mortality, prematurity, and low birth weight.[173,174] Dizygous twinning has been observed to be nearly two-fold (1.6% vs 1.0%) increased in women who conceive soon after cessation of oral contraception.[170] This effect was greater with greater duration of use.

The only reason (and it is a good one) to recommend that women defer attempts to conceive for a month or two after stopping the pill is to improve the accuracy of gestational dating by allowing accurate identification of the last menstrual period.

Breastfeeding

Oral contraception has been demonstrated to diminish the quantity and quality of lactation in postpartum women. Also of concern is the potential hazard of transfer of contraceptive steroids to the infant (a significant amount of the progestational component is transferred into breast milk);[175] however, no adverse effects have thus far been identified. Women who use oral contraception have a lower incidence of breastfeeding after the 6th postpartum month, regardless of whether oral contraception is started at the first, second, or third postpartum month.[176–178]

In adequately nourished women, no impairment of infant growth can be detected; presumably compensation is achieved either through supplementary feedings or increased suckling.[179] In an 8-year follow-up study of children breastfed by mothers using oral contraceptives, no effect could be detected on diseases, intelligence, or psychological behavior.[180] This study also found that mothers on birth control pills lactated a significantly shorter period of time than controls, a mean of 3.7 months vs 4.6 months in controls.

Because the above considerations indicate that oral contraception shortens the duration of breastfeeding, it is worthwhile to consider the contraceptive effectiveness of lactation. In Scotland, no ovulation could be detected in women during exclusive breastfeeding.[181] However, in Chile, 14% of women ovulated during full breastfeeding, although full nursing provided effective contraception up to 3 months postpartum.[182,183] It has been argued that the threshold for suppression of ovulation is at least 5 feedings for a total of at least 65 minutes per day of suckling duration.[184] However in the studies from Chile, the frequency of nursing was the same in breastfeeders who ovulated and those who did not.

In Mexico, a study of 29 breastfeeding mothers and 10 nonbreastfeeders observed that in the absence of bleeding and supplementary feedings, 100% of the breastfeeders remained anovulatory for 3 months postpartum, and 96% up to 6 months.[185] The median time from delivery to first ovulation was 259 days for breastfeeders compared to 119 days for nonbreastfeeders. However, by the third postpartum month, 18% of the breastfeeders had ovulated. Only amenorrheic women who exclusively breastfeed at regular intervals, including nighttime, during the first 6 months have the contraceptive protection equivalent to that provided by oral contraception; with menstruation or after 6 months, the risk of ovulation increases.[186] Supplemental feeding increases the risk of ovulation (and pregnancy) even in amenorrheic women.[187] Total protection against pregnancy is achieved by the exclusively breastfeeding woman for a duration of only 10 weeks. Our reommendations (the Rule of 3's) are provided below under "The Postpartum Visit."

It is apparent that while lactation provides a contraceptive effect, it is variable and not reliable for every woman. Furthermore, because frequent suckling is required to maintain full milk production, women who use oral contraception and also breastfeed less frequently (e.g., because they work outside their home) have two reasons for decreased milk volume. This combination can make it especially difficult to continue nursing.

Because of the concerns regarding the impact of oral contraceptives on breastfeeding, a useful alternative is to combine the contraceptive effect of lactation with the progestin-only minipill. (See Chapters 3 and 8) This low-dose of progestin has no negative impact on breast milk, and some studies document an increase in milk quantity and nutritional quality. Highly effective (near total) protection can be achieved with the combination of lactation and the minipill.

Other Considerations

Prolactin-Secreting Adenomas

Because estrogen is known to stimulate prolactin secretion and to cause hypertrophy of the pituitary lactotrophs, it is appropriate to be concerned over a possible relationship between oral contraception and olactin-secreting adenomas. Several case-control studies have uniformly concluded that no such relationship exists.[188,189] Data from both the RCGP and the OFPA studies indicated no increase in the incidence of pituitary adenomas.[154,190] Previous use of oral contraceptives is not related to the size of prolactinomas at presentation and diagnosis.[96,190] Oral contraception can be prescribed to patients with pituitary microadenomas without fear of subsequent tumor growth.[97] *We have routinely prescribed oral contraception to patients with pituitary microadenomas and have never observed evidence of tumor growth.*

Postpill Amenorrhea

The approximate incidence of "postpill amenorrhea" is 0.7–0.8%, which is equal to the incidence of spontaneous secondary amenorrhea,[174,191,192] and there is no evidence to support the idea that oral contraception caus secondary amenorrhea. If a cause and effect relationship exists between oral contraception and subsequent amenorrhea, one would expect the incidence of infertility to be increased after a given population discontinues use of oral contraception. In those women who discontinue oral contraception in order to get pregnant, 50% conceive by 3 months, and after 2 years, a maximum of 15% of nulliparous women and 7% of parous women fail to conceive,[174] figures comparable to those quoted for the prevalence of spontaneous infertility. Attempts to document a cause and effect relationship between oral contraceptive use and secondary amenorrhea have failed.[193] While patients with this problem come more quickly to our attention because of previous oral contraceptive use and follow-up, there is no cause and effect relationship. Women who have not resumed menstrual function within 12 months should be evaluated as any other patient with secondary amenorrhea.

Use During Puberty

An important related question is: should oral contraception be advised for a young woman with irregular menses and oligoovulation or anovulation? The fear of subsequent infertility should not be a deterrent to providing appropriate contraception. Women who have irregular menstrual periods are more likely to develop secondary amenorrhea whether they use oral contraception or not. The possibility of subsequent secondary amenorrhea is less of a risk and a less urgent problem for a young woman than leaving her unprotected. The need for contraception takes precedence.

There is no evidence that the use of oral contraceptives in the pubertal, sexually active girl impairs growth and development of the reproductive system.[169] Again, the most important concern is and should be the prevention of an unwanted pregnancy. For most teenagers oral contraception, dispensed in the 28-day package for better compliance, is the contraceptive method of choice.

The Postpartum Visit

The individual woman is in need of contraception early in the postpartum period. In a careful study of 22 postpartum, nonbreastfeeding women, the mean time from delivery to the first menses was 45 ± 10.1 days, and no woman ovulated before 25 days after delivery.[194] A high proportion of the first cycles (81.8%) and the subsequent cycles (37%) were not normal; however, this is certainly not predictable in individual women. Others have documented a mean delay of 7 weeks before resumption of ovulation, but half of the women studied ovulated before the 6th week, the time of the traditional postpartum visit. *The obstetrical tradition of scheduling the postpartum visit at 6 weeks should be changed. A 3-week visit would be more productive in avoiding postpartum surprises.*

The Rule of 3's:

In the presence of FULL breastfeeding, a contraceptive method should be used beginning in the *3rd postpartum month*.

With PARTIAL breastfeeding or NO breastfeeding, a contraceptive method should begin during the *3rd postpartum week*.

After the termination of a pregnancy of less than 12 weeks, oral contraception can be started immediately. After a pregnancy of 12 or more weeks, oral contraception has traditionally been started 2 weeks after delivery to avoid an increased risk of thrombosis during the initial postpartum period. This practice has been based on a theoretical concern which is probably no longer an issue with low-dose oral contraception. We believe that oral contraception can be started immediately after a second trimester abortion or premature delivery.

Infections and Oral Contraception

Bacterial STDs

Sexually transmitted diseases (STDs) are one of the most common public health problems in the United States. Approximately 1 million cases of pelvic inflammatory disease (PID) occur annually in the United States.[195] This upper genital tract infection is usually a consequence of STDs. The best estimate of subsequent tubal infertility is derived from an excellent Swedish report; approximately 12% after one episode of PID, 23% after 2 episodes, and 54% after 3 episodes.[196] Because pelvic infection is the single greatest threat to the reproductive future of a young woman, the now recognized protection offered by oral contraception against pelvic inflammatory disease is highly important.[197–200] *The risk of hospitalization for PID is reduced by approximately 50%–60%, but at least 12 months of use are necessary, and the protection is limited to current users.*[198,201] Furthermore, if a patient does get a pelvic infection, the severity of the salpingitis found at laparoscopy is decreased.[202] The mechanism of this protection remains unknown. Speculation includes thickening of the cervical mucus to prevent movement of pathogens and bacteria-laden sperm into the uterus and tubes, and decreased menstrual bleeding reducing movement of pathogens into the tubes as well as a reduction in "culture medium."

The argument has been made that this protection is limited to gonococcal disease, and chlamydial infections may even be enhanced. Fifteen of 17 published studies by 1985 reported a positive association of oral contraceptives with lower genital tract chlamydial cervicitis.[203] Because lower genital tract infections caused by chlamydia are on the rise (now the most prevalent bacterial STD in the U.S.) and the rate of hospitalization for PID is also increased, it is worthwhile for both patients and clinicians to be alert for symptoms of cervicitis or salpingitis in women on oral contraception who are at high risk of sexually transmitted disease (multiple sexual partners, a history of STD, or cervical discharge). The mechanism for the association between chlamydial cervicitis and oral contraceptives may be the well-recognized extension of the columnar epithelium from the endocervix out over the cervix (ectopia) that occurs with oral contraceptive use.[204]

Despite this potential relationship between oral contraception and chlamydial infections, it should be emphasized that there is no evidence for an impact of oral contraceptives increasing the incidence of tubal infertility.[205] In fact, a case-control study indicated that oral contraceptive users with chlamydia infection are protected against symptomatic PID.[206] Thus, the influence of oral contraception on the upper reproductive tract may be different than on the lower tract. These observations on fertility are derived mostly, if not totally, from women using oral contraceptives containing 50 μg of estrogen. The continued progestin dominance of the lower-dose formulations, however, should produce the same protective impact, and evidence indicates that this is so.[201]

Viral STDs

The viral STDs include human immunodeficiency virus (HIV), human papillomavirus (HPV), herpes simplex virus (HSV), and hepatitis B (HBV). At the present time, no known associations exist between oral contraception and the viral STDs. Of course, significant prevention includes barrier methods of contraception (see Chapter 6). Thus far, most studies have found no association between oral contraceptive use and HIV seropositivity, and some have indicated a protective effect.[207,208] *For women not in a stable, monogamous relationship, a dual approach is recommended, combining the contraceptive efficacy and protection against PID offered by oral contraception with the use of a barrier method (and spermicide) for prevention of viral STDs.*

Other Infections

In the British prospective studies, urinary tract infections were increased in users of oral contraception by 20%, and a correlation was noted with estrogen dose. An increased incidence of cervicitis was also reported, an effect related to the progestin dose. The incidence of cervicitis increased with the length of time the pill was used, from no higher after 6 months to 3 times higher by the 6th year of use. A significant increase in a variety of viral diseases, e.g., chickenpox, was observed, suggesting steroid effects on the immune system. The prevalence of these effects with low-dose oral contraception is unknown.

Oral contraception is not linked to bacterial vaginosis, but appears to protect against infections with *Trichomonas*.[209] Evidence is lacking to convincingly implicate oral contraception with vaginal infections with *Candida* species,[209] however, clinical experience is sometimes impressive when recurrence and cure repeatedly follow use and discontinuation of oral contraception.

Patient Management

Absolute Contraindications to the Use of Oral Contraception

1. Thrombophlebitis, thromboembolic disorders, cerebral vascular disease, coronary occlusion, or a past history of these conditions, or conditions predisposing to these problems.
2. Markedly impaired liver function. Steroid hormones are contraindicated in patients with hepatitis until liver function tests return to normal.
3. Known or suspected breast cancer.
4. Undiagnosed abnormal vaginal bleeding.
5. Known or suspected pregnancy.
6. Smokers over the age of 35.

Relative Contraindications Requiring Clinical Judgment and Informed Consent

1. Migraine headaches. In retrospective studies of high-dose pills, migraine headaches have been associated with an increased risk of stroke, however some women report an improvement in their headaches.
2. Hypertension. A woman under 35 who is otherwise healthy and whose blood pressure is controlled by medication can elect to use oral contraception.
3. Uterine leiomyoma. This is no longer a contraindication with the low-dose formulations. There is evidence that the risk of leiomyomas was decreased by 31% in women who used higher dose oral contraception for 10 years.[210] However, a case-control study with lower dose oral contraceptives found neither a decrease nor an increase in risk.[211] The administration of low-dose oral contraceptives to women with leiomyomata does not stimulate fibroid growth, and is associated with a reduction in menstrual bleeding.[212]
4. Gestational diabetes. Low-dose formulations do not produce a diabetic glucose tolerance response in women with previous gestational diabetes, and there is no evidence that oral contraception increases the inci-

dence of overt diabetes mellitus.[86] We believe that women with previous gestational diabetes can use oral contraception with annual assessment of the fasting glucose level.

5. Elective surgery. The recommendation that oral contraception should be discontinued 4 weeks before elective surgery to avoid an increased risk of postoperative thrombosis is based upon data derived from high-dose pills. If possible, it is safer to follow this recommendation, but it is probably less critical with low-dose oral contraceptives. It is prudent to maintain contraception right up to the performance of a sterilization procedure, and this short, outpatient operation probably carries very minimal risk.

6. Epilepsy. Oral contraceptives do not exacerbate epilepsy, and in some women, improvement in seizure control has occurred.[213] Antiepileptic drugs, however, may decrease the effectiveness of oral contraception.

7. Obstructive jaundice in pregnancy. Not all patients with this history will develop jaundice on oral contraception, especially with the low-dose formulations.

8. Sickle cell disease or sickle C disease. Patients with sickle cell trait can use oral contraception. The risk of thrombosis in women with sickle cell disease or sickle C diseases is theoretical (and medical-legal). We believe effective protection against pregnancy in these patients warrants the use of low-dose oral contraception.

9. Diabetes melllitus. Effective prevention of pregnancy outweighs the small risk of complicating vascular disease in diabetic women who are under age 35 and otherwise healthy.

10. Gallbladder disease. Oral contraceptives do not cause gallstones, but may accelerate the emergence of symptoms when gallstones are already present.

Clinical Decisions

Surveillance

In view of the increased safety of low-dose preparations for healthy young women with no risk factors, patients need be seen only every 12 months for exclusion of problems by history, measurement of the blood pressure, urinalysis, breast examination, palpation of the liver, and pelvic examination with Pap smear. Women with risk factors should be seen every 6 months by appropriately trained personnel for screening of problems by history and blood pressure measurement. Breast and pelvic examinations are necessary only yearly. It is worth emphasizing that better continuation is achieved by reassessing new users within 3 months. It is at this time that subtle fears and unvoiced concerns need to be confronted and resolved.

Oral contraception is safer than we thought it was, and the low-dose preparations are extremely safe. Health care providers should make a significant effort to get this message to our patients (and our colleagues). We must make sure our patients receive adequate counseling, either from ourselves or our professional staff. The major reason why patients discontinue oral contraception is fear of side effects.[214] Let's take time to put the risks into proper perspective, and to emphasize the benefits as well as the risks.

Laboratory surveillance should be used only when indicated. Routine biochemical measurements fail to yield sufficient information to warrant the expense. Assessing the cholesterol-lipoprotein profile and carbohydrate metabolism should follow the same guidelines applied to all patients, users and nonusers of contraception. The following is a useful guide as to who should be monitored with blood screening tests for glucose, lipids, and lipoproteins:

> Young women, at least once.
> Women 35 years or older.
> Women with a strong family history of heart disease, diabetes mellitus, or hypertension.
> Women with gestational diabetes melllitus.
> Women with xanthomatosis.
> Obese women.
> Diabetic women.

Choice of Pill

The therapeutic principle remains: utilize the formulations which give effective contraception and the greatest margin of safety. The multiphasic preparations do have a reduced progestin dosage compared to some of the existing monophasic products; however, based on currently available information there is little difference between the low-dose monophasics and the multiphasics. It remains to be seen whether formulations with the new progestins will provide protection against cardiovascular disease, nevertheless the new progestin combinations offer minimal metabolic impact (although it is by no means certain yet that this impact is better than the available low-dose formulations). The one exception is monophasic preparations containing relatively high-doses of levonorgestrel, 150–250 µg; these should be avoided in favor of low-dose formulations.

You and your patients are urged to choose a low-dose preparation containing less than 50 µg of estrogen, combined with low-doses of new or old progestins, avoiding the high-doses of levonorgestrel. Current data support the view that there is greater safety with preparations containing less than 50 µg of estrogen. The arguments in this chapter indicate that all patients should begin oral contraception with low-dose products, and that patients on higher-dose oral contraception should be changed to the low-dose preparations. Stepping down to a lower dose can be accomplished immediately with no adverse reactions such as increased bleeding or failure of contraception.

The pharmacologic effects in animals of various formulations have been used as a basis for therapeutic recommendations in selecting the optimal oral contraceptive pill. *These recommendations (tailor-making the pill to the patient) have not been supported by appropriately controlled clinical trials. All too often this leads to the prescribing of a pill of excessive dosage with its attendant increased risk of serious side effects.* It is worth repeating our earlier comments on potency. Oral contraceptive potency (specifically progestin potency) is no longer a consideration when it comes to prescribing birth control pills. The potency of the various progestins has been accounted for by appropriate adjustments of dose. Clinical advice based on potency is an artificial exercise which has not stood the test of time. The biologic effect of the various progestational components in current low-dose oral contraceptives is approximately the same. Our progress in lowering the doses of the steroids contained in oral contraceptives has yielded products with little serious differences.

Pill Taking

Effective contraception is present during the first cycle of pill use, provided the pills are started no later than the 5th day of the cycle, and no pills are missed. Thus, starting oral contraception on the first day of menses assures immediate protection. In the United States, most clinicians and patients prefer the Sunday start packages, beginning on the first Sunday following menstruation. This can be easier to remember, and it usually avoids menstrual bleeding on weekends. It is probable, but not totally certain, that even if a dominant follicle should emerge in occasional patients after a Sunday start, an LH surge and ovulation would still be prevented.[215] Some clinicians prefer to advise patients to use added protection in the first week of use.

Occasionally patients would like to postpone a menstrual period, e.g., for a wedding, holiday, or vacation. This can be easily achieved by omitting the 7-day hormone-free interval. Simply start a new package of pills the next day after finishing the series of 21 pills in the previous package. Remember, when using a 28 pill package, the patient would start a new package after using the 21 *active* pills.

The use of oral contraception shortens the duration of breastfeeding. For this reason, oral contraception is best deferred until lactation is discontinued. A good alternative is the progestin-only minipill which has no negative impact on breast milk (See Chapters 3 and 8). The minipill has a failure rate of 3%, but when it is combined with the contraceptive action of prolactin due to lactation, nearly total protection can be achieved.

The obstetrical tradition of scheduling the postpartum visit at 6 weeks should be changed. A visit during the 3rd week allows the institution of effective contraception before ovulation resumes. After the termination of a pregnancy of less than 12 weeks, oral contraception should be started immediately. After a pregnancy of 12 or more weeks, the start of oral contraception has traditionally been delayed. The latter delay has been based on theoretical concern over an increased risk of thrombosis early in the postpartum period. This is probably no longer an issue with low-dose oral contraception. We believe that oral contraception can be started immediately after a second trimester abortion or premature delivery.

There is no rationale for recommending a pill-free interval "to rest." The serious side effects are not eliminated by pill-free intervals. This practice all too often results in unwanted pregnancies.

What to do when pills are missed. *If a woman misses 1 pill,* she should take that pill as soon as she remembers and take the next pill as usual. No back-up is needed.

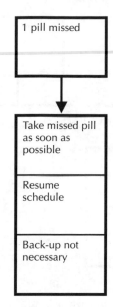

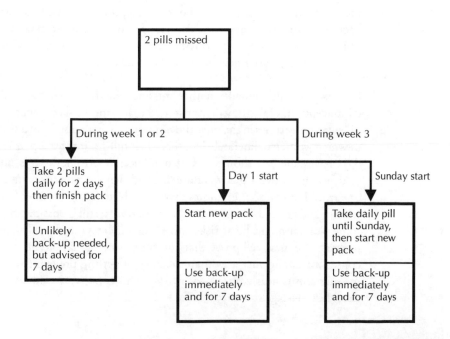

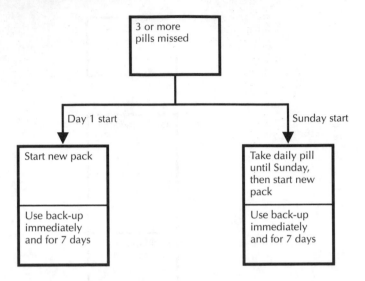

If she misses 2 pills in the first two weeks, she should take two pills on each of the next two days; it is unlikely that a back-up method is needed, but the official consensus is to recommend back-up for the next 7 days.

If 2 pills are missed in the third week, or if more than active 2 pills are missed at any time, another form of contraception should be used as back-up immediately and for 7 days; if a Sunday starter, keep taking a pill every day until Sunday, on Sunday start a new package; if a non-Sunday starter, start a new package the same day.

Studies have questioned whether missing pills has an impact on contraception. One study demonstrated that skipping 4 consecutive pills at varying times in the cycle did not result in ovulation.[215] Studies in which women deliberately lengthen their pill-fee interval up to 11 days have failed to show signs of ovulation.[216] So far there is no evidence that moving to lower doses has had an impact on the margin of error. However, the studies have involved small numbers of women and given the large individual variation, it still is possible that some women might be at risk with a small increase in the pill-free interval. We may well prove that current recommendations are too conservative, and that a woman's chance of getting pregnant with missing pills is nearly zero. Nevertheless, this conservative advice is the safest message to convey.

Clinical Problems

Breakthrough Bleeding

A major continuation problem is breakthrough bleeding. Breakthrough bleeding gives rise to fears and concerns; it is aggravating, and even embarrassing. Therefore, upon starting oral contraception, patients need to be fully informed regarding breakthrough bleeding.

There are two characteristic breakthrough bleeding problems: irregular bleeding in the first few months after starting oral contraception, and unexpected bleeding after many months of use. Effort should be made to manage the bleeding problem in a way that allows the patient to remain on low-dose oral contraception. *There is no evidence that the onset of bleeding is associated with decreased efficacy, no matter what oral contraceptive formulation is used, even the lowest-dose products.* Indeed, in a careful study, breakthrough bleeding did not correlate with changes in the blood levels of the contraceptive steroids.[217]

The most frequently encountered breakthrough bleeding is that which occurs in the first few months of use. The incidence is greatest in the first 3 months, ranging from 10–30% in the first month to lesss than 10% in the third. It is best managed by encouragement and reassurance. This bleeding usually disappears by the third cycle in the majority of women. If necessary, even this early pattern of breakthrough bleeding can be treated as outlined below. It is helpful to explain to the patient that this bleeding represents tissue breakdown as the endometrium adjusts from its usual thick state to the relatively thin state allowed by the hormones in oral contraceptives.

Breakthrough bleeding which occurs after many months of oral contraceptive use is a consequence of the progestin-induced decidualization. This endometrium is shallow and tends to be fragile and prone to breakdown and asynchronous bleeding.

If bleeding occurs just before the end of the pill cycle, it can be managed by having the patient stop the pills, wait 7 days and start a new cycle. If breakthrough bleeding is prolonged or if it is aggravating for the patient, regardless of the point in the pill cycle, control of the bleeding can be achieved with a short course of exogenous estrogen. Conjugated estrogen, 1.25 mg, or estradiol, 2 mg, is administered daily for 7 days when the bleeding is present, no matter where the patient is in her pill cycle. The patient continues to adhere to the schedule of pill taking. Usually one course of estrogen solves the problem, and recurrence of bleeding is unusual (but if it does recur, another 7-day course of estrogen is effective).

Responding to irregular bleeding by having the patient take 2 or 3 pills is not effective. The progestin component of the pill will always dominate, hence doubling the number of pills will also double the progestational impact and its decidualizing, atrophic effect on the endometrium. The addition of extra estrogen while keeping the progestin dose unchanged is logical and effective. This allows the patient to remain on the low-dose formulation with its advantage of greater safety. Breakthrough bleeding, in our view, is not sufficient reason to expose patients to the increased risks associated with higher-dose oral contraceptives. Any bleeding which is not handled by this routine requires investigation for the presence of pathology.

There is no evidence that any oral contraceptive formulations that are approximately equivalent in estrogen and progestin dosage are significantly different in the rates of breakthrough bleeding. Clinicians often become impressed that switching to another product effectively stops the breakthrough bleeding. It is more likely that the passage of time is the responsible factor, and bleeding would have stopped regardless of switching and regardless of product.

Amenorrhea

With low-dose pills, the estrogen content is not sufficient in some women to stimulate endometrial growth. The progestational effect dominates to such a degree that a shallow atrophic endometrium is produced, lacking sufficient tissue to yield withdrawal bleeding. It should be emphasized that permanent atrophy of the endometrium does not occur, and resumption of normal ovarian function will restore endometrial growth and development. Indeed, there is no harmful, permanent consequence of amenorrhea while on oral contraception.

The major problem with amenorrhea while on oral contraception is the anxiety produced in both patient and clinician because the lack of bleeding may be a sign of pregnancy. The patient is anxious because of the uncertainty regarding pregnancy, and the clinician is anxious because of the medical-legal concerns stemming from the old studies which indicated an increased risk of congenital abnormalities among the offspring of women who inadvertently used oral contraception in early pregnancy. We reviewed this problem earlier, and emphatically stated that there is no association between oral contraception and an increased risk of congenital malformation, and there is no increased risk of having abnormal children.

The incidence of amenorrhea in the first year of use with low-dose oral contraception is less than 1%. This incidence increases with duration, reaching perhaps 5% after several years of use. It is important to alert patients upon starting oral contraception that diminished bleeding and possibly no bleeding may ensue.

Amenorrhea is a difficult management problem. A pregnancy test will allow reliable assessment for the presence of pregnancy even at this early stage. However, routine, repeated use of such testing is expensive and annoying, and may lead to discontinuation of oral contraception. *A simple test for pregnancy is to assess the basal body temperature during the END of the pill-free week; a basal body temperature less than 98 degrees is not consistent with pregnancy and oral contraception can be continued.*

Many women are reassured with an understanding of why there is no bleeding and are able to continue on the pill despite the amenorrhea. Some women cannot reconcile themselves to a lack of bleeding, and this is an indication for trying other formulations (a practice unsupported by any clinical trials, and therefore, the expectations are uncertain). But again, this problem does not warrant exposing patients to the greater risks of major side effects associated with higher-dose products.

Some clinicians have observed that the addition of extra estrogen for 1 month (1.25 mg conjugated estrogens or 2 mg estradiol daily throughout the 21 days while taking the oral contraceptive) will rejuvenate the endometrium, and withdrawal bleeding will resume, persisting for many months.

Weight Gain

The complaint of weight gain is frequently cited as a major problem with compliance. Yet studies of the low-dose preparations fail to demonstrate a significant weight gain with oral contraception, and no major differences among the various products.[218] This is obviously a problem of perception. The clinician has to carefully reinforce the lack of association between low-dose oral contraceptives and weight gain and focus the patient on the real culprit: diet and level of exercise. Most women gain a moderate amount of weight as they age, whether they take oral contraceptives or not.

Acne

Low-dose oral contraceptives improve acne regardless of which product is used.[219,220] The low progestin doses (including levonorgestrel formulations) currently used are insufficient to stimulate an androgenic response.

Ovarian Cysts

Anecdotal reports suggested that ovarian cysts are encountered more frequently and suppress less easily with multiphasic formulations. This observation failed to withstand careful scrutiny.[221] Functional ovarian cysts occurred less frequently in women on higher-dose oral contraception.[222] This protection appears to be reduced with the current lower dose products. Thus, the risk of such cysts is not eliminated and therefore, clinicians can encounter such cysts in patients taking any of the oral contraceptive formulations.

Drugs That Affect Efficacy

There are many anecdotal reports of patients who conceived on oral contraceptives whle taking antibiotics. There is little evidence, however, that antibiotics such as ampicillin, metronidazole, quinolone, and tetracycline, which reduce the bacterial flora of the gastrointestinal tract, affect oral contraceptive efficacy. Studies indicate that while antibiotics can alter the excretion of contraceptive steroids, plasma levels are unchanged, and there is no evidence of ovulation.[223,224]

There is good reason to believe that drugs which stimulate the liver's metabolic capacity can affect oral contraceptive efficacy. Othe other hand, a search of a large database failed to discover any evidence that lower-dose oral contraceptives are more ikely to fail or to have more drug interaction problems when other drugs are used.[225]

To be cautious, patients on medications that affect liver metabolism should choose an alternative contraceptive. These drugs are as follows:

Rifampin.
Phenobarbital.
Phenytoin (Dilantin).
Primidone (Mysoline).
Carbamazepine (Tegretol).
Possibly ethosuximide, and griseofulvin.

Other Drug Interactions

Although not extensively documented, there is reason to believe that oral contraceptives potentiate the action of diazepam (Valium), chlordiazepoxide (Librium), tricyclic antidepressants, and theophylline.[226–228] Thus, lower doses of these agents may be effective in oral contraceptive users. Because of an influence on clearance rates, oral contraceptive users may require larger doses of acetaminophen and aspirin.[229,230]

Migraine Headaches

True migraine headaches are morcommon in men, while tension headachesccur equallin men and men. There ve been no wellone studies to deterne the impact of ol contraception on migraine headaches. Patients may report that their headaches are worse or better.

Studies with high-dose pills indicated that migraine headaches were linked to a risk of stroke. More recent studies reflecting the use of low-dose formulations yield mixed results. One failed to find a further increase in stroke in patients with migraine who use oral contraception, another concluded that the use of oral contraception by migraineurs was associated with a 4-fold increase of the already increased risk of ischemic stroke.[231,232] Because of the seriousness of this potential complication, the onset of visual symptoms or severe headaches requires a response. If the patient is at a higher dose, a move to a low-dose formulation may relieve the headaches. Switching to a different brand is worthwhile, if only to evoke a placebo response. True vascular headaches (classic migraine) are an indication to avoid or discontinue oral contraception. If a patient insists on using oral contraception, a product containing 20 µg estrogen should be used.

Clues to severe vascular headaches:

- Headaches that last a long time.
- Dizziness, nausea, or vomiting with headaches.
- Scotomata or blurred vision.
- Episodes of blindness.
- Unilateral, unremitting headaches.
- Headaches that continue despite medication.

In some women, a relationship exists between their fluctuating hormone levels during a menstrual cycle and migraine headaches, with the onset of headaches characteristically coinciding with menses. We have had personal success (anecdotal to be sure) alleviating headaches by eliminating the menstrual cycle, either with the use of *daily* oral contraceptives or the daily administration of a progestational agent (such as 10 mg medroxyprogesterone acetate). Some women with migraine headaches have extremely gratifying responses. Women who experience an exacerbation of their headaches with oral contraception should consider one of the progestin-only methods.

Summary: Oral Contraceptive Use and Medical Problems

Gestational Diabetes. There is no contraindication to oral contraceptive use following gestational diabetes.[86]

Diabetes Mellitus. Oral contraception can be used by diabetic women less than 35 years old who do not smoke and are otherwise healthy (especially an absence of diabetic vascular complications). A case-control study of young women with insulin-dependent diabetes mellitus could detect no differences comparing oral contraceptive users (for 1 to 7 years) to non-users in the following important measures: longitudinal hemoglobin A1c levels, cholesterol levels, evidence of retinopathy or nephropathy.[87]

Hypertension. Low-dose oral contraception can be used in women less than age 35 years old with hypertension controlled by medication, and who are otherwise healthy and do not smoke. We recommend the lowest-dose estrogen formulation.

Pregnancy-Induced Hypertension. Women with pregnancy-induced hypertension can use oral contraception as soon as the blood pressure is normal in the postpartum period.

Hemorrhagic Disorders. Women with hemorrhagic disorders and women taking anticoagulants can use oral contraception. Inhibition of ovulation can avoid the real problem of a hemorrhagic corpus luteum in these patients. A reduction in menstrual blood loss is another benefit of importance.

Gallbladder Disease. Oral contraception use may precipitate a symptomatic attack in women known to have stones or a positive history for gallbladder disease and, therefore, should either be used very cautiously or not at all.

Obesity. An obese woman who is otherwise healthy can use low-dose oral contraception.

Hepatic Disease. Oral contraception can be utilized when liver function tests return to normal. Follow-up liver function tests should be obtained after 2–3 months of use.

Seizure Disorders. There is no impact of oral contraceptives on pattern or frequency of seizures. The concern is that anticonvulsant-induced hepatic enzyme activity can increase the risk of contraceptive failure. Some clinicians advocate the use of higher dose (50 µg estrogen) products; however, no studies have been performed to demonstrate that this higher dose is necessary.

Mitral Valve Prolapse. Oral contraception use is limited to non-smoking patients who are asymptomatic (no clinical evidence of regurgitation). There is a small subset of patients with mitral valve prolapse who are at increased risk of thromboembolism. Patients with atrial fibrillation, migraine headaches, or clotting factor abnormalities should consider progestin-only methods or the IUD (prophylactic antibiotics should cover IUD insertion if mitral regurgitation is present).

Systemic Lupus Erythematosus. Oral contraceptive use can exacerbate systemic lupus erythematous, and the vascular disease associated with lupus represents a contraindication to estrogen-containing oral contraceptives.[233] The progestin-only methods can be considered.

Migraine Headaches. Low-dose oral contraception (the lowest estrogen dose formulation) can be tried with careful surveillance in women with common migraine headaches. Daily administration can prevent menstrual migraine headaches. Oral contraception is best avoided in women with classic migraine headaches associated with neurologic symptoms.

Sickle Cell Disease. Patients with sickle cell trait can use oral contraception. The risk of thrombosis in women with sickle cell disease or sickle C diseases is theoretical (and medical-legal). We believe effective protection against pregnancy in these patients warrants the use of low-dose oral contraception.

Benign Breast Disease. Benign breast disease is not a contraindication for oral contraception; with 2 years of use, the condition may improve.

Congenital Heart Disease or Valvular Heart Disease. Oral contraception is contraindicated only if there is marginal cardiac reserve or a condition that predisposes to thrombosis.

Hyperlipidemia. Because low-dose oral contraceptives have negligible impact on the lipoprotein profile, hyperlipidemia is not an absolute contraindication, with the exception of very high levels of triglycerides (which can be made worse by estrogen). If vascular disease is already present, oral contraception should be avoided. If other risk factors are present, especially smoking, oral contraception is not recommended. Dyslipidemic patients who begin oral contraception should have their lipoprotein profiles monitored monthly for a few visits to ensure no adverse impact. If the lipid abnormality cannot be held in control, an alternative method of contraception should be used.[234] Oral contraceptives containing desogestrel, noregestimate, or gestodene can increase HDL levels, but it is not known if this change is clinically significant.

Depression. Low-dose oral contraceptives have minimal, if any, impact on mood.

Smoking. Oral contraception is absolutely contraindicated in smokers over the age of 35. In patients 35 years old and younger, heavy smoking (15 or more cigarettes per day) is a relative contraindication. The relative risk of cardiovascular events is increased for women of all ages who smoke and use oral contraceptives; however, because the actual incidence of cardiovascular events is so low at a young age, the real risk is very low for young women, although it increases with age. An ex-smoker (for at least one year) should be regarded as a non-smoker. Risk is only linked to active smoking. Is there room for judgment? Given the right circumstances, low-dose oral contraceptives might be appropriate for a light smoker or the user of a nicotine patch. A 20 µg estrogen formulation may benefit smoking women, regardless of age (because this dose of estrogen has no impact on clotting factors and platelet activation in smokers).[45,46]

Pituitary Prolactin-Secreting Adenomas. Low-dose oral contraception can be used in the presence of microadenomas.

Infectious Mononucleosis. Oral contraception can be used as long as liver function tests are normal.

Ulcerative Colitis. There is no association between oral contraception and ulcerative colitis. Women with this problem can use oral contraceptives.[235] Oral contraceptives are absorbed mainly in the small bowel.

An Alternative Route of Administration

Occasionally a situation may be encountered when an alternative to oral administration of contraceptive pills is required. For example, patients receiving chemotherapy can either have significant nausea and vomiting, or mucositis, both of which would prevent oral drug administration. The low-dose oral contraceptives can be administered vaginally. Initially it was claimed that two pills must be placed high in the vagina daily in order to produce contraceptive steroid blood levels comparable to the oral administration of one pill.[236,237] However, a large clinical trial has demonstrated typical contraceptive efficacy with one pill per day.[238]

Noncontraceptive Benefits

The Noncontraceptive Benefits of Oral Contraception

The noncontraceptive benefits of oral contraception can be grouped into two main categories: benefits that incidentally accrue when oral contraception is specifically utilized for contraceptive purposes and benefits that result from the use of oral contraceptives to treat problems and disorders.

The noncontraceptive incidental benefits can be listed as follows:

Effective Contraception.
  • less need for induced abortion.
  • less need for surgical sterilization.
Less Endometrial Cancer.
Less Ovarian Cancer.
Fewer Ectopic Pregnancies.
More Regular Menses.
  • less flow.
  • less dysmenorrhea.
  • less anemia.
Less Salpingitis.
Less Rheumatoid Arthritis.
Increased Bone Density.
Probably Less Endometriosis.
Possibly Less Benign Breast Disease.
Possibly Protection against Atherosclerosis.
Possibly Fewer Fibroids.
Possibly Fewer Ovarian Cysts.

Many of these benefits have been previously discussed. Protection against pelvic inflammatory disease is especially noteworthy and a major contribution to not only preservation of fertility but to lower health care costs. Also important is the prevention of ectopic pregnancies. Ectopic pregnancies have increased in incidence (partly due to an increase in STDs) and represent a major cost for our society and a threat to both fertility and life for individual patients.

Of course, prevention of benign and malignant neoplasia is an outstanding feature of oral contraception. High-dose oral contraceptive use decreased the incidence of benign breast disease diagnosed clinically as well as fibrocystic disease and fibroadenomas diagnosed by biopsy; hopefully the same impact will become evident with current lower dose formulations. A 40% reduction in ovarian cancer and a 50% reduction in endometrial cancer represent substantial protection. Studies with higher-dose formulations documented in long-term users a 31% reduction in uterine leiomyomata and in current users a 78% reduction in corpus luteum cysts and a 49% reduction in functional ovarian cysts.[210,222] The impact of low-dose preparations on these problems remains to be accurately measured and may be less. A case-control study with low-dose oral contraceptives found no impact on the risk of uterine fibroids, neither increased nor decreased.[211] Two epidemiologic studies have indicated that a progressive decline in the incidence of ovarian cysts is proportional to the steroid doses in oral contraceptives.[239,240] In one of these studies, current low-dose monophasic and multiphasic formulations provided no protection against functional ovarian cysts.[240] This apparent weaker protection afforded by the current low-dose formulations makes it very likely that clinicians will encounter such cysts in their patients on oral contraceptives.

The low-dose contraceptives are as effective as higher-dose preparations in reducing menstrual flow and the prevalence and severity of dysmenorrhea.[241,242] The use of oral contraception is associated with a lower incidence of endometriosis.[243] These benefits involving two common gynecologic problems have an important, positive impact on compliance.

An Austrian study concluded that osteoporosis occurs later and is less frequent in women who have used long-term oral contraception.[244] Cross-sectional studies of postmenopausal women indicate that prior use of oral contraception is associated with higher levels of bone density and that the degree of protection is related to duration of exposure.[245,246] Because women who have had the opportunity to use oral contraception are just now entering the postmenopausal years, it will be several years before we know if previous oral contraceptive users have fewer fractures. However, the bone density effects certainly make it probable that previous users of oral contraception will have fewer fractures due to osteoporosis late in life.

The literature on rheumatoid arthritis has been controversial, with studies in Europe finding evidence of protection and studies in North America failing to demonstrate such an effect. An excellent Danish case-control study was designed to answer criticisms of shortcomings in the previous literature.[247] Ever-use of oral contraception reduced the relative risk of rheumatoid arthritis by 60%, and the strongest protection was present in women with a positive family history. A meta-analysis concluded that the evidence consistently indicated a protective effect, but that rather than preventing the development of rheumatoid arthritis, oral contraception may modify the course of disease, inhibiting the progression from mild to severe disease.[248]

Oral contraceptives are frequently utilized to manage the following problems and disorders:

Definitely Beneficial:
- dysfunctional uterine bleeding.
- dysmenorrhea.
- mittelschmerz.
- endometriosis prophylaxis.
- acne and hirsutism.
- hormone therapy for hypothalamic amenorrhea.
- prevention of menstrual porphyria.
- control of bleeding (dyscrasias, anovulation).

Probably Beneficial:
- functional ovarian cysts.
- premenstrual syndrome.

Oral contraceptives have been a cornerstone for the treatment of anovulatory, dysfunctional uterine bleeding. For patients who need effective contraception, oral contraceptives are a good choice to provide hormone therapy to amenorrheic patients, as well as to treat dysmenorrhea. Oral contraceptives are also a good choice to provide prophylaxis against the recurrence of endometriosis in a woman who has already undergone more vigorous treatment with surgery or the GnRH analogues. To protect against endometriosis, oral contraceptives should be taken daily, with no break and no withdrawal bleeding.

The low-dose oral contraceptives are effective in treating acne and hirsutism. Suppression of free testosterone levels is comparable to that achieved with higher dosage.[219,220] The beneficial clinical effect is the same with low-dose preparations containing levonorgestrel, previously recognized to cause acne at high dosage.[220] Formulations with desogestrel, gestodene, and norgestimate are associated with greater increases in sex hormone binding globulin and significant decreases in free testosterone levels. Theoretically these products would be more effective in the treatment of acne and hirsutism; however, this is yet to be documented by clinical studies. It is possible that all low-dose formulations through the combined effects of an increase in sex hormone binding globulin and a decrease in testosterone production produce an overall similar clinical response, especially over time (a year or more).[219]

Oral contraceptives have long been used to speed the resolution of ovarian cysts, but the efficacy of this treatment has not been established. In a small study, 24 patients who had persistent cysts after exogenous gonadotropin treatment were randomized to receive an oral contraceptive or expectant management.[249] No advantage for the contraceptive treatment could be demonstrated. The cysts resolved completely and equally fast in both groups. Of course, these were functional cysts secondary to ovulation induction, and this experience may not apply to spontaneously appearing cysts. Oral contraception does provide protection in women who repetitively form ovarian cysts.

Conclusion. Oral contraceptives are associated with a collection of effects which yield an overall improvement in individual health. From a public health point of view, the combined impact leads to a decrease in the cost of health care. For both individual and public health, these impacts are especially significant in older women. These considerations allow the clinician to present oral contraception with a very positive attitude, an approach which makes an important contribution to a patient's ability to make appropriate health choices.

Continuation: Failure or Success?

Despite the fact that oral contraception is highly effective, hundreds of thousands of unintended pregnancies (close to 1 million) occur each year in the United States because of the failure of oral contraception. Worldwide, literally millions of unintended pregnancies result from poor compliance. In general, young, unmarried, poor, and minority women are more likely to have failures, reaching rates of 10–20%.[250] Overall, the failure rate with actual use ranges from 3 to 6%. This difference between the theoretical efficacy and actual use reflects compliance and noncompliance. Noncompliance includes a wide variety of behavior: failure to fill the initial prescription, failure to continue on the medication, and incorrectly taking oral contraception. Compliance (continuation) is an area in which personal behavior, biology, and pharmacology come together. Oral contraceptive continuation reflects the interaction of these influences. Unfortunately, women who discontinue oral contraception often utilize a less effective method or, worse, fail to substitute another method.

There are 3 major factors that affect continuation:

1. Fears and concerns regarding cancer, cardiovascular disease, and the impact of oral contraception on future fertility.
2. The experience of side effects such as breakthrough bleeding and amenorrhea, and perceived experience of "minor" problems such as headaches, nausea, and weight gain.
3. Non-medical issues such as inadequate instructions on pill-taking, complicated pill packaging, and difficulties arising from the patient package insert.

The information in this chapter is the foundation for good continuation, but the clinician must go beyond the presentation of information and develop an effective means of communicating that information. We recommend the following approach to the clinician-patient encounter as one way to improve continuation with oral contraception.

1. Explain how oral contraception works.
2. Review briefly the risks and benefits of oral contraception, but be careful to put the risks in proper perspective, and to emphasize the safety and noncontraceptive benefits of low-dose oral contraceptives.
3. Show and demonstrate to the patient the package of pills she will use.
4. Explain how to take the pills:
   • When to start.
   • The importance of developing a daily routine to avoid missing pills.
   • What to do if pills are missed.
5. Review the side effects that can affect continuation: amenorrhea, breakthrough bleeding, headaches, weight gain, nausea, etc., and what to do if one or more occurs.
6. Explain the warning signs of potential problems: abdominal or chest pain, trouble breathing, severe headaches, visual problems, leg pain or swelling.
7. Ask the patient to be sure to call if another clinician prescribes other medications.
8. Ask the patient to repeat critical information to make sure she understands what has been said. Ask if the patient has any questions.

9. Schedule a return appointment in 2–3 months to review understanding and address fears and concerns.
10. Make sure a line of communication is open to clinician or office personnel. Ask the patient to call for any problem or concern before she stops taking the oral contraceptives.

References

1. **Perone N,** The progestins, in Goldzieher JW, editor, *Pharmacology of the Contraceptive Steroids,* Raven Press, Ltd., New York, 1994, pp 5–20.

2. **Asbell B,** *The Pill: A Biography of the Drug that Changed the World,* Random House, New York, 1995.

3. **Djerassi C,** *The Pill, Pygmy Chimps, and Degas' Horse,* Basic Books, 1992.

4. **Pincus G,** *The Control of Fertility,* Academic Press, New York, 1965.

5. **Goldzieher JW,** Selected aspects of the pharmacokinetics and metabolism of ethinyl estrogens and their clinical implications, Am J Obstet Gynecol 163:318, 1990.

6. **Stanczyk FZ, Roy S,** Metabolism of levonorgestrel, norethindrone, and structurally related contraceptive steroids, Contraception 42:67, 1990.

7. **Edgren RA,** Progestagens, in Givens J, editor, *Clinical Uses of Steroids,* Yearbook, Chicago, 1980, pp 1–29.

8. **Speroff L, DeCherney A,** Evaluation of a new generation of oral contraceptives, Obstet Gynecol 81:1034, 1993.

9. **Jung-Hoffman C, Kuhl H,** Interaction with the pharmacokinetics of ethinylestradiol and progestogens contained in oral contraceptives, Contraception 40:299, 1989.

10. **Hümpel M, Täuber U, Kuhnz W, Pfeffer M, Brill K, Heithecker R, Louton T, Steinberg B, Seifert W, Schütt B,** Protein binding of active ingredients and comparison of serum ethinyl estradiol, sex hormone-binding globulin, corticosteroid-binding globulin, and cortisol levels in women using a combination of gestodene/ethinyl estradiol (Femovan) or a combination of desogestrel/ethinyl estradiol (Marvelon) and single dose ethinyl estradiol bioequivalence from both oral contraceptives, Am J Obstet Gynecol 163:329, 1990.

11. **Dibbelt L, Knuppen R, Jütting G, Heimann S, Klipping CO, Parikka-Olexik H,** Group comparison of serum ethinyl estradiol, SHBG and CBG levels in 83 women using two low-dose oral contraceptives for three months, Contraception 43:1, 1991.

12. **Trussell J, Hatcher RA, Cates W Jr, Stewart FH, Kost K,** Contraceptive failure in the United States: an update, Stud Fam Plann 21:51, 1990.

13. **Royal College of General Practitioners,** *Oral Contraceptives and Health,* Pitman Publishing, New York, 1974.

14. **Royal College of General Practitioners,** Oral contraception study: mortality among oral contraceptive users, Lancet 2:727, 1977.

15. **Royal College of General Practitioners,** Oral contraceptive study: oral contraceptives, venous thrombosis, and varicose veins, J Roy Coll Gen Pract 28:393, 1978.

16. Royal College of General Practitioners Oral Contraceptive Study, Further analyses of mortality in oral contraceptive users, Lancet 1:541, 1981.

17. Royal College of General Practitioners Oral Contraceptive Study, Incidence of arterial disease among oral contraceptive users, J Roy Coll Gen Pract 33:75, 1983.

18. Vessey MP, McPherson K, Johnson B, Mortality among women participating in the Oxford/Family Planning Association contraceptive study, Lancet 2:731, 1977.

19. Vessey MP, McPherson K, Yeates D, Mortality in oral contraceptive users, Lancet 1:549, 1981.

20. Vessey MP, Lawless M, Yeates D, Oral contraceptives and stroke: findings in a large prospective study, Br Med J 289:530, 1984.

21. Ramcharan S, Pellegrin FA, Ray RM, Hsu J-P, The Walnut Creek Contraceptive Drug Study. A prospective study of the side effects of oral contraceptives, J Reprod Med 25:366,360, 1980.

22. Porter JB, Hershel J, Walker AM, Mortality among oral contraceptive users, Obstet Gynecol 70:29, 1987.

23. Ory HW, Association between oral contraceptives and myocardial infarction, JAMA 237:2619, 1977.

24. Shapiro S, Slone D, Rosenberg L, Kaufman DW, Stolley PD, Miettinen OS, Oral contraceptive use in relation to myocardial infarction, Lancet 1:743, 1979.

25. Hennekens CH, Evans D, Peto R, Oral contraceptive use, cigarette smoking and myocardial infarction, Br J Fam Plann 5:66, 1979.

26. Rosenberg L, Hennekens CH, Rosner B, Belanger C, Rothman KH, Speizer FE, Oral contraceptive use in relation to nonfatal myocardial infarction, Am J Epidemiol 11:59, 1980.

27. Meade TW, Greenburg G, Thompson SG, Progestogens and cardiovascular reactions associated with oral contraceptives and a comparison of the safety of 50- and 30- μg estrogen preparations, Br Med J 280:1157, 1980.

28. Kay CR, The happiness pill, J Roy Coll Gen Pract 30:8, 1980.

29. Vessey MP, Villard-Mackintosh I, McPherson K, Yeates D, Mortality among oral contraceptive users: 20 year follow up of women in a cohort study, Br Med J 299:1487, 1989.

30. Bottinger LE, Boman G, Eklund G, Westerholm B, Oral contraceptives and thromboembolic disease: effects of lowering oestrogen content, Lancet 1:1097, 1980.

31. Gerstman BB, Piper JM, Tomita DK, Ferguson WJ, Stadel BV, Lundin FE, Oral contraceptive estrogen dose and the risk of deep venous thromboembolic disease, Am J Epidemiol 133:32, 1991.

32. **Lidegaard Ø,** Oral contraception and risk of a cerebral thromboembolic attack: results of a case-control study, Br Med J 306:956, 1993.

33. **Hannaford PC, Croft PR, Kay CR,** Oral contraception and stroke: evidence from the Royal College of General Practitioners' Oral Contraception Study, Stroke 25:935, 1994.

34. **Thorogood M, Mann J, Murphy M, Vessey M,** Risk factors for fatal venous thromboembolism in young women: a case-control study, Int J Epidemiol 21:48, 1992.

35. **Farmer RDT, Preston TD,** The risk of venous thromboembolism associated with low estrogen oral contraceptives, J Obstet Gynaecol 15:195, 1995.

36. **WHO Collaborative Study of Cardiovascular Disease and Steroid Hormone Contraception,** Venous thromboembolic disease and combined oal contraceptives: results of international multicentre case-control study, Lancet 348:1575, 1995.

37. **Barrett DH, Anda RF, Escobedo LG, Croft JB, Williamson DF, Marks JS,** Trends in oral contraceptive use and cigarette smoking, Arch Fam Med 3:438, 1994.

38. **Hajjar KA,** Factor V Leiden: an unselfish gene? New Engl J Med 331:1585, 1994.

39. **Svensson PJ, Dahlbäck B,** Resistance to activated protein C as a basis for venous thrombosis, New Engl J Med 330:517, 1994.

40. **Hellgren M, Svensson PJ, Dahlbäck B,** Resistance to activated protein C as a basis for venous thromboembolism associated with pregnancy and oral contraceptives, Am J Obstet Gynecol 173:210, 1995.

41. **Rees DC, Cox M, Clegg JB,** World distribution of factor V Leiden, Lancet 346:1133, 1995.

42. **Jespersen J, Petersen KR, Skouby SO,** Effects of newer oral contraceptives on the inhibition of coagulation and fibrinolysis in relation to dosage and type of steroid, Am J Obstet Gynecol 163:396, 1990.

43. **Notelovitz M, Kitchens CS, Khan FY,** Changes in coagulation and anticoagulation in women taking low-dose triphasic oral contraceptives: a controlled comparative 12-month clinical trial, Am J Obstet Gynecol 167:1255, 1992.

44. **Schlit AF, Grandjean P, Donnez J, Lavenne E,** Large increase in plasmatic 11-dehydro-TXB$_2$ levels due to oral contraceptives, Contraception 51:53, 1995.

45. **Fruzzetti F, Ricci C, Fioretti P,** Haemostasis profile in smoking and nonsmoking women taking low-dose oral contraceptives, Contraception 49:579, 1994.

46. Basdevant A, Conard J, Pelissier C, Guyene T-T, Lapousterle C, Mayer M, Guy-Grand B, Degrelle H, Hemostatic and metabolic effects of lowering the ethinyl-estradiol dose from 30 mcg to 20 mcg in oral contraceptives containing desogestrel, Contraception 48:193, 1993.

47. Vandenbroucke JP, Koster T, Briët E, Reitsma PH, Bertina RM, Rosendaal FR, Increased risk of venous thrombosis in oral-contraceptive users who are carriers of factor V Leiden mutation, Lancet 344:1453, 1994

48. Pabinger I, Schneider B, and the GTH Study Group, Thrombotic risk of women with hereditary antithrombin III, protein C, and protein S deficiency taking oral contraceptive medication, Thromb Haemost 5:548, 1994.

49. Stampfer MJ, Willett WC, Colditz GA, Speizer FE, Hennekens CH, Past use of oral contraceptives and cardiovascular disease: a meta-analysis in the context of the Nurses' Health Study, Am J Obstet Gynecol 163:285, 1990.

50. Rosenberg L, Palmer JR, Lesko SM, Shapiro S, Oral contraceptive use and the risk of myocardial infarction, Am J Epidemiol 131:1009, 1990.

51. Croft P, Hannaford PC, Risk factors for acute myocardial infarction in women: evidence from the Royal College of General Practitioners' oral contraception study, Br Med J 298:165, 1989.

52. Colditz, GA and the Nurses' Health Study Research Group, Oral contraceptive use and mortality during 12 years of follow-up: the Nurses' Health Study, Ann Intern Med 120:821, 1994.

53. WHO Collaborative Study of Cardiovascular Disease and Steroid Hormone Contraception, Effect of different progestagens in low oestrogen oral contraceptives on venous thromboembolic disease, Lancet 348:1582, 1995.

54. Jick H, Jick SS, Gurewich V, Myers MW, Vasilakis C, Risk of idiopathic cardiovascular death and nonfatal venous thromboembolism in women using oral contraceptives with differing progestagen components, Lancet 348:1589, 1995.

55. Bloemenkammp KWM, Rosendaal FR, Helmerhorst FM, Buller HR, Vandenbroucke JP, Enhancement by factor V Leiden mutation of risk of deep-vein thrombosis associated with oral contraceptives containing a third-generation progestagen, Lancet 348:1593, 1995.

56. Spitzer WO, Lewis MA, Heinemann LAJ, Thorogood M, MacRae KD, on behalf of Transitional Reasearch Group on Oral Contraceptives and the Health of Young Women, Third generation oral contraceptives and risk of venous thromboembolic disorders: an international case-control study, Br Med J, 312:83,1996.

57. Wahl P, Walden C, Knopp R, Hoover J, Wallace R, Heiss G, Refkind B, Effect of estrogen/progestin potency on lipid/lipoprotein cholesterol, New Engl J Med 308:862, 1983.

58. **Burkman RT, Robinson JC, Kruszon-Moran D, Kimball AW, Kwiterovich P, Burford RG,** Lipid and lipoprotein changes associated with oral contraceptive use: a randomized clinical trial, Obstet Gynecol 71:33, 1988.

59. **Patsch W, Brown SA, Grotto AM Jr, Young RL,** The effect of triphasic oral contraceptives on plasma lipids and lipoproteins, Am J Obstet Gynecol 161:1396, 1989.

60. **Gevers Leuven JA, Dersjant-Roorda MC, Helmerhorst FM, de Boer R, Neymeyer-Leloux A, Havekes L,** Estrogenic effect of gestodene-desogestrel-containing oral contraceptives on lipoprotein metabolism, Am J Obstet Gynecol 163:358, 1990.

61. **Kloosterboer HJ, Rekers H,** Effects of three combined oral contraceptive preparations containing desogestrel plus ethinyl estradiol on lipid metabolism in comparison with two levonorgestrel preparations, Am J Obstet Gynecol 163:370, 1990.

62. **Notelovitz M, Feldmand EB, Gillespy M, Gudat J,** Lipid and lipoprotein changes in women taking low-dose, triphasic oral contraceptives: a controlled, comparative, 12-month clinical trial, Am J Obstet Gynecol 160:1269, 1989.

63. **Engel JH, Engel E, Lichtlen PR,** Coronary atherosclerosis and myocardial infarction in young women — role of oral contraceptives, Eur Heart J 4:1, 1983.

64. **Jugdutt BI, Stevens GF, Zacks DJ, Lee SJK, Taylor RF,** Myocardial infarction, oral contraception, cigarette smoking, and coronary aratery spasm in young women, Am Heart J 106:757, 1983.

65. **Croft P, Hannaford PC,** Risk factors for acute myocardial infarction in women, Br Med J 298:674, 1989.

66. **Adams MR, Clarkson TB, Koritnik DR, Nash HA,** Contraceptive steroids and coronary artery atherosclerosis in cynomolgus macaques, Fertil Steril 47:1010, 1987.

67. **Clarkson TB, Adams MR, Kaplan JR, Shively CA, Koritnik DR,** From menarche to menopause: coronary artery atherosclerosis and protection in cynomolgus monkeys, Am J Obst Gynecol 160:1280, 1989.

68. **Clarkson TB, Shively CA, Morgan TM, Koritnik DR, Adams MR, Kaplan JR,** Oral contraceptives and coronary artery atherosclerosis of cynomolgus monkeys, Obstet Gynecol 75:217, 1990.

69. **Kushwaha RS, Hazzard WR,** Exogenous estrogens attenuate dietary hypercholesterolemia and atherosclerosis in the rabbit, Metabolism 30:57, 1981.

70. **Hough JL, Zilversmit DB,** Effect of 17 beta estradiol on aortic cholesterol content and metabolism in cholesterol-fed rabbits, Arteriosclerosis 6:57, 1986.

71. Henriksson P, Stamberger M, Eriksson M, Rudling M, Diczfulusy U, Berglund L, Angelin B, Oestrogen-induced changes in lipoprotein metabolism: role in prevention of atherosclerosis in the cholesterol-fed rabbit, Eur J Clin Invest 19:395, 1989.

72. Hirvonen E, Heikkila-Idanpaan J, Cardiovascular death among women under 40 years of age using low-estrogen oral contraceptives and intrauterine devices in Finland from 1975 to 1984, Am J Obstet Gynecol 163:281, 1990.

73. Mant D, Villard-Mackintosh L, Vessey MP, Yeates D, Myocardial infarction and angina pectoris in young women, J Epidemiol Community Health 41:215, 1987.

74. Thorogood M, Mann J, Murphy M, Vessey M, Fatal stroke and use of oral contraceptives: findings from a case-control study, Am J Epidemiol 136:35, 1992.

75. Kovacs L, Bartfai G, Apro G, Annus J, Bulpitt C, Belsey E, Pinol A, The effect of the contraceptive pill on blood pressure: a randomized controlled trial of three progestogen-oestrogen combinations in Szeged, Hungary, Contraception 33:69, 1986.

76. Nichols M, Robinson G, Bounds W, Newman B, Guillebaud J, Effect of four combined oral contraceptives on blood pressure in the pill-free interval, Contraception 47:367, 1993.

77. Qifang S, Deliang L, Xiurong J, Haifang L, Zhongshu Z, Blood pressure changes and hormonal contraceptives, Contraception 50:131, 1994.

78. Darney P, Safety and efficacy of a triphasic oral contraceptive containing desogrestrel: results of three multicenter trials, Contraception 48:323, 1993.

79. Pritchard JA, Pritchard SA, Blood pressure response to estrogen-progestin oral contraceptives after pregnancy-induced hypertension, Am J Obstet Gynecol 129:733, 1977.

80. Gaspard UJ, Lefebvre PJ, Clinical aspects of the relationship between oral contraceptives, abnormalities in carbohydrate metabolism, and the development of cardiovascular disease, Am J Obstet Gynecol 163:334, 1990.

81. Bowes WA, Katta LR, Droegemueller W, Braight TG, Triphasic randomized clinical trial: comparison of effects on carbohydrate metabolism, Am J Obstet Gynecol 161:1402, 1989.

82. van der Vange N, Kloosterboer HJ, Haspels AA, Effect of seven low-dose combined oral contraceptive preparations on carbohydrate metabolism, Am J Obstet Gynecol 156:918, 1987.

83. Godsland IF, Crook D, Simpson R, Proudler T, Gelton C, Lees B, Anyaoku V, Devenport M, Wynn V, The effects of different formulations of oral contraceptive agents on lipid and carbohydrate metabolism, New Engl J Med 323:1375, 1990.

105

84. Duffy TJ, Ray R, Oral contraceptive use: prospective follow-up of women with suspected glucose intolerance, Contraception 30:197, 1984.

85. Hannaford PC, Kay CR, Oral contraceptives and diabetes mellitus, Br Med J 299:315, 1989.

86. Kjos SL, Shoupe D, Douyan S, Friedman RL, Bernstein GS, Mestman JH, Mishell DR Jr, Effect of low-dose oral contraceptives on carbohydrate and lipid metabolism in women with recent gestational diabetes: results of a controlled, randomized, prospective study, Am J Obstet Gynecol 163:1822, 1990.

87. Garg SK, Chase HP, Marshall G, Hoops SL, Holmes DL, Jackson WE, Oral contraceptives and renal and retinal complications in young women with insulin-dependent diabetes mellitus, JAMA 271:1099, 1994.

88. Petersen KR, Skouby SO, Sidelmann J, Mølsted-Pedersen L, Jespersen J, Effects of contraceptive steroids on cardiovascular risk factors in women with insulin-dependent diabetes mellitus, Am J Obstet Gynecol 171:400, 1994.

89. Royal College of General Practitioners' Oral Contraception Study, Oral contraceptives and gallbladder disease, Lancet 2:957, 1982.

90. Bennion LJ, Ginsberg RL, Garnick MB, Bennett PH, Effects of oral contraceptives on the gallbladder bile of normal women, New Engl J Med 294:189, 1976.

91. Grodstein F, Colditz GA, Hunter DJ, Manson JE, Willett WC, Stampfer MJ, A prospective study of symptomatic gallstones in women: relation with oral contraceptives and other risk factors, Obstet Gynecol 84:207, 1994.

92. La Vecchia C, Negri E, D'Avanzo B, Parazzini F, Genitle A, Franceschi S, Oral contraceptives and noncontraceptive oestrogens in the risk of gallstone disease requiring surgery, J Epidemiol Community Health 46:234, 1992.

93. Vessey M, Painter R, Oral contraceptive use and benign gallbladder disease; revisited, Contraception 50:167, 1994.

94. Vessey MP, Villard-Mackintosh L, Painter R, Oral contraceptives and pregnancy in relation to peptic ulcer, Contraception 46:349, 1992.

95. Lashner BA, Kane SV, Hanauer SB, Lack of association between oral contraceptive use and ulcerative colitis, Gastroenterology 99:1032, 1990.

96. Hulting A-L, Werner S, Hagenfeldt K, Oral contraceptives do not promote the development or growth of prolactinomas, Contraception 27:69, 1983.

97. Corenblum B, Donovan L, The safety of physiological estrogen plus progestin replacement therapy and with oral contraceptive therapy in women with pathological hyperprolactinemia, Fertil Steril 59:671, 1993.

98. **The Cancer and Steroid Hormone Study of the CDC and NICHD,** Combination oral contraceptive use and the risk of endometrial cancer, JAMA 257:796, 1987.

99. **Schlesselman JJ,** Oral contraceptives and neoplasia of the uterine corpus, Contraception 43:557, 1991.

100. **Vessey MP, Painter R,** Endometrial and ovarian cancer and oral contraceptives — findings in a large cohort study, Br J Cancer 71:1340, 1995.

101. **Mant JWF, Vessey MP,** Ovarian and endometrial cancers, Cancer Surveys 19:287, 1994.

102. **The Cancer and Steroid Hormone Study of the CDC and NICHD,** The reduction in risk of ovarian cancer associated with oral-contraceptive use, New Engl J Med 316:650, 1987.

103. **Hankinson SE, Colditz GA, Hunter DJ, Spencer TL, Rosner B, Stampfer MJ,** A quantitative assessment of oral contraceptive use and risk of ovarian cancer, Obstet Gynecol 80:708, 1992.

104. **Whittemore AS, Harris R, Itnyre J, and the Collaborative Ovarian Cancer Group,** Characteristics relating to ovarian cancer risk: collaborative analysis of 12 US case-control studies. II. Invasive epithelial ovarian cancers in white women, Am J Epidemiol 136:1184, 1992.

105. **Rosenberg L, Palmer JR, Zauber AG, Warshauer ME, Lewis JL Jr, Strom BL, Harlap S, Shapiro S,** A case-control study of oral contraceptive use and invasive epithelial ovarian cancer, Am J Epidemiol 139:654, 1994.

106. **Brinton LA,** Oral contraceptives and cervical neoplasia, Contraception 43:581, 1991.

107. **Delgado-Rodriguez M, Sillero-Arenas M, Martin-Moreno JM, Galvez-Vargas R,** Oral contraceptives and cancer of the cervix uteri. A meta-analysis, Acta Obstet Gynecol Scand 71:368, 1992.

108. **Gram IT, Macaluso M, Stalsberg H,** Oral contraceptive use and the incidence of cervical intraepithelial neoplasia, Am J Obstet Gynecol 167:40, 1992.

109. **Irwin KL, Rosero-Bixby L, Oberle MW, Lee NC, Whatley AS, Fortney JA, Bonhomme MG,** Oral contraceptives and cervical cancer risk in Costa Rica: detection bias or causal association? JAMA 259:59, 1988.

110. **Ye Z, Thomas DB, Ray Rm, and the WHO Collaborative Study of Neoplasia and Steroid Contraceptives,** Combined oral contraceptives and risk of cervical carcinoma *in situ*, Int J Epidemiol 24:19, 1995.

111. **Brinton LA, Reeves WC, Brenes MM, Herrero R, de Britton RC, Gaitan E, Tenorio F, Garcia M, Rawls WE,** Oral contraceptive use and risk of invasive cervical cancer, Int J Epidemiol 19:4, 1990.

112. **Ursin G, Peters RK, Henderson BE, d'Ablaing G III, Monroe KR, Pike MC,** Oral contraceptive use and adenocarcinoma of cervix, Lancet 344:1390, 1994.

113. **Neuberger J, Forman D, Doll R, Williams R,** Oral contraceptives and hepatocellular carcinoma, Br Med J 292:1355, 1986.

114. **Palmer JR, Rosenberg L, Kaufman DW, Warshauer ME, Stolley P, Shapiro S,** Oral contraceptive use and liver cancer, Am J Epidemiol 130:878, 1989.

115. **WHO Collaborative Study of Neoplasia and Steroid Contraceptives,** Combined oral contraceptives and liver cancer, Int J Cancer 43:254, 1989.

116. **Brinton LA, Vessey MP, Flavel R, Yeates D,** Risk factors for benign breast disease, Am J Epidemiol 113:203, 1981.

117. **Charreau I, Plu-Bureau G, Bachelot A, Contesso G, Guinebretiere JM, L"e, MG,** Oral contraceptive use and risk of benign breast disease in a French case-control study of young women, Eur J Cancer Prev 21:47, 1993.

118. **Vessey M, Baron J, Doll R, McPherson K, Yeates D,** Oral contraceptives and breast cancer: final report of an epidemiological study, Br J Cancer 47:455, 1982.

119. **Vessey M, McPherson K, Villard-Mackintosh L, Yeates D,** Oral contraceptives and breast cancer: latest findings in a large cohort study, Br J Cancer 59:613, 1989.

120. **Romieu I, Willett WC, Colditz GA, Stampfer MJ, Rosner B, Hennekens, CH, Speizer FE,** Prospective study of oral contraceptive use and risk of breast cancer in women, J Natl Cancer Inst 81:1313, 1989.

121. **La Vecchia C, Decarli A, Fasoli M, Franceschi S, Gentile A, Negri E, Parazzini F, Tognomi G,** Oral contraceptives and cancers of the breast and of the female genital tract. Interim results from a case-control study, Br J Cancer 54:311, 1986.

122. **Meirik O, Dami H, Christoffersen T, Lund E, Bergstrom R, Bergsjo P,** Oral contraceptive use and breast cancer in young women, Lancet 2:650, 1986.

123. **Kay CR, Hannaford PC,** Breast cancer and the pill — further report from the Royal College of General Practitioners' oral contraceptive study, Br J Cancer 58:675, 1988.

124. **Miller DR, Rosenberg L, Kaufman DW, Stolley P, Warshauer ME, Shapiro S,** Breast cancer before age 45 and oral contraceptive use: new findings, Am J Epidemiol 129:269, 1989.

125. **UK National Case-Control Study Group,** Oral contraceptive use and breast cancer risk in young women, Lancet 1:973, 1989.

126. **WHO Collaborative Study of Neoplasia and Steroid Contraceptives,** Breast cancer and combined oral contraceptives: Results from a multinational study, Br J Cancer 61:110, 1990.

127. **McPherson K, Neil A, Vessey MP,** Oral contraceptives and breast cancer, Lancet 2:414, 1983.

128. Hennekens CH, Speizer FE, Lipnik RJ, Rosner B, Bain C, Belanger C, Stampfer MJ, Willett W, Peto R, Case-control study of oral contraceptive use and breast cancer, J Natl Cancer Inst 72:39, 1984.

129. Rosenberg L, Miller DR, Kaufman DW, Helmrich SP, Stolley PD, Schoffenfeld D, Shapiro S, Breast cancer and oral contraceptive use, Am J Epidemiol 119:167, 1984.

130. Stadel BV, Rubin GL, Webster LA, Schlesselman JJ, Wingo PA, Oral contraceptives and breast cancer in young women, Lancet 2:970, 1985.

131. Paul C, Skegg DCG, Spears GFS, Kaldor JM, Oral contraceptives and breast cancer: a national study, Br Med J 293:723, 1986.

132. McPherson K, Vessey MP, Neil A, Doll R, Jones L, Roberts M, Early oral contraceptive use and breast cancer: Results of another case-control study, Br J Cancer 56:653, 1987.

133. Stadel BV, Lai SL, Oral contraceptives and premenopausal breast cancer in nulliparous women, Contraception 38:287, 1988.

134. Lipnick RJ, Buring JE, Hennekens CH, Rosner B, Willett W, Bain C, Stampfer MJ, Colditz GA, Peto R, Speizer FE, Oral contraceptives and breast cancer: a prospective cohort study, JAMA 255:58, 1986.

135. Pike MC, Krailo MD, Henderson BE, Duke A, Roy S, Breast cancer in young women and use of oral contraceptives: possible modifying effect of formulation and age at use, Lancet 2:926, 1983.

136. Ursin G, Aragaki CC, Paganini-Hill A, Siemiatycki J, Thompson WD, Haile RW, Oral contraceptives and premenopausal bilateral breast cancer: a case-control study, Epidemiology 3:414, 1992.

137. Rookus MA, Leeuwen FE, for the Netherlands Oral Contraceptives and Breast Cancer Study Group, Oral contraceptives and risk of breast cancer in women aged 20–54 years, Lancet 344:844, 1994.

138. White E, Malone KE, Weiss NS, Daling JR, Breast cancer among young U.S. women in relation to oral contraceptive use, J Natl Cancer Inst 86:505, 1994.

139. Brinton LA, Daling JR, Liff JM, Schoenberg JB, Malone KE, Stanford JL, Coates RJ, Gammon MD, Hanson L, Hoover RN, Oral contraceptives and breast cancer risk among younger women, J Natl Cancer Inst 87:827, 1995.

140. Stanford JL, Brinton LA, Hoover RN, Oral contraceptives and breast cancer: results from an expanded case-control study, Br J Cancer 60:375, 1989.

141. Schildkraut JM, Hulka BS, Wilkinson WE, Oral contraceptives and breast cancer: a case-control study with hospital and community controls, Obstet Gynecol 76:395, 1990.

142. Cancer and Steroid Hormone Study, CDC and NICHD, Oral contraceptive use and the risk of breast cancer, New Engl J Med 315:405, 1986.

143. Murray P, Schlesselman JJ, Stadel BV, Shenghan L, Oral contraceptives and breast cancer risk in women with a family history of breast cancer, Am J Obstet Gynecol 73:977, 1989.

144. Schlesselman JJ, Stadel BV, Murray P, Shenghan L, Breast cancer risk in relation to type of estrogen contained in oral contraceptives, Contraception 36:595, 1987.

145. Schlesselman JJ, Stadel BV, Murray P, Lai S, Breast cancer in relation to early use of oral contracpetives. No evidence of a latent effect, JAMA 259:1828, 1988.

146. Wingo PA, Lee NC, Ory HW, Beral V, Peterson HB, Rhodes P, Age-specific differences in the relationship between oral contraceptive use and breast cancer, Obstet Gynecol 78:161. 1991.

147. La Vecchia C, Negri E, Franceschi S, Talamini R, Amadori D, Filiberti R, Conti E, Montella M, Veronesi A, Parazzini F, Ferraroni M, Decarli A, Oral contraceptives and breast cancer: a cooperative Italian study, Int J Cancer 60:163, 1995.

148. Paul C, Skegg DCG, Spears GFS, Oral contraceptives and risk of breast cancer, Int J Cancer 46:366, 1990

149. National Cancer Institute, Annual cancer statistics review, including cancer trends: 1950–1985, National Institutes of Health, Bethesda, 1989.

150. Rushton L, Jones DR, Oral contraceptive use and breast cancer risk: a meta-analysis of variations with age at diagnosis, parity and total duration of oral contraceptive use, Br J Obstet Gynaecol 99:239, 1992.

151. Stadel BV, Schlesselman JJ, Oral contraceptive use and the risk of breast cancer in women with a "prior" history of benign breast disease, Am J Epidemiol 123:373, 1986.

152. Green A, Oral contraceptives and skin neoplasia, Contraception 43:653, 1991.

153. Hannaford PC, Villard-Mackintosh L, Vessey MP, Kay CR, Oral contraceptives and malignant melanoma, Br J Cancer 63:430, 1991.

154. Milne R, Vessey M, The association of oral contraception with kidney cancer, colon cancer, gallbladder cancer (including extrahepatic bile duct cancer) and pituitary tumors, Contraception 43:667, 1991.

155. Berkowitz RS, Bernstein MR, Harlow BL, Rice LW, Lage JM, Goldstein DP, Cramer DW, Case-control study of risk factors for partial molar pregnancy, Am J Obstet Gynecol 173:788, 1995.

156. Janerich DT, Dugan JM, Standfast SJ, Strite L, Congenital heart disease and prenatal exposure to exogenous sex hormones, Br Med J 1:1058, 1977.

157. Nora JJ, Nora AH, Blu J, Ingram J, Foster D, Exogenous progestogen and estrogen implicated in birth defects, JAMA 240:837, 1978.

110

158. **Heinonen OP, Slone D, Monson RR, et al,** Cardiovascular birth defects in antenatal exposure to female sex hormones, New Engl J Med 296:67, 1976.

159. **Simpson JL, Phillips OP,** Spermicides, hormonal contraception and congenital malformations, Adv Contracept 6:141, 1990.

160. **Savolainen E, Saksela E, Saxen L,** Teratogenic hazards of oral contraceptives analyzed in a national malformation register, Am J Obstet Gynecol 140:521, 1981.

161. **Michaelis J, Michaelis H, Gluck E, Koller S,** Prospective study of suspected associations between certain drugs administered during early pregnancy and congenital malformations, Teratology 27:57, 1983.

162. **Bracken MB,** Oral contraception and congenital malformations in offspring: a review and meta-analysis of the prospective studies, Obstet Gynecol 76:552, 1990.

163. **Ressequie LJ, Hick JF, Bruen JA, Noller KL, O'Fallon WM, Kurland LT,** Congenital malformations among offspring exposed in utero to progestins, Olsted County, Minnesota, 1936–1974, Fertil Steril 43:514, 1985.

164. **Katz Z, Lancet M, Skornik J, Chemke J, Mogilemer B, Klinberg M,** Teratogenicity of progestogens given during the first trimester of pregnancy, Obstet Gynecol 65:775, 1985.

165. **Vessey MP, Wright NH, McPherson K, Wiggins P,** Fertility after stoping different methods of contraception, Br Med J 1:265, 1978.

166. **Vessey MP, Smith MA, Yates D,** Return of fertility after discontinuation of oral contraceptives: influence of age and parity, Br J Fam Plann 11:120, 1986.

167. **Linn S, Schoenbaum SC, Monson RR, Rosner B, Ryan KJ,** Delay in conception for former 'pill' users, JAMA 247:629, 1982.

168. **Bracken MB, Hellenbrand KG, Holford TR,** Conception delay after oral contraceptive use: the effect of estrogen dose, Fertil Steril 53:21, 1990.

169. **Bagwell MA, Coker AL, Thompson SJ, Baker ER, Addy CL,** Primary infertility and oral contraceptive steroid use, Fertil Steril 63:1161, 1995.

170. **Rothman KJ,** Fetal loss, twinning, and birth weight after oral-contraceptive use, New Engl J Med 297:468, 1977.

171. **Rothman KJ, Liess J,** Gender of offspring after oral-contraceptive use, New Engl J Med 295:859, 1976.

172. **Magidor S, Poalti H, Harlap S, Baras M,** Long-term follow-up of children whose mothers used oral contraceptives prior to contraception, Contraception 29:203, 1984.

173. **Vessey M, Doll R, Peto R, Johnson B, Wiggins P,** A long-term follow-up study of women using different methods of contraception — an interim report, J Biosoc Sci 8:373, 1976.

174. **Royal College of General Practitioners,** The outcome of pregnancy in former oral contraceptive users, Br J Obstet Gynaecol 83:608, 1976.

175. **Betrabet SS, Shikary ZK, Toddywalla VS, Toddywalla SP, Patel D, Saxena BN,** Transfer of norethisterone (NET) and levonorgestrel (LNG) from a single tablet into the infant's circulation through the mother's milk, Contraception 35:517, 1987.

176. **Diaz S, Peralta O, Juez G, Herreros C, Casado ME, Salvatierra AM, Miranda P, Durn E, Croxatto HB,** Fertility regulation in nursing women: III. Short-term influence of a low-dose combined oral contraceptive upon lactation and infant growth, Contraception 27:1, 1982.

177. **Croxatto HB, Diaz S, Peralta O, Juez G, Herreros C, Casado ME, Salvatierra AM, Miranda P, Durn E,** Fertility regulation in nursing women: IV. Long-term influence of a low-dose combined oral contraceptive initiated at day 30 postpartum upon lactation and child growth, Contraception 27:13, 1983.

178. **Peralta O, Diaz S, Juez G, Herreros C, Casado ME, Salvatierra AM, Miranda P, Durn E, Croxatto HB,** Fertility regulation in nursing women: V. Long-term influence of a low-dose combined oral contraceptive initiated at day 90 postpartum upon lactation and infant growth, Contraception 27:27, 1983.

179. **WHO Task Force on Oral Contraceptives,** Effects of hormonal contraceptives on milk volume and infant growth, Contraception 30:505, 1984.

180. **Nilsson S, Mellbin T, Hofvander Y, Sundelin C, Valentin J, Nygren KG,** Long-term follow-up of children breast-fed by mothers using oral contraceptives, Contraception 34:443, 1986.

181. **Howie PW, McNeilly AS, Houston MJ, Cook A, Boyle H,** Effect of supplementary food on suckling patterns and ovarian activity during lactation, Br Med J 283:757, 1981.

182. **Perez A, Vela P, Masnick GS, Potter RG,** First ovulation after childbirth: the effect of breastfeeding, Am J Obstet Gynecol 114:1041, 1972.

183. **Diaz S, Peralta O, Juez G, Salvatierra AM, Casado ME, Duran E, Croxatto HB,** Fertility regulation in nursing women. I. The probablity of conception in full nursing women living in an urban setting, J Biosoc Sci 14:329, 1982.

184. **McNeilly AS, Glasier A, Howie PW,** Endocrine control of lactational infertility, in Dobbing J, editor, *Maternal Nutrition and Lactational Infertility,* Nevey/Raven Press, New York, 1985, p. 177.

185. **Rivera R, Kennedy KI, Ortiz E, Barrera M, Bhiwandiwala PP,** Breastfeeding and the return to ovulation in Durango, Mexico, Fertil Steril 49:780, 1988.

186. **Gray RH, Campbell OM, Apelo R, Eslami SS, Zacur H, Ramos RM, Gehret JC, Labbok MH,** Risk of ovulation during lactation, Lancet 335:25, 1990.

187. Diaz S, Aravena R, Cardenas H, Casado ME, Miranda P, Schiappacasse V, Croxatto HB, Contraceptive efficacy of lactational amenorrhea in urban Chilean women, Contraception 43:335, 1991.

188. Pituitary Adenoma Study Group, Pituitary adenomas and oral contraceptives: a multicenter case-control study, Fertil Steril 39:753, 1983.

189. Shy FKK, McTiernan AM, Daling JR, Weiss NS, Oral contraceptive use and the occurrence of pituitary prolactinomas, JAMA 249:2204, 1983.

190. Wingrave SJ, Kay CR, Vessey MP, Oral contraceptives and pituitary adenomas, Br Med J 280:685, 1980.

191. Furuhjelm M, Carlstrom K, Amenorrhea following use of combined oral contraceptives, Acta Obstet Gynecol Scand 52:373, 1973.

192. Shearman RP, Smith ID, Statistical analysis of relationship between oral contraceptives, secondary amenorrhea and galactorrhea, J Obstet Gynecol Br Comwlth 79:654, 1972.

193. Jacobs HS, Knuth UA, Hull MGR, Franks S, Post "pill" amenorrhea — cause or coincidence? Br Med J 2:940, 1977.

194. Gray RH, Campbell OM, Zacur HA, Labbok MH, MacRae SL, Postpartum return of ovarian activity in nonbreastfeeding women monitored by urinary assays, J Clin Endocrinol Metab 64:645, 1987.

195. Washington AE, Cates W, Zaidi AA, Hospitalizations for pelvic inflammatory disease: epidemiology and trends in the United States, 1975 to 1981, JAMA 251:2529, 1984.

196. Westrom I, Incidence, prevalence, and trends of acute pelvic inflammatory disease and its consequences in industrialized countries, Am J Obstet Gynecol 138:880, 1980.

197. Westrom L, Bengtsson LP, Mardh PA, The risk of pelvic inflammatory disease in women using intrauterine contraceptive devices as compared to non-users, Lancet 2:221, 1976.

198. Eschenbach DA, Harnisch JP, Holmes KK, Pathogenesis of acute pelvic inflammatory disease: role of contraception and other risk factors, Am J Obstet Gynecol 128:838, 1977.

199. Rubin GL, Ory WH, Layde PM, Oral contraceptives and pelvic inflammatory disease, Am J Obstet Gynecol 140:630, 1980.

200. Senanayake P, Kramer DG, Contraception and the etiology of pelvic inflammatory diseases: new perspectives, Am J Obstet Gynecol 138:852, 1980.

201. Panser LA, Phipps WR, Type of oral contraceptive in relation to acute, initial episodes of pelvic inflammatory disease, Contraception 43:91, 1991.

202. Svensson L, Westrom L, Mardh P, Contraceptives and acute salpingitis, JAMA 251:2553, 1984.

203. **Cates W Jr, Washington AE, Rubin GL, Peterson HB,** The pill, chlamydia and PID, Fam Plann Perspect 17:175, 1985.

204. **Critchlow CW, Wölner-Hanssen P, Eschenbach DA, Kiviat NB, Koutsky LA, Stevens CE, Holmes KK,** Determinants of cervical ectopia and of cervicitis: age, oral contraception, specific cervical infection, smoking, and douching, Am J Obstet Gynecol 173:534, 1995.

205. **Cramer DW, Goldman MB, Schiff I, Belisla S, Albrecht B, Stadel B, Gibson M, Wilson E, Stillman R, Thompson I,** The relationship of tubal infertility to barrier method and oral contraceptive use, JAMA 257:2446, 1987.

206. **Wolner-Hanssen P, Eschenbach DA, Paavonen J, Kiviat N, Stevens CE, Critchlow C, DeRouen T, Holmes KK,** Decreased risk of symptomatic chlamydial pelvic inflammatory disease associated with oral contraceptive use, JAMA 263:54, 1990.

207. **Lazzarin A, Saracco A, Musicco M, Nicolosi A,** Man-to-woman sexual transmission of the human immunodeficiency virus: risk factors related to sexual behaviour, man's infectiousness, and woman's susceptibility, Arch Intern Med 151:2411, 1991.

208. **Costello Daly C, Helling-Giese GE, Mati JK, Hunter DJ,** Contraceptive methods and the transmission of HIV: implications for family planning, Genitourin Med 70:110, 1994.

209. **Barbone F, Austin H, Louv WC, Alexander WJ,** A follow-up study of methods of contraception, sexual activity, and rates of trichomoniasis, candidiasis, and bacterial vaginosis, Am J Obstet Gynecol 163:510, 1990.

210. **Ross RK, Pike MC, Vessey MP, Bull D, Yeates D, Casagrande JT,** Risk factors for uterine fibroids: reduced risk associated with oral contraceptives, Br J Med 293:359, 1986.

211. **Parazzini F, Negri E, Lavecchia C, Fedele L, Rabaiotti M, Luchini L,** Oral contraceptive use and risk of uterine fibroids, Obstet Gynecol 79:430, 1992.

212. **Friedman AJ, Thomas PP,** Does low-dose combination oral contraceptive use affect uterine size or menstrual flow in premenopausal women with leiomyomas? Obstet Gynecol 85:631, 1995.

213. **Mattson RH, Cramer JA, Darney PD, Naftolin F,** Use of oral contraceptives by women with epilepsy, JAMA 256:238, 1986

214. **Milsom I, Sundell G, Andersch B,** A longitudinal study of contraception and pregnancy outcome in a representative sample of young Swedish women, Contraception 43:111, 1991.

215. **Letterie GS, Chow GE,** Effect of "missed" pills on oral contraceptive effectiveness, Obstet Gynecol 79:979, 1992.

216. **Killick SR, Bancroft K, Oelbaum S, Morris J, Elstein M,** Extending the duration of the pill-free interval during combined oral contraception, Adv Contraception 6:33, 1990.

217. **Jung-Hoffman C, Kuhl H,** Intra- and interindividual variations in contraceptive steroid levels during 12 treatment cycles: no relation to irregular bleedings, Contraception 42:423, 1990.

218. **Carpenter S, Neinstein LS,** Weight gain in adolescent and young adult oral contraceptive users, J Adol Health Care 7:342, 1986.

219. **van der Vange N, Blankenstein MA, Kloosterboer HJ, Haspels AA, Thijssen JHH,** Effects of seven low-dose combined oral contraceptives on sex hormone binding globulin, corticosteroid binding globulin, total and free testosterone, Contraception 41:345, 1990.

220. **Lemay A, Dewailly SD, Grenier R, Huard J,** Attenuation of mild hyperandrogenic activity in postpubertal acne by a triphasic oral contraceptive containing low doses of ethynyl estradiol and d,l-norgestrel, J Clin Endocrinol Metab 71:8, 1990.

221. **Grimes DA, Hughes JM,** Use of multiphasic oral contraceptives and hospitalizations of women with functional ovarian cysts in the United States, Obstet Gynecol 73:1037, 1989.

222. **Vessey M, Metcalfe A, Wells C, McPherson K, Westhoff C, Yeates D,** Ovarian neoplasms, functional ovarian cysts, and oral contraceptives, Br Med J 294:1518, 1987.

223. **Neely JL, Abate M, Swinker M, D'Angio R,** The effect of doxycycline on serum levels of ethinyl estradiol, norethindrone, and endogenous progesterone, Obstet Gynecol 77:416, 1991.

224. **Murphy AA, Zacur HA, Charache P, Burkman RT,** The effect of tetracycline on levels of oral contraceptives, Am J Obstet Gynecol 164:28, 1991.

225. **Szoka PR, Edgren RA,** Drug interactions with oral contraceptives: compilation and analysis of an adverse experience report database, Fertil Steril 49(Suppl):31S, 1988.

226. **Abernethy DR, Greenblatt DJ, Divoll M, et al,** Impairment of diazepam metabolism by low-dose estrogen-containing oral-contraceptive steroids, New Engl J Med 306:791, 1982.

227. **Baciewicz AM,** Oral contraceptive drug interactions, Ther Drug Monit 7:26, 1985.

228. **Tornatore KM, Kanarkowski R, McCarthy TL, et al,** Effect of chronic oral contraceptive steroids on theophylline disposition, Eur J Clin Pharmacol 23:129, 1982.

229. **Mitchell MC, Hanew T, Meredith CG, et al,** Effects of oral contraceptive steroids on acetaminophen metabolism and elimination, Clin Pharmacol Ther 34:48, 1983.

230. **Gupta KC, Joshi JV, Hazari K, et al,** Effect of low estrogen combination oral contraceptives on metabolism of aspirin and phenylbutazone, Int J Clin Pharmacol Ther Toxicol 20:511, 1982.

231. Tzourio C, Tehindrazanarierelo A, Iglésias S, Alpérovitch A, Chgedru F, d'Anglejan-Chatillon J, Bousser M-G, Case-control study of migraine and risk of ischaemic stroke in young women, Br Med J 310:830, 1995.

232. Lidegaard Ø, Oral contraceptives, pregnancy and the risk of cerebral thromboembolism: the influence of diabetes, hypertension, migraine and previous thrombotic disease, Br J Obstet Gynaecol 102:153, 1995.

233. Jungers P, Dougados M, Pelissier L, Kuttenn F, Tron F, Lesavre P, Bach JF, Influence of oral contraceptive therapy on the activity of systemic lupus erythematosus, Arthritis Rheum 25:618, 1982.

234. Knopp RH, LaRosa JC, Burkman RT Jr, Contraception and dyslipidemia, Am J Obstet Gynecol 168:1994, 1993.

235. Lashner BA, Kane SV, Hanauer SB, Lack of association between OC use and ulcerative colitis, Gastroenterology 99:1032, 1990.

236. Coutinho EM, da Silva AR, Carreira C, Rodrigues V, Goncalves MT, Conception control by vaginal administration of pills containing ethinyl estradiol and dl-norgestrel, Fertil Steril 42:478, 1984.

237. Sullivan-Nelson M, Kuller JA, Zacur HA, Clinical use of oral contraceptives administered vaginally: a case report, Fertil Steril 52:864, 1989.

238. Coutinho EM, de Souza JC, da Silva AR, de Acosta OM, et al, Comparative study on the efficacy and acceptability of two contraceptive pills administered by the vaginal route: an international multicenter clinical trial, Clin Pharmacol Ther 53:65, 1993.

239. Lanes SF, Birmann B, Walker AM, Singer S, Oral contraceptive type and functional ovarian cysts, Am J Obstet Gynecol 166:956, 1992.

240. Holt VL, Daling JR, McKnight B, Moore D, Stergachis A, Weiss NS, Functional ovarian cysts in relation to the use of monophasic and triphasic oral contraceptives, Obstet Gynecol 79:529, 1992.

241. Milsom E, Sundell G, Andersch B, The influence of different combined oral contraceptives on the prevalence and severity of dysmenorrhea, Contraception 42:497, 1990.

242. Larsson G, Milsom I, Lindstedt G, Rybo G, The influence of a low-dose combined oral contraceptive on menstrual blood loss and iron status, Contraception 46:327, 1992.

243. Sangi-Haghpeykar H, Poindexter AN III, Epidemiology of endometriosis among parous women, Obstet Gynecol 85:983, 1995.

244. Enzelsberger H, Metka M, Heytmanek G, Schurz B, Kurz C, Kusztrich M, Influence of oral contraceptive use on bone density in climacteric women, Maturitas 9:375, 1988.

245. Kleerekoper M, Brienza RS, Schultz LR, Johnson CC, Oral contraceptive use may protect against low bone mass, Arch Intern Med 151:1971, 1991.

116

246. **Kritz-Silverstein D, Barrett-Connor E,** Bone mineral density in post-menopausal women as determined by prior oral contraceptive use, Am J Public Health 83:100, 1993.

247. **Hazes JMW, Dijkmans BAC, Vandenbroucke JP, De Vries RRP, Cats A,** Reduction of the risk of rheumatoid arthritis among women who take oral contraceptives, Arthritis Rheum 33:173, 1990.

248. **Spector TD, Hochberg MC,** The protective effect of the oral contraceptive pill on rheumatoid arthritis: an overview of the analytical epidemiological studies using meta-analysis, J Clin Epidemiol 43:1221, 1990.

249. **Steinkampf MP, Hammond KR, Blackwell RE,** Hormonal treatment of functional ovarian cysts: a randomized, prospective study, Fertil Steril 54:775, 1990.

250. **Jones EF, Forrest JD,** Contraceptive failure in the United States: revised estimates from the 1982 National Survey of Family Growth, Fam Plann Perspect 21:103, 1989.

3

Special Uses of Oral Contraception:
The Progestin-Only Minipill
Emergency Contraception

O RAL CONTRACEPTION is a phrase which appropriately denotes a vast body of knowledge (Chapter 2)
pertaining to the combined estrogen-progestin "birth
control pill." However, there are two special types of oral contraception which deserve separate consideration, the progestin-only minipill
and emergency contraception.

The Progestin-Only Minipill

The minipill contains a small dose of a progestational agent and must
be taken daily, in a continuous fashion.[1,2] There is no evidence for any
difference in clinical behavior among these.

Minipills available worldwide:

1. Micronor, Nor-QD, Noriday, Norod ---- 0.350 mg
   norethindrone
2. Microval, Noregeston, Microlut ---------- 0.030 mg
   norgestrel
3. Ovrette, Neogest ----------------------------- 0.075 mg
   levonorgestrel
4. Exluton --- 0.500 mg
   lynestrenol
5. Femulen --- 0.500 mg
   ethynodial diacetate

Mechanism of Action

The small amount of progestin in the circulation (about 25% of that in combined oral contraceptives) will have a significant impact only on those tissues very sensitive to the female sex steroids, estrogen and progesterone. The contraceptive effect is more dependent upon endometrial and cervical mucus effects, since gonadotropins are not consistently suppressed. The endometrium involutes and becomes hostile to implantation, and the cervical mucus becomes thick and impermeable. Approximately 40% of patients will ovulate normally. Tubal physiology may also be affected, but this is speculative.

Because of the low dose, the minipill must be taken every day at the same time of day. The change in the cervical mucus requires 2–4 hours to take effect, and most importantly, the impermeability diminishes 22 hours after administration, and by 24 hours sperm penetration is essentially unimpaired.

Ectopic pregnancy is not prevented as effectively as intrauterine pregnancy. Although the overall incidence of ectopic pregnancy is not increased (it is still much lower than the incidence in women not using a contraceptive method), when pregnancy occurs, the clinician must suspect that it is more likely to be ectopic. A previous ectopic pregnancy should not be regarded as a contraindication to the minipill.

There are no significant metabolic effects (lipid levels, carbohydrate metabolism, and coagulation factors remain unchanged),[3] and there is an immediate return to fertility upon discontinuation (unlike the delay seen with the combination oral contraceptive).

Efficacy

Failure rates have been documented to range from 1.1 to 9.6 per 100 women in the first year of use.[4] The failure rate is higher in younger women (3.1 per 100 woman-years) compared to women over age 40 (0.3 per 100 woman-years).[5] In motivated women, the failure rate is comparable to the rate (less than 1 per 100 woman-years) with combination oral contraception.[6–8]

Pill Taking

The minipill should be started on the first day of menses, and a back-up method must be used for the first 7 days because some women (very few) ovulate as early as 7–9 days after the onset of menses. The pill should be keyed to a daily event to ensure regular administration at the same time of the day. If pills are forgotten or gastrointestinal illness impairs absorption, the minipill should be resumed as soon as possible, and a back-up method should be used immediately and until the pills have been resumed for at least 2 days. If 2 or more pills are missed in a row and there is no menstrual bleeding in 4–6 weeks, a pregnancy test should be obtained. *If more than 3 hours late in taking a pill, a back-up method should be used for 48 hours.*

Problems

In view of the unpredictable effect on ovulation, it is not surprising that irregular menstrual bleeding is the major clinical problem. The daily progestational impact on the endometrium also contributes to this problem. Patients can expect to have normal, ovulatory cycles (40%), short, irregular cycles (40%), or a total lack of cycles ranging from irregular bleeding to spotting and amenorrhea (20%). This is the major reason why women discontinue the minipill method of contraception.[6]

Women on progestin-only contraception develop more functional, ovarian follicular cysts.[9] Nearly all, if not all, regress. This is not a clinical problem of any significance. Women who have experienced frequent ovarian cysts would be happier with methods that effectively suppress ovulation (combined oral contraceptives and Depo-Provera).

The levonorgestrel minipill may be associated with acne. The mechanism is similar to that seen with Norplant. The androgenic activity of levonorgestrel decreases the circulating levels of sex hormone binding globulin (SHBG). Therefore free steroid levels (levonorgestrel and testosterone) will be increased despite the low dose. This is in contrast to the action of combined oral contraception where the effect of the progestin is countered by the estrogen-induced increase in SHBG.

The incidence of the other minor side effects is very low, probably at the same rate which would be encountered with a placebo.

121

Clinical Decisions

There are two situations where excellent efficacy, probably near total effectiveness, is achieved: lactating women and women over age 40. In lactating women, the contribution of the minipill is combined with prolactin-induced suppression of ovulation, adding up to very effective protection.[10] In women over age 40, reduced fecundity adds to the minipill's effects.

There is another reason why the minipill is a good choice for the breastfeeding woman. There is no evidence for any adverse effect on breastfeeding as measured by milk volume and infant growth and development.[11–13] In fact, there is a modest positive impact; women using the minipill breastfeed longer and add supplementary feeding at a later time.[14] Because of the slight positive impact on lactation, the minipill can be started immediately after delivery.

The minipill is a good choice in situations where estrogen is contraindicated, such as patients with serious medical conditions (diabetes with vascular disease, severe systemic lupus erythematosus, cardiovascular disease). It should be noted that the freedom from estrogen effects, although likely, is presumptive. Substantial data, for example on associations with vascular disease, blood pressure, and cancer, are not available because relatively small numbers have chosen to use this method of contraception. On the other hand, it is logical to conclude that any of the progestin effects associated with the combination oral contraceptives can be related to the minipill according to a dose-response curve; all effects should be reduced.

No impact can be measured on the coagulation system.[15] The minipill can probably be used in women with previous episodes of thrombosis, but the package insert in the United States carries the same precautions and warnings that combined oral contraceptives carry. This is not appropriate in view of the absence of estrogen and the lower dose of progestin. Theoretically, minipills should be free of serious complications. Unfortunately, the overly cautious package insert injects an element of medical-legal risk for the clinician.

The minipill is a good alternative for the occasional woman who reports diminished libido on combination oral contraceptives, presumably due to decreased androgen levels. The minipill should also be considered for the few patients who report minor side effects (gastrointestinal upset, breast tenderness, headaches) of such a degree that the combination oral contraceptive is not acceptable.

Because of the relatively low doses of progestin administered, patients using medications that increase liver metabolism should avoid this method of contraception. These drugs include the following:

Rifampin.
Phenobarbital.
Phenytoin (Dilantin).
Primidone (Mysoline).
Carbamazepine (Tegretol).
Possibly ethosuximide and griseofulvin.

Do the noncontraceptive benefits associated with combination oral contraception apply to the minipill? Studies are unable to help us with this issue, again because of relatively small numbers of users. However, the progestin impact on cervical mucus, endometrium, and ovulation leads one to think the benefits will be present (reduced risks of pelvic infection, endometrial cancer, and ovarian cancer), but probably at reduced levels.

Good efficacy with the minipill requires regularity, taking the pill at the same time each day. There is less room for forgetting, and therefore, the minipill is probably not a good choice for a disorganized adult or for the average adolescent.

Emergency Contraception

The use of large doses of estrogen to prevent implantation was pioneered by Morris and van Wagenen at Yale in the 1960s. The initial work in monkeys led to the use of high doses of diethylstilbestrol (25–50 mg/day) and ethinyl estradiol in women.[16] It was quickly appreciated that these extremely large doses of estrogen were associated with a high rate of gastrointestinal side effects. Yuzpe developed a method utilizing a combination oral contraceptive, resulting in an important reduction in dosage.[17] The following treatment regimens have been documented to be effective:

Ovral: 2 tablets followed by 2 tablets 12 hours later.
Lo Ovral, Nordette, Levlen, Triphasil, Trilevlen:
    4 tablets followed by 4 tablets 12 hours later.

This method has been more commonly called postcoital contraception, or the "morning after" treatment. Emergency contraception is a more accurate and appropriate name, indicating the intention to be one-time protection. It is an important option for patients, and should be considered when condoms break, sexual assault occurs, if diaphragms or cervical caps dislodge, or with the lapsed use of any method. In studies at abortion units, 50–60% of the patients would have been suitable for emergency contraception and would have used it if readily available.[18,19] In the U.S., it is estimated that emergency contraception could prevent 1.7 million unintended pregnancies and the number of induced abortions would decrease from 1.5 million to 800,000.[20]

Many women do not know of this method, and it has been difficult to obtain.[19] In Europe, special packages with printed instructions are marketed specifically for emergency contraception. Even if women are aware of this method, accurate and detailed knowledge is lacking.[21] A favorable attitude towards this method requires knowledge and availability.

Clinicians should consider providing emergency contraceptive kits to patients (a kit can be a simple envelope containing instructions and the appropriate number of oral contraceptives) to be taken when needed. It would be a major contribution to our efforts to avoid unwanted pregnancies, for all patients without contraindications to oral contraceptives to have emergency contraception available for use when needed. In our view, this would be much more effective in reducing the need for abortion than waiting for patients to call.

Mechanism and Efficacy

The mechanism of action is not known with certainty, but it is believed with justification that this treatment interferes with implantation and survival of the embryo.[22] The efficacy has been confirmed in large clinical trials and summarized in a complete review of the literature.[23,24] Treatment with high doses of estrogen yields a failure rate of approximately 1%, with the combination oral contraceptive, about 2%. The failure rate is lowest with high doses of ethinyl estradiol given within 72 hours (0.1%), but the side effects make the combination oral contraceptive a better choice.

Treatment Method

Treatment should be initiated as soon after exposure as possible, but no later than 72 hours. Because of possible, but unlikely, harmful effects of these high doses to a fetus, an already existing pregnancy should be ruled out prior to use of postcoital hormones. Furthermore, the patient should be offered therapeutic abortion if the method fails. This patient encounter also provides an important opportunity to screen for STDs.

The combination oral contraceptive method delivers significantly less steroid hormone, and this reduction in the total dose and the number of doses reduces the side effects and limits them to a shorter time period. It is worth adding an antiemetic, oral or suppository, to the treatment. Side effects reflect the high doses used: nausea, vomiting, breast tenderness, headache, and dizziness. If a patient vomits within an hour after taking pills, additional pills must be administered as soon as possible. The usual contraindications for oral contraception apply to this use. **In view of the high dose of estrogen, emergency contraception with steroid hormones should not be provided to women with either a personal or family history of idiopathic thrombotic disease.**

A 3-week follow-up visit should be scheduled to assess the result, and to counsel for routine contraception.

Could other combination oral contraceptive products be used? Since other doses and other formulations have never been tested, the efficacy is unknown. It would not be appropriate to expose patients to an unknown failure rate. Levonorgestrel in a dose of 0.75 mg given twice, 12 hours apart, is as successful as the combination oral contraceptive method, but this dose is equivalent to 20 pills of the levonorgestrel progestin-only minipill.[25] The use of danazol for this purpose is relatively untested, but RU486, the progesterone antagonist, has been without failures and with lower side effects in preliminary trials.

The 3 major problems with the available methods of emergency contraception are the high rate of side effects, the need to start treatment within 72 hours after intercourse, and the small, but important, failure rate. Mifepristone (RU486) in a single oral low dose of 50 mg is associated with markedly less nausea and vomiting and an efficacy rate of nearly 100%.[26,27] Because the next menstrual cycle is delayed after mifepristone, contraception should be initiated immediately after treatment. Ironically, RU 486, around which swirls the abortion controversy, can make an effective contribution to preventing unwanted pregnancies and induced abortions.

Another method of emergency contraception is the insertion of a copper IUD, up to 5 days after unprotected intercourse. The failure rate (in a small number of studies) is very low, 0.1%.[23,24] This method definitely prevents implantation, but it is not suitable for women who are not candidates for intrauterine contraception, e.g., multiple sexual partners, rape victim.

References

1. **Chi I,** The safety and efficacy issues of progestin-only oral contraceptives — an epidemiologic perspective, Contraception 47:1, 1993.

2. **McCann MF, Potter LS,** Progestin-only oral contraception: a comprehensive review, Contraception 50(Suppl 1):S9-S195, 1994.

3. **Ball MJ, Gillmer AE,** Progestagen-only oral contraceptives: comparison of the metabolic effects of levonorgestrel and norethisterone, Contraception 44:223, 1991.

4. **Trussell J, Kost K,** Contraceptive failure in the United States: a critical review of the literature, Stud Fam Plann 18:237, 1987.

5. **Vessey MP, Lawless M, Yeates D, McPherson K,** Progestogen-only contraception: findings in a large prospective study with special reference to effectiveness, Br J Fam Plann 10:117, 1985.

6. **Broome M, Fotherby K,** Clinical experience with the progestogen-only pill, Contraception 42:489, 1990.

7. **Bisset AM, Dingwall-Fordyce I, Hamilton MJK,** The efficacy of the progestogen-only pill as a contraceptive method, Br J Fam Plann 16:84, 1990.

8. **Seth A, Jain U, Sharma S, et al,** A randomized, double-blind study of two combined and two progestogen-only oral contraceptives, Contraception 25:243, 1982.

9. **Tayob Y, Adams J, Jacobs HS, Guillebaud J,** Ultrasound demonstration of increased frequency of functional ovarian cysts in women using progestogen-only oral contraception, Br J Obstet Gynaecol 92:1003, 1985.

10. **Dunson TR, McLaurin VL, Grubb GS, Rosman AW,** A multicenter clinical trial of a progestin-only oral contraceptive in lactating women, Contraception 47:23, 1993.

11. **WHO Special Programme of Research, Development, and Research Training in Human Reproduction, Task Force on Oral Contraceptives,** Effects of hormonal contraceptives on milk volume and infant growth, Contraception 30:505, 1984.

12. **WHO Task Force for Epidemiological Research on Reproductive Health; Special Programme of Research, Development and Research Training in Human Reproduction,** Progestogen-only contraceptives during lactation. I. Infant growth, Contraception 50:35, 1994.

13. **WHO Task Force for Epidemiological Research on Reproductive Health; Special Programme of Research, Development and Research Training in Human Reproduction,** Progestogen-only contraceptives during lactation. II. Infant development, Contraception 50:55, 1994.

14. **McCann MF, Moggia AV, Hibbins JE, Potts M, Becker C,** The effects of a progestin-only oral contraceptive (levonorgestrel 0.03 mg) on breast-feeding, Contraception 40:635, 1989.

15. **Fotherby K,** The progestogen-only pill and thrombosis, Br J Fam Plann 15:83, 1989.

16. **Morris J McL, van Wagenen G,** Compounds interfering with ovum implantation and development. III. The role of estrogens, Am J Obstet Gynecol 96:804, 1966.

17. **Yuzpe AA, Smith RP, Rademaker AW,** A multicenter clinical investigation employing ethinyl estradiol combined with dl-norgestrel as a postcoital contraceptive agent, Fertil Steril 37:508, 1982.

18. **Burton R, Savage W, Reader F,** The "morning after pill." Is this the wrong name for it? Br J Fam Plann 15:119, 1990.

19. **Young L, McCowan LM, Roberts HE, Farquhar CM,** Emergency contraception — why women don't use it, N Z Med J 108:145, 1995.

20. **Harper CC, Ellerton CE,** The emergency contraceptive pill: a survey of knowledge and attitudes among students at Princeton, Am J Obstet Gynecol 173:1438, 1995.

21. **Trussell J, Stewart F, Guest F, Hatcher RA,** Emergency contraceptive pills: a simple proposal to reduce unintended pregnancies, Fam Plann Perspect 24:269, 1992.

22. **Young DC, Wiehle RD, Joshi SG, Pindexter AN III,** Emergency contraception alters progesterone-associated endometrial protein in serum and uterine luminal fluid, Obstet Gynecol 84:266, 1994.

23. **Fasoli M, Parazzini F, Cecchetti G, La Vecchia C,** Post-coital contraception: an overview of published studies, Contraception 39:459, 1989.

24. **Haspels AA,** Emergency contraception: a review, Contraception 50:101, 1994.

25. **Ho PC, Kwan MSW,** A prospective randomized comparison of levonorgestrel with the Yuzpe regimen in post-coital contraception, Hum Reprod 8:389, 1993.

26. **Webb AMC, Russell J, Elstein M,** Comparison of Yuzpe regimen, danazol, and mifepristone (RU486) in oral postcoital contraception, Br Med J 305:927, 1992.

27. **Glasier A, Thong KJ, Dewar M, Mackie M, Baird DT,** Mifepristone (RU 486) compared with high-dose estrogen and progestogen for emergency postcoital contraception, New Engl J Med 327:1041, 1992.

4

Implant Contraception: Norplant

PROGESTIN-ONLY IMPLANT contraception is the first new contraceptive available in the United States since oral contraception was introduced and IUDs were re-discovered in the 1960s.[1] Norplant is a "sustained release" system using Silastic tubing permeable to steroid molecules to provide stable circulating levels of synthetic progestin over years of use. Norplant was first introduced into clinical trials in Chile in 1972. Assessment of this method was completed in more than 45 countries, and in 1990, Norplant was approved for marketing in the U.S., the 20th country to do so.[2]

The progestin, circulating at levels one-fourth to one-tenth of those obtained with combined oral contraceptives, prevents conception by suppressing ovulation and thickening cervical mucus to inhibit sperm penetration so that fertilization rarely occurs.[3] Because serum levels of progestin remain low and because no estrogen is administered, this long-acting contraceptive method does not cause any serious health effects.[2] This method does, however, cause some bothersome side effects attributable to sustained administration of progestin, such as changes in menstrual pattern, weight gain, headache, and effects on mood.

The long-acting progestin methods (including Norplant and Depo-Provera) are as effective as sterilization and IUDs, and more effective than oral and barrier contraception.[4] An important reason for this high efficacy in actual use is the nature of the delivery systems themselves which require little effort on the part of the user. Since compliance does not require frequent resupply or instruction in use, as with oral contraception, theoretical (lowest expected) effectiveness is very close to the actual or typical (use) effectiveness.

Sustained-release methods require less of the user but they demand more of the clinician. Norplant involves minor operative procedures for placement and for discontinuation. Clinicians have a special responsibility to become skillful in the operations required to remove implants and to be available to women when those skills are required to terminate use. Disturbances of menstrual patterns and other side effects prompt many more questions from patients about these methods than about use of the familiar oral, intrauterine, and barrier contraceptives.[5]

The Norplant System

The Norplant subdermal implant system is a long-acting, low-dose, reversible, progestin-only method of contraception for women. It was developed by the Population Council. The implants are manufactured, under license of the Population Council, by Huhtamaki Oy/Leiras Pharmaceuticals in Finland.

The currently available Norplant system consists of 6 capsules, each measuring 34 mm in length with a 2.4 mm outer diameter and containing 36 mg crystalline levonorgestrel. The capsules are made of flexible, medical grade Silastic (polydimethylsiloxane and methylvinyl siloxane copolymer) tubing which is sealed shut with Silastic medical adhesive (polydimethylsiloxane). The cavity of the capsule has an inner diameter of 1.57 mm, with an inner length of 30 mm. The 6 capsules contain a total of 216 mg levonorgestrel which is very stable and has remained unchanged in capsules examined after more than 9 years of use.

The implants come packaged in heat-sealed pouches that have a shelf life of 5 years from the date of manufacture and have an additional 5-year effective life once inserted. Storage at room temperature with uncontrolled humidity has not altered their composition or lifespan after 4 years, but optimally the implants should be stored in a cool, dry area away from direct sunlight. The implants can be ethylene oxide sterilized, but cannot be sterilized by ionizing radiation, dry heat, or autoclaving.

The components of Norplant are not new. The Silastic in the tubing has been used in surgical applications such as prosthetic devices, heart valves, and drainage tubes, since the 1950s, and in the most common method of female sterilization (Fallope Rings) since 1970. The progestin, levonorgestrel, has been widely used in oral contraceptives since the 1960s. The toxicology, teratogenicity, and pharmacology of levonorgestrel have been well studied. What is new is the way the system delivers a sustained level of levonorgestrel for a long time — in ongoing trials, up to 7 years, although currently approved for 5 years.

Mechanism of Action

The release rate of the capsule is determined by its total surface area and the thickness of the capsule wall. The levonorgestrel diffuses through the wall of the tubing into the surrounding tissues where it is absorbed by the circulatory system and distributed systemically, avoiding an initial high level in the circulation as with orally or injected steroids. Within 24 hours after insertion, plasma concentrations of levonorgestrel range from 0.4 to 0.5 ng/mL, high enough to prevent conception.[6]

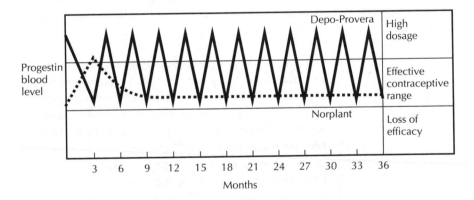

The capsules release approximately 80 μg of levonorgestrel per 24 hours during the first 6–12 months of use. This rate declines gradually to 50 μg daily by 9 months and 30 μg per day for the remaining duration of use. The 80 μg of hormone released by the implants during the first few months of use is about equivalent to the daily dose of levonorgestrel delivered by the progestin-only, minipill oral contraceptive, and 25–50% of the dose delivered by low-dose combined oral contraceptives.

Mean plasma concentrations below 0.20 ng/mL are associated with increased pregnancy rates. After 6 months of use, daily levonorgestrel concentrations are about 0.35 ng/mL; at 2.5 years, the levels decrease to 0.25–0.35 ng/mL. Until the 5-year mark, mean levels remain above 0.25 ng/mL.[7]

Body weight affects the circulating levels of levonorgestrel. The greater the weight of the user, the lower the levonorgestrel concentrations at any time during Norplant use. The greatest decrease over time occurs in women weighing more than 70 kg (154 pounds), but even for heavy women, the release rate is high enough to prevent pregnancy at least as reliably as oral contraceptives.

Levonorgestrel levels may also be affected by the levels of sex hormone binding globulin (SHBG). Levonorgestrel has a high affinity for SHBG. In the week after Norplant insertion, SHBG levels decline rapidly, then return to about half of preinsertion levels by 1-year of use. This effect on SHBG is not uniform and may account for some of the individual variations in plasma levonorgestrel concentrations.[8]

The mechanism by which Norplant prevents conception is only partially explained. There are 3 probable modes of action, which are similar to those attributed to the contraceptive effect of the progestin-only, minipills.

1. The levonorgestrel suppresses at both the hypothalamus and the pituitary the luteinizing hormone (LH) surge necessary for ovulation. As determined by progesterone levels in many users over several years, about one-third of all cycles are ovulatory.[7,9] During the first 2 years of use, only about 10% of women are ovulatory, but by 5 years of use, more than 50% are.

2. The constant level of levonorgestrel has a marked effect on the cervical mucus. The mucus thickens and decreases in amount, forming a barrier to sperm penetration.[6,10]

3. The levonorgestrel suppresses the estradiol-induced cyclic maturation of the endometrium, and eventually causes atrophy. These changes could prevent implantation should fertilization occur; however, no evidence of fertilization can be detected in Norplant users.[11]

Advantages

Norplant is a safe, highly effective, continuous method of contraception that requires little user effort or motivation and, unlike injectable contraception, is rapidly reversible. Because this is a progestin-only method, it can be utilized by women who have contraindications for the use of estrogen-containing oral contraceptives. The sustained release of low doses of progestin avoids the high initial dose delivered by injectables and the daily hormone surge associated with oral contraceptives. Norplant is not a coitus-related contraceptive method. The use-effectiveness closely approximates the theoretical effectiveness. Norplant is an excellent choice for a breastfeeding woman (there is no effect on breastfeeding) and can be inserted immediately postpartum.

Disadvantages

There are some disadvantages associated with the use of the Norplant system.

1. Norplant causes disruption of bleeding patterns in up to 80% of users, especially during the first year of use, and some women or their partners find these changes unacceptable.[5] Endogenous estrogen is nearly normal, and unlike the combined oral contraceptives, progestin is not regularly withdrawn to allow endometrial sloughing. Consequently, the endometrium sheds at unpredictable intervals.

2. The implants must be inserted and removed in a surgical procedure performed by trained personnel. Women cannot initiate or discontinue the method without the assistance of a clinician. The incidence of complicated removals is approximately 5%, an incidence that can be best minimized by good training and experience in Norplant insertion.[12]

3. Because the insertion and removal of Norplant requires a minor surgical procedure, initiation and discontinuation costs will be higher than with oral contraceptives or barrier methods.

4. The implants can be visible under the skin. This sign of the use of contraception may be unacceptable for some women, and for some partners.[5]

133

5. Norplant is not known to provide protection against sexually transmitted diseases (STDs) such as herpes, human papillomavirus, HIV, gonorrhea, or chlamydia. Users at risk for STDs must consider adding a barrier method to prevent infection.

Indications

The Norplant system is indicated for use by women of reproductive age who are sexually active and desire continuous contraception. Norplant should be considered for women who:

1. Desire spacing of future pregnancies.
2. Desire a highly effective, long-term method of contraception.
3. Experience serious or minor estrogen-related side effects with oral contraception.
4. Have difficulty remembering to take pills every day, have contraindications or difficulty using IUDs, or desire a non-coitus-related method of contraception.
5. Have completed their childbearing but do not desire permanent sterilization.
6. Have a history of anemia with heavy menstrual bleeding.
7. Are considering sterilization, but are not yet ready to undergo surgery.
8. Women with chronic illnesses, whose health will be threatened by pregnancy.

Absolute Contraindications

Norplant use is contraindicated in women who have:

1. *ACTIVE* thrombophlebitis or thromboembolic disease.
2. Undiagnosed genital bleeding.
3. *ACUTE* liver disease.
4. Benign or malignant liver tumors.
5. Known or suspected breast cancer.

Relative Contraindications

Based on clinical judgment and appropriate medical management,

Norplant *MAY BE USED* by women with a history of or current diagnosis of the following conditions:

1. Heavy cigarette smoking (15 or more daily) in women older than 35 years.
2. History of ectopic pregnancy.
3. Diabetes mellitus. Because multiple studies have failed to observe a significant impact on carbohydrate metabolism, Norplant, in our view, is particularly well-suited for diabetic women.
4. Hypercholesterolemia.
5. Hypertension.
6. History of cardiovascular disease, including myocardial infarction, cerebral vascular accident, coronary artery disease, angina, or a previous thromboembolic event. Patients with artificial heart valves.
7. Gallbladder disease.
8. Chronic disease, such as immunocompromised patients.

Norplant is not contraindicated in the following situations, but other methods are probably preferable:

1. Severe acne.
2. Severe vascular or migraine headaches.
3. Severe depression.
4. Concomitant use of medications that induce microsomal liver enzymes (phenytoin, phenobarbital, carbamazepine, rifampin). In this case, we do not recommend the use of Norplant because of a likely increased risk of pregnancy due to lower blood levels of levonorgestrel.[2]

Efficacy

Norplant is a highly effective method of birth control. In studies conducted in 11 countries, totaling 12,133 woman-years of use, the pregnancy rate was 0.2 pregnancies per 100 woman-years of use.[2,13] All but one of the pregnancies that occurred during this evaluation were present at the time of implant insertion. If these luteal phase insertions are excluded from analysis, the first year pregnancy rate was 0.01 per 100 woman-years.

Failure Rates During the First Year of Use, United States [4]

Method	Percent of Women with Pregnancy Lowest Expected	Typical
No method	85.0%	85.0%
Combination Pill	0.1	3.0
Progestin only	0.5	3.0
IUDs		3.0
Progesterone IUD	2.0	<2.0
Copper T 380A	0.8	<1.0
Norplant	0.2	0.2
Female sterilization	0.2	0.4
Male sterilization	0.1	0.15
Depo-Provera	0.3	0.3
Spermicides	3.0	21.0
Periodic abstinence		20.0
Calendar	9.0	
Ovulation method	3.0	
Symptothermal	2.0	
Post–ovulation	1.0	
Withdrawal	4.0	18.0
Cervical cap	6.0	18.0
Sponge		
Parous women	9.0	28.0
Nulliparous women	6.0	18.0
Diaphragm and spermicides	6.0	18.0
Condom	2.0	12.0

The overall pregnancy rate after 2 years of use in 9 countries was 0.2 per 100 woman-years of use.[2] The pregnancy rate achieved in the U.S. trials during the second year of use was higher (2.1 per 100 woman-years). Two factors may account for this difference. First, users in the U.S. weighed, on the average, more than study participants in other countries. Clinical trials have demonstrated a direct correlation between weight greater than 70 kg (154 pounds) and an increased risk of pregnancy, but even for heavy women, pregnancy rates are lower than with oral contraception. Second, two different types of Silastic tubing were used in the manufacture of Norplant capsules.[14] The first type contained a larger proportion of inert filler and was more dense, while the second type contained less filler and was less dense. Higher pregnancy rates have been observed among women using the more dense capsules, and in the U.S. trials, capsules were more often of the more dense variety. The less dense tubing is now the only one used in the manufacture of Norplant and has a 15% higher release rate than denser tubing.

Pregnancy Rates According to Years of Use [2,13]

First Year	Second Year	Third Year	Fourth Year	Fifth Year
0.2%	0.2%	0.9%	0.5%	1.1%

Using the less dense tubing, there now are no weight restrictions for Norplant users, but heavier women (more than 70 kg) may experience slightly higher pregnancy rates in the fourth and fifth years of use compared to lighter women. Even in the later years, however, pregnancy rates for heavier women using Norplant are lower than with oral contraception. The differences in pregnancy rates by weight are probably due to the dilutional effect of larger body size on the low, sustained serum levels of levonorgestrel. Heavier women should not rely on Norplant beyond the 5-year limit. For slender women the duration of Norplant's efficacy may extend well into the fifth year of use. In some extended trials, no pregnancies have occurred into the 7th year.

Norplant is less effective in women who are also using drugs which accelerate hepatic microsomal metabolism. These drugs include phenytoin (Dilantin), carbamazepine (Tegretrol), phenobarbitol, and rifampin. Since serum levels are already low, rapid metabolism can push them under the contraceptive level. For women with compromised hepatic function, the low serum levels of levonorgestrel present no metabolic problem because even if excretion is impaired, levels will not become very high.

Ectopic Pregnancy

The ectopic pregnancy rate during Norplant use has been 0.28 per 1,000 woman-years.[2] *Although the risk of developing an ectopic pregnancy during use of Norplant is low, when pregnancy does occur, ectopic pregnancy should be suspected. because about 30% of Norplant pregnancies are ectopic.*

Ectopic Pregnancy Rates per 1,000 Woman-Years [2, 15, 16]

Non-contraceptive users, all ages	3.0–4.5
Copper T-380 IUD	0.20
Norplant	0.28

Menstrual Effects

Menstrual bleeding patterns are highly variable among users of Norplant. Some alteration of menstrual patterns will occur during the first year of use in approximately 80% of users.[17,18] The changes include alterations in the interval between bleeding, the duration and volume of menstrual flow, and spotting. Oligomenorrhea and amenorrhea also occur, but are less common, less than 10% after the first year. Irregular and prolonged bleeding usually occurs during the first year. Although bleeding problems occur much less frequently after the second year, they can occur at any time.[18,19]

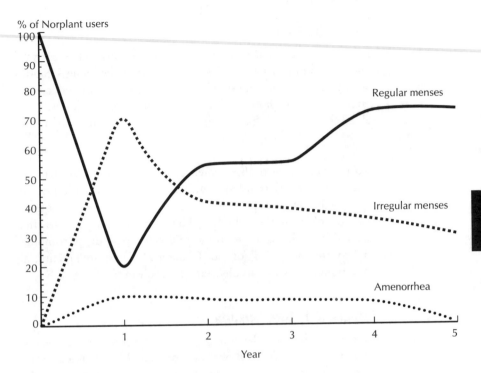

% of Norplant users

Despite an increase in the number of spotting and bleeding days over preinsertion menstrual patterns, hemoglobin concentrations rise in Norplant users because of a decrease in the average amount of menstrual blood loss.[20,21]

Patients who can no longer tolerate the presence of prolonged bleeding will benefit from a short course of oral estrogen: conjugated estrogens, 1.25 mg, or estradiol, 2 mg, administered daily for 7 days. A therapeutic dose of one of the prostaglandin inhibitors given during the bleeding will help to diminish flow, but estrogen is the most effective.[22]

Although the Norplant system is very effective, pregnancy must be considered in women reporting amenorrhea who have been ovulating previously, as evidenced by regular menses prior to an episode of amenorrhea. A sensitive urine pregnancy test should be obtained. Women who remain amenorrheic throughout their use of Norplant are unlikely to become pregnant.[18] It is important to explain to patients the mechanism of the amenorrhea: the local progestational effect causing decidualization and atrophy.

Metabolic Effects

Exposure to the sustained, low dose of levonorgestrel delivered by the implants is not associated with significant metabolic changes. Studies of carbohydrate metabolism,[23,24] liver function,[25,26] blood coagulation,[27,28] immunoglobulin levels,[23,29] serum cortisol levels,[30] and blood chemistries[23,26] have failed to detect changes outside of normal ranges.

No major impact on the lipoprotein profile can be demonstrated.[3,31,32] Minor changes are transient, and with prolonged duration of use, lipoproteins return to preinsertion levels. Long-term exposure to the low dose of levonorgestrel released by Norplant is unlikely to affect users' risk of atherogenesis, just as prolonged exposure to combined oral contraception has not (See Chapter 2). There are no clinically important effects on carbohydrate metabolism.[23,24,33]

Effects on Future Fertility

Circulating levels of levonorgestrel become too low to measure within 48 hours after removal of Norplant. Most women resume normal ovulatory cycles during the first month after removal. The pregnancy rates during the first year after removal are comparable to those of women not using contraceptive methods and trying to become pregnant. There are no long-term effects on future fertility, nor are there any effects on sex ratios, rates of ectopic pregnancy, spontaneous abortion, stillbirth, or congenital malformations,[2,13] The return of fertility after Norplant removal is prompt and pregnancy outcomes are within normal limits. The rate and outcome of subsequent pregnancies are not influenced by duration of use.

For women who are spacing their pregnancies, the difference between Norplant and Depo-Provera in the timing of the return to fertility can be critical. Norplant allows precise timing of pregnancy because the return of ovulation after Norplant removal is so prompt. Depo-Provera, on the other hand, can cause up to 18 months delay in return to fertility. By that time, 90% of users of either method will have ovulated, but in the first several months, the difference is dramatic. By 3 months after removal, half of Norplant users will have ovulated, but 10 months must elapse before half of Depo-Provera users are ovulatory.

Side Effects

The occurrence of serious side effects is very rare, no different in incidence than that observed in the general population. In addition to the menstrual changes, the following side effects have been reported: headache, acne, weight change, mastalgia, hyperpigmentation over the implants, hirsutism, depression, mood changes, anxiety, nervousness, ovarian cyst formation, and galactorrhea.[2,13,17,19,34]

It is difficult, of course, to be certain which of these effects were actually caused by the levonorgestrel. Although most of these side effects are minor in nature, they can cause patients to discontinue the method. Patients often find common side effects tolerable after assurance that they do not represent a health hazard.[5] Many complaints respond to reassurance; others can be treated with simple therapies. The most common side effect experienced by users is headache; about 20% of women who discontinue use do so because of headache.[5,34]

Stroke, thrombotic thrombocytopenic purpura, thrombocytopenia, and pseudotumor cerebri have been reported with Norplant.[35] However, it is by no means established that the incidence of these problems is increased, and there is little reason to suspect a cause and effect relationship.

Weight Change. Women using Norplant more frequently complain of weight gain than of weight loss, but findings are variable. In the Dominion Republic, 75% of those who changed weight lost, while in San Francisco, two-thirds gained. Assessment of weight change in Norplant users is confounded by changes in exercise, diet, and aging. Although an increase in appetite can be attributed to the androgenic activity of levonorgestrel, it is unlikely that the low levels with Norplant have any clinical impact. Counseling for weight changes should include dietary review and focus on dietary changes. Indeed, a 5-year follow-up of 75 women with Norplant implants could document no increase in the body mass index (nor was there a correlation between irregular bleeding and body weight).[36]

Mastalgia. Bilateral mastalgia, often occurring premenstrually, is usually associated with complaints of fluid retention. After pregnancy has been ruled out, reassurance and therapy aimed at symptomatic relief are indicated. This symptom decreases with increasing duration of Norplant use. Most Norplant users respond

141

to treatment and do not elect to remove the implants. Careful assessments of the relationship between methylxanthines and mastalgia have failed to demonstrate a link. The most effective treatments are the following: danazol (200 mg/day), vitamin E (600 units/day), bromocriptine (2.5 mg/day), or tamoxifen (20 mg/day), but there are no studies of these treatments in Norplant users.

Galactorrhea. Galactorrhea is more common among women who have had insertion of the implants upon discontinuation of lactation. Pregnancy and other possible causes should be ruled out by performing a pregnancy test and a thorough breast examination. Patients should be reassured that this is a common occurrence among implant and oral contraceptive users. Decreasing the amount of breast and nipple stimulation during sexual relations might alleviate the symptom, but if amenorrhea accompanies persistent galactorrhea, a prolactin level should be obtained.

Acne. Acne, with or without an increase in oil production, is the most common skin complaint among Norplant users. The acne is caused by the androgenic activity of the levonorgestrel which produces a direct impact and also causes a decrease in sex hormone binding globulin (SHBG) levels leading to an increase in free steroid levels (both levonorgestrel and testosterone). This is in contrast to combined oral contraceptives which contain levonorgestrel, where the estrogen effect on SHBG (an increase) produces a decrease in unbound, free androgens. Common therapies for complaints of acne include dietary change, practice of good skin hygiene with the use of soaps or skin cleansers, and application of topical antibiotics (e.g., 1% clindamycin solution or gel, or topical erythromycin). Use of local antibiotics helps most users to continue Norplant.

Ovarian Cysts. Unlike oral contraception, the low serum progestin levels maintained by Norplant do not suppress FSH which continues to stimulate ovarian follicle growth in most users. The LH peak during the first two years of use, on the other hand, is usually abolished so that these follicles do not ovulate.[9] However, some continue to grow and cause pain or be palpated at the time of pelvic examination.[37] Adnexal masses are approximately 8 times more frequent in Norplant users compared to normally cycling women. Because these are simple cysts (and most regress spontaneously within one month of detection), they need not be sonographically or laparoscopically evaluated. Further evaluation is indicated if they became large and painful or fail to regress. Regular ovulators are less likely to form cysts so the situation is likely to improve after two years of Norplant use.

Herpes Simplex. Some users have complained of outbreaks of genital herpes simplex lesions occurring more frequently than prior to insertion. Most commonly, the lesions develop during periods of prolonged spotting or bleeding with the wearing of sanitary napkins. Use of vaginal tampons for bleeding and suppression of the virus with oral acyclovir (200 mg tid for up to 6 months) have been sucessful in dealing with this problem.

Cancer. Levonorgestrel and Silastic have been thoroughly evaluated in animals and humans for their carcinogenic effects, and none has been found. Epidemiologic evaluation awaits long-term use by large numbers of women. We can speculate on possible effects of Norplant based on our experience with oral contraceptives and Depo-Provera. The risk of endometrial cancer ought to be reduced. A study of the endometrial effects of Norplant failed to find any evidence of hyperplasia, even when levonorgestrel levels were low and endogenous estradiol production normal.[38] The risk of ovarian cancer is also probably reduced, but not as much as with methods that completely suppress ovulation. Breast and cervical cancer effects will be as difficult to assess because of confounding variables as they are with oral contraception and Depo-Provera. The low dose of Norplant, however, would be unlikely to have effects different from other hormonal contraceptives.

Patient Evaluation

The usual personal and family medical history and physical examination should concentrate on factors that might contraindicate use of the various contraceptive options. If a patient elects to use Norplant, a detailed description of the method, including effectiveness, side effects, risks, benefits, as well as insertion and removal procedures, should be provided. Before insertion, the patient should read and sign a written consent for the surgical placement of Norplant. It should include a review of the potential complications of the procedure which include reaction to the local anesthetic, infection, expulsion of the implants, superficial phlebitis, bruising, and the possibility of a subsequent difficult removal.

Insertion can be performed at any time during the menstrual cycle as long as pregnancy can be ruled out. If the patient's last menstrual period was abnormal, if she has recently had sexual intercourse without contraception, or if there are reasons to suspect pregnancy, a sensitive urine pregnancy test should be performed. Norplant can be inserted immediately postpartum, but certainly should be initiated no later than the third postpartum week. Acne and headache are less common in women who receive Norplant immediately postpartum, and there is no difference in post pregnancy weight loss compared to women who receive it 4–6 weeks later.[39]

Patients should be questioned regarding allergies to local anesthetics, antiseptic solutions, and tape. A discussion about the technique of insertion and anticipated sensations is an important part of preparing the patient for the experience. All patients approach insertion with some degree of apprehension which can be decreased by detailed explanations and preparation.[14,40]

Selection of the site for placement of Norplant is based on both functional and aesthetic factors. Various sites (the upper leg, forearm, and upper arm) have been used in clinical trials. The nondominant, upper, inner arm is usually the best site. This area is easily accessible to the clinician with minimal exposure of the patient. It is well protected during most normal activities. It is not highly visible, and imigration of the implants from this site has not been documented. The site of placement does not affect circulating levonorgestrel levels.

Insertion Technique

Insertion is carried out under local anesthesia in the office or clinic by someone, usually a physician or nurse practitioner, trained in the technique described here.[41] The procedure takes 5–10 minutes.

Proper insertion is important for easy removal later. If the implants are placed just under and parallel to the skin (subdermally) with the tips near the insertion site close together and with their opposite ends far apart in a fan-shaped distribution, removal will be easier than if they are deeply placed and not fanned out.

Required Equipment.

- 6 cc syringe.
- 1.5 inch, 18-gauge needle for drawing up the anesthetic.
- 1.5 inch, 22-gauge needle for injecting the anesthetic.
- Sterile 4 x 4 gauze sponges.
- 1% chloroprocaine or lidocaine without epinephrine.
- Antiseptic solution.
- No. 11 scalpel.
- Steristrips or butterfly closures.
- Elastic bandage.
- A specially marked 10-gauge trocar with a blunt obturator,
- The 6 implants,
- Sterile gloves,
- 3 sterile drapes (under the arm, fenestrated over the arm, sterile field for supplies).

145

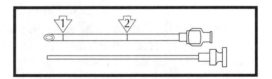

The specially marked trocar bears two marks along the length of the barrel to aid in the correct placement of the implants. The first mark is close to the bevel and indicates how far the trocar should be retracted before redirecting it for placement of subsequent implants. The second mark is close to the hub and indicates the length of the trocar that must be inserted under the skin prior to loading the implants for placement.

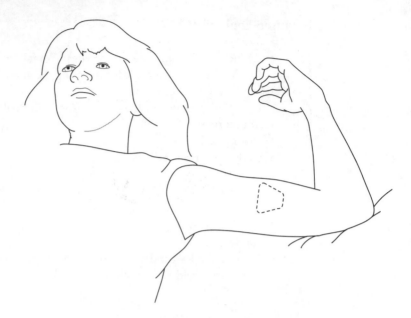

Positioning the Patient. The patient is placed in a supine position with the full length of her arm exposed. The upper inner arm is positioned by bending the elbow to 90 degrees and rotating the arm out, allowing full exposure of the insertion site at the medial aspect of the bicep. Adequate support under the arm should be provided to ensure comfort. To minimize the risk of infection, strict aseptic technique should be maintained throughout the procedure. A sterile drape is placed under the arm, and a 10 x 10 cm area of skin on the upper arm is cleaned with an antiseptic such as povidone-iodine. An insertion site approximately 4 fingerbreadths (8–12 cm) superior and lateral to the medial epicondyle of the humerus is identified.

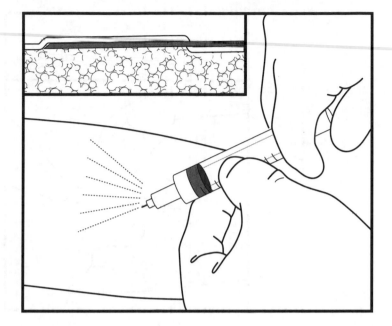

Anesthesia. Local anesthesia for the incision is obtained by raising a wheal of 1% chloroprocaine or lidocaine using a 22-gauge needle. The needle is then advanced under the skin its full length to its hub, and 1 mL of anesthetic is injected as it is withdrawn. The needle is advanced 5 more times to create, in the shape of a fan, an anesthetic field with 6 channels along which the implants will be placed. This requires about 6 mL of anesthetic. Injection of the anesthetic along these channels raises the dermis from the underlying tissue and allows easier introduction of the trocar.

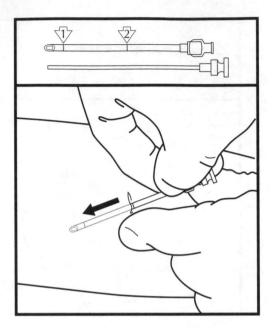

Incision and Placement. The no. 10 trocar and its obturator can usually be pushed directly through the skin without first making an incision, but if the skin is tough, a 2 mm skin incision is made with the no. 11 scalpel at the selected site 8–12 cm above the medial humeral epicondyle. The trocar with obturator in place is advanced as superficially as possible under the skin by maintaining an upward angle on the trocar. The trocar should elevate the skin at all times, and it should not be forced into the skin. If resistance is met, a slightly different angle to the left or right should be tried, along with a rotation of the trocar under the skin. If dimpling is seen, the trocar is not sufficiently underneath the skin.

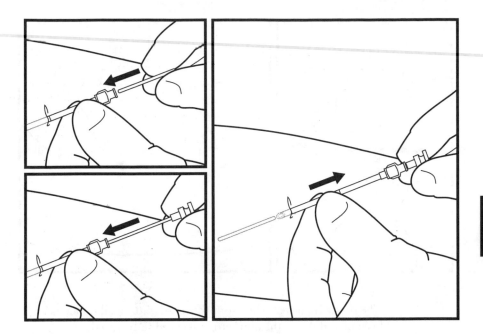

Once the trocar has been advanced to the mark nearest the hub (4.5 cm), the obturator is removed, and the first implant is loaded into the trocar. The obturator is replaced and used to advance the implant to the end of the trocar until slight, initial resistance is met. Holding the obturator stationary, the trocar is completely retracted over the obturator leaving the implant behind. Pushing on the obturator while withdrawing the trocar will advance the implant too far into the tissue, resulting in poor alignment with the distal tips of the other implants. After the trocar is completely retracted on the obturator, gentle downward pressure is exerted on the proximal end of the implant while retracting the trocar and obturator together to the mark closest to the bevel. This will ensure that the distal tip of the implant lies at least 0.5 cm above the incision.

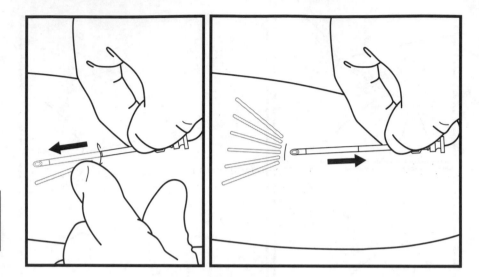

The trocar is not removed from the incision until all implants have been placed. With the obturator advanced fully into the trocar, the direction of the trocar is changed so that the next implant will lie at a 15 degree angle from the previous implant, forming a fanlike distribution of the 6 implants. A finger is placed on the previous implant and with gentle downward pressure, its position is fixed while advancing the trocar to the mark near the hub for placement of the next implant. Placement of a finger over the previous implant will ensure adequate spacing and prevent inadvertent puncture of the implant already placed. The obturator is removed, and the second implant is loaded and placed. The procedure is repeated for each implant to be inserted.

Most women experience little pain during the insertion.[14] The most commonly reported discomfort is a burning sensation during the injection of the local anesthetic. This effect of local anesthetic can be eliminated for most patients by adding 1 meq of sodium bicarbonate to each 10 mL of anesthetic (this shortens shelf life to 24 hours).[42] After the onset of anesthesia in 2–3 minutes, most women feel no more than a pressure sensation.

Closure. After all the implants have been inserted, the skin is closed with an adhesive strip. Sutures are not required. The insertion site is covered with two sterile 4 x 4 gauze sponges. An elastic bandage is wrapped around the upper arm to create a pressure dressing that should be left in place for 24 hours if there has been no trauma, 72 hours if a hematoma has formed.

After completing the insertion, the placement of the implants should be documented with a drawing in the medical record, indicating the relationship of each implant to the others. The patient should be advised that there may be bruising around the implants. The pressure dressing should be kept in place for 24 hours (longer if an obvious hematoma develops during insertion), and the adhesive strip until it falls off (usually in 3–5 days). Pain is unusual, but if it occurs it can be relieved with aspirin, acetaminophen, or nonsteroidal anti-inflammatory agents. Infection or expulsion of the implants is rare (less than 1%), and usually occurs when an implant is left pressing against the wound.[43] The clinician should be called for local pain, discharge, swelling, or fever.

Complications of Insertion

Potential complications include infection, hematoma formation, local irritation or rash over the implants, expulsion of one or more of the implants, and allergic reactions to adhesives or the dressing. The incidence of complications is minimized by clinician training and experience, and the use of strict aseptic technique.

Infection. The rate of infection varies among clinics and countries. The overall risk of infection after Norplant insertion is 0.8%.[43] Infections usually occur within the first week after insertion, but can present as long as 4–5 months later. Infection can be treated either by the removal of the implants or the administration of oral antibiotics while the implants remain in place. One-third of insertion site infections treated with antibiotics are unresponsive to therapy and require removal.[43] There have been no reports of infections leading to serious injury. Rarely, a superficial phlebitis develops. If it resolves over 1–2 weeks with heat and elevation of the arm, the implants need not be removed.

Expulsion. Expulsion of one or more of the implants occurs in 0.4% of users, usually within the first few months of use.[43] The majority of expulsions are associated with concurrent infection at the insertion site. Another cause of expulsion is failure to advance the implants far enough from the incision, causing pressure on the incision by the distal tip of the implant. If an implant is expelled without evidence of infection, a new one can be inserted. If a new implant cannot be inserted within a few weeks, then the remaining implants should be removed. Remember to remind the patient that another method of contraception must be used while waiting for reinsertion.

Local Reactions. Although not common, hematomas can form when Norplant is inserted. The use of a pressure dressing for 72 hours will prevent enlargment. Application of an ice pack for 30 minutes immediately after insertion also helps. Local irritation, rash, pruritus, and pain occur in 4.7% of users, usually during the first month of use.[43] These problems resolve spontaneously, but itching can be relieved by topical corticoid steroids.

Removal Techniques

Although Norplant removal is an office procedure requiring only a small amount of local anesthesia and a few simple instruments, instruction and practice are necessary.[41] Practicing on a model arm after viewing an instructional video makes first removals faster and less uncomfortable for both clinician and patient. A removal kit containing a model arm, removal forceps, and a manual and video tape illustrating basic technique is available at no charge from Wyeth-Ayerst, P.O. Box 8299, Philadelphia, PA 19101. As for insertion, the patient should read and sign an informed consent to be filed in her medical record. We recommend that the patient be given a copy.

Proper positioning of the implants at the time of insertion is the most important factor influencing ease of removal. If the implants have been inserted with the distal tips (those away from the axilla) far apart or with the implants crossing or touching one another, or too deeply, a larger incision and more time are required. Removal is easiest when the implants are just under the skin with their distal tips close together in a fan shape. The fibrous sheaths that form around implants can also make removal more difficult, especially if they are dense.

Most removals are not painful (80% of our patients reported pain as "none" or "slight"), and systemic analgesia is not required.[44] Time for removal ranges from 5 to 40 minutes, with an average of 20 minutes. The most common cause of discomfort during the procedure is injection of the local anesthetic. Again, this stinging sensation can be relieved if one meq sodium bicarbonate is added to each 10 mL of local anesthetic.[43] Patients may feel pressure or tugging from manipulation of the fibrous sheaths and the implants, but these sensations are not severe if the clinician waits a few minutes after injection of the local anesthetic.

Removal with Instruments. This approach to removal is the one described in the package insert and has been used around the world for 15 years. The technique requires 3 small sterile drapes (one fenestrated), sterile gloves, antiseptic solution such as povidone-iodine, 25-gauge 1.5 inch needle with a 3 mL syringe, local anesthetic (1% lidocaine with 1:100,000 epinephrine, buffered with 1 meq sodium bicarbonate per 10 mL lidocaine), one curved and one straight mosquito clamp, 4 x 4 sterile gauze sponges, and a no. 11 blade scalpel.

The patient is placed in a supine position with her arm flexed and externally rotated as for insertion. A thick book positioned under the patient's arm can make her more comfortable and provide a better operating field. A sterile towel is placed under the arm. The implants are best seen by stretching the skin above and below the implants. Palpate all 6 of the implants before starting; if some portion of every implant cannot be felt, it may be better to sonographically or radiographically image (see below) the impalpable ones before removal because when the palpable implants are gone, they are lost as landmarks.

The skin is cleansed with the antiseptic solution, preparing a wide area above and below the implants so that the incision won't be contaminated during manipulations for removal. Scrape the antiseptic solution from the skin lying over the implants (the sterile stick of a cotton tipped applicator can be used) and let the arm dry. This will leave an impression of the implants that helps find them for removal. Drape the arm with a fenestrated towel and use a third towel to create a sterile field for instruments on a Mayo stand or table.

Wearing sterile gloves, an incision site is selected by pressing down on the proximal ends of the capsules and palpating their distal tips with a finger. Careful selection of the incision site is the most critical step for easy removal. The best incision site is right at the distal tips, midway between the most medial and lateral implants. This can be the same as the insertion site, but generally the removal incision is made a few millimeters higher up on the arm to ensure placing it as close as possible to the tips of all the implants.

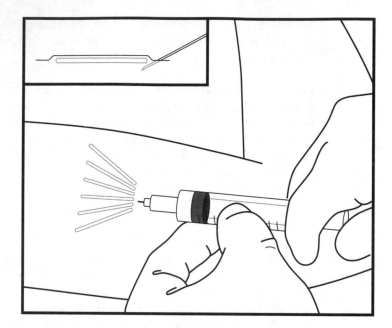

A local anesthetic containing 1:100,000 epinephrine reduces bleeding and allows better visualization of the implants. The 25-gauge needle is used to raise a 1 cm wheal of local anesthetic just under the tips of the implants. About 2 mL are sufficient, although more may be required later. Injection of too much anesthetic over the implants can obscure the tips and make removal more difficult. A 3–5 mm incision is made with the no. 11 scalpel right at the mid point of the cluster of implant tips. A larger incision is not usually required and can cause bleeding that can obscure the implants. Implants can be removed by the clinician either sitting or standing, but if sitting, a wheeled stool allows repositioning as needed.

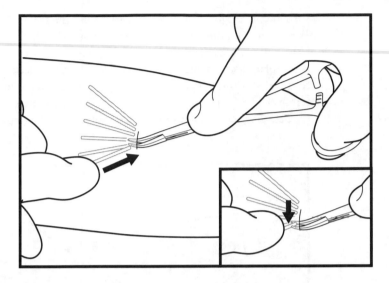

The implant that is most superficial and closest to the incision is removed first. This implant is pushed gently toward the incision with the fingers until the tip is visible and can be grasped with a curved mosquito clamp.

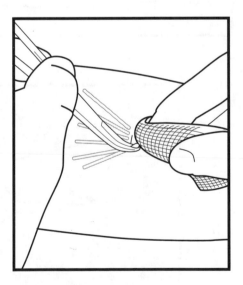

The fibrous sheath covering the implant is dissected away using a finger covered with an opened gauze sponge. If the sheath is too dense for the sponge, it can be cautiously dissected with the straight clamp, a needle tip, or, for really dense sheaths, with the scalpel, taking care not to cut open the implant. If the point of the scalpel blade is used to nick the sheath over the thick Silastic plug at the tip of the implant, the implant itself will not be cut, but if the sheath is incised across the thin walls of the implant, the implant can be severed and require removal in two portions. If the sheath must be incised with the scalpel, the incision should be along, not across, the implant.

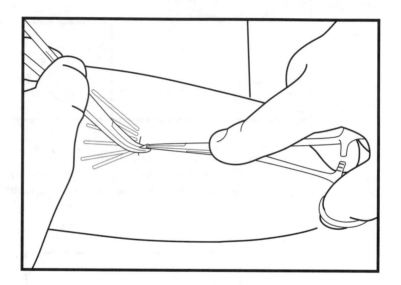

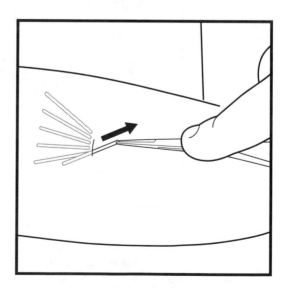

Once the sheath is opened and the white tip of the first implant is exposed, it is grasped with the straight clamp. The curved clamp is released and the implant is gently pulled out. This procedure is repeated with the remaining implants.

If the implant tips cannot be guided to the incision with digital pressure on the skin above the implants, the jaws of the straight mosquito are inserted into the incision and opened just beneath the skin to separate the tissue layers. The straight clamp is removed, and the curved clamp is inserted with the tips pointing upward toward the skin. The clamp is opened and the implant is guided down between the jaws with a forefinger on the skin above the implant. This downward pressure on the tips of the clamp is often the most painful part of the removal procedure. When the implant is pushed between the jaws of the clamp, the clamp is secured at the first or second ratchet. Too much pressure on the implant can fracture the Silastic capsule, making removal more difficult. The implant should not be pulled out with the curved clamp.

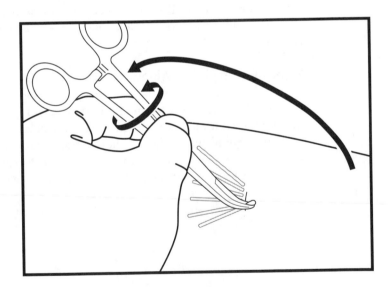

If the implant cannot be seen, after gentle traction, the clamp handle is flipped 180 degrees until it points in the opposite direction, toward the patient's head. A portion of the sheath is cleared with an opened sponge, or if necessary, the scalpel tip, incising longitudinally, not across the implant. The exposed portion is then grasped with the straight clamp, the curved clamp is released, and the implant is removed with gentle traction. The procedure is repeated until all the implants are removed.

At the completion of the procedure, the implants should be counted to ensure that all have been removed. If any of the implants have been broken, the pieces should be aligned and compared with an intact capsule to determine that all of the implant has been removed. An adhesive strip is used to close the incision while pinching the skin edges together. A pressure dressing is then applied as after insertion, and removed the next day. The fibrous sheaths can remain for months causing the patient to think that implants were left behind. For that reason, it is important to show the implants to the patient at the time of removal.

If removal of some of the implants is difficult, painful, or prolonged, the procedure should be interrupted and the patient should return in a few weeks to complete the removal. The remaining implants will be easier to remove after bleeding and swelling have subsided. A new incision can be made closer to the implants that were difficult to remove the first time. Even if some of the implants remain, the patient should immediately begin to use another method of contraception.

Removal with Fingers Alone. Implants can be removed with less pain and bleeding, and through a smaller incision if the use of instruments is avoided. The amount of trauma and bruising in the surrounding tissues is decreased, the scar is less visible, and the risk of breaking the implants is reduced. The disadvantages of this approach are that it can take longer, and that it may not be successful for implants that were poorly aligned or too deep at placement.

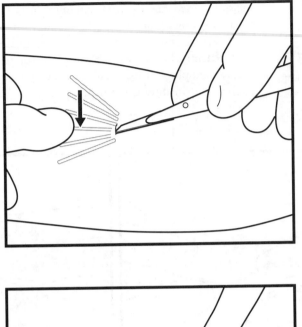

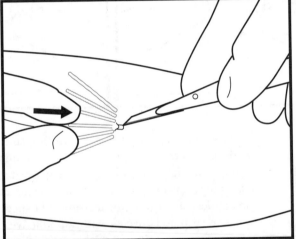

After preparation of the patient, the distal tips of the implants are palpated to identify the implant that is most centrally located and equidistant from the other tips. No more than 0.5 mL of buffered lidocaine with epinephrine is injected into the dermis immediately over the most prominent cluster of implant tips, raising a wheal of about 1 cm in diameter. Too much anesthetic makes it difficult to locate the implant tips under the skin. The area of the injection should be massaged for a minute or two to disperse the anesthetic. Pressure is applied with fingers on the proximal (axillary) ends of the implants so that the distal tips press up against the skin. A 3–4 mm incision is made through the skin onto the tips of the implants until the rubbery sensation of the Silastic plugs at the tips of the implants can be felt against the point of the scalpel blade. The fibrous sheath is incised by nicking the sheath with the tip of the scalpel blade against the implant plugs. It may take several passes across the tips with the scalpel held in different directions to fully open the ends of the sheaths.

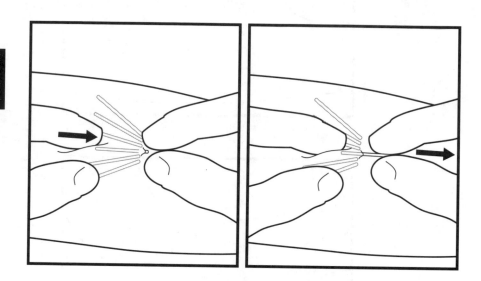

As the sheath is opened, the end of the implant will come into view. With finger pressure on its other end, the implant can be pushed through the incision until it can be grasped and pulled out. The remaining implants can be removed using the same technique if they are not deep or far from the incision. The incision is closed with an adhesive strip and covered with an adhesive dressing. A pressure dressing is not required with this technique because there is little subcutaneous trauma.

Holding the implant up against the incision with finger pressure is critical for success with this technique. If pressure is released, the implant will slip back to the position defined by the fibrous sheath around it. As the implants are manipulated using the fingers of both hands, the scalpel must be held so that it is immediately available to incise the sheaths without releasing the implants. It is best to keep the scalpel in one hand with thumb and index finger while manipulating the implants, holding the implants with the rest of the fingers of both hands.

If the implants will not move toward the incision with finger pressure, they can be grasped with a hemostatic clamp, but the incision will usually have to be lenghthened 2–3 mm in order to admit the clamp. The procedure followed is then as described for instrumental removals above. It may be necessary to inject more local anesthetic, but not more than 1 mL at a time where the clamp will be applied to the implant.

Difficult Removals. Removal is more difficult if the implants are broken during attempts to extract them. Once an implant is damaged, it can fracture repeatedly with further attempts to grasp it with clamps. To decrease this risk, the implants should be grasped by the Silastic plugs at their ends whenever possible and as little traction as possible should be used for exposure and removal. If the scalpel is required to open the fibrous sheath around the implant, care should be taken to avoid slicing the capsule. If it has not been possible to grasp the Silastic plug at the end of implant, in order to open the fibrous sheath, incise along the length of the implant; cut longitudinally, not across, the implant. Rarely, removal of cut or broken implants will require an additional incision at the proximal end of the implant so that the remaining piece can be removed. Even more rarely, an implant can neither be palpated under the skin nor found through an incision. Such "lost" implants are most easily located with a high frequency (7–10 megahertz), short focus ultrasound just prior to the removal procedure to help place the incision directly over the implant.[45] Use a transverse orientation to identify the 6 shadows (the implants themselves are more difficult to see), measure the depth, and draw lines representing their locations on the surface of the skin after using beads or a paper clip as a marker.

Standard radiography will identify implants but will not locate them precisely enough for removal and cannot be used during the procedure. Compression "mammography" of the upper arm with grid, bead, or needle localization is a better radiographic technique.[46]

161

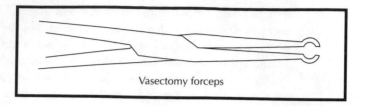

Vasectomy forceps

Another instrumental technique employs a modified vasectomy forceps and is very useful for removing deeply or assymmetrically placed capsules. It requires a larger incision made in the center of the field of implants. The vasectomy forceps is advanced under the skin toward the mid portion of the implants. Those in the center are grasped first (in the middle of each implant), pulled into the incision, and cleaned free of their fibrous sheath as in the standard technique. The implant is then extracted, bending it in the middle in a "U" shape. The implants furthest away from the incision are removed last by advancing the forcep under the skin.[47]

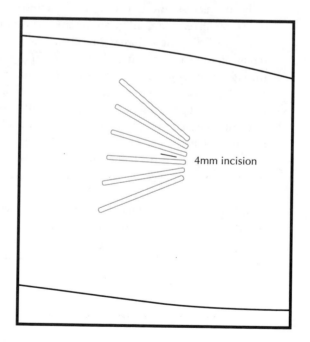

4mm incision

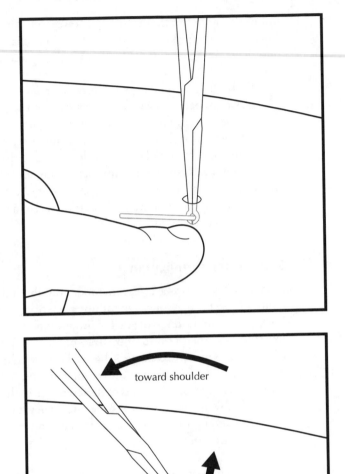

toward shoulder

We have found this approach to be especially useful for deeply placed, single capsules that are otherwise difficult to remove. The incision is made directly above the mid portion of the implant as determined by sonography or compression radiography. The scalpel blade (or a 25-gauge needle) is advanced to the depth of the implant as determined by imaging to feel for the capsule. The vasectomy forceps is advanced along the same track until the capsule can be grasped and elevated into the incision, freed from its fibrous sheath, and extracted.

It is likely that additional procedures for removing contraceptive implants have been, or will be, developed, but for all procedures, removals are easier, faster, and less painful when the implants are properly inserted in the first place, in a symmetric arc just under, but not in, the skin.[12,48] Experienced clinicians agree that about half of difficult removals are due to improper placement.[12] When one and two implant systems become available over the next few years, removals will be easier, but careful insertion will remain the real secret to trouble-free removal.

Reasons for Termination

Although Norplant is a 5-year method, only about 30% of women continue use for that long. Discontinuation occurs at a rate of 10–15% yearly, about the same as for intrauterine contraception, but lower than for barrier or oral contraception.[2,14,19] Bothersome side effects such as menstrual changes, headache, or weight change are the primary reasons for termination of implant use.[5,34,49] Users who cannot tolerate these symptoms request removal in the first two years of use while women who want another pregnancy, the most common personal reason for removal, are more likely to terminate use in the third or fourth year.

Menstrual changes are the most common cause for discontinuation of Norplant in the first year of use. The next most common reasons for discontinuing Norplant are headache, weight change, mood change, anxiety or nervousness, depression, ovarian cyst formation, and lower abdominal pain. Presence of ovarian cysts is not usually an indication for removal of Norplant and is almost never a reason for surgery. Most will resolve spontaneously within 4 weeks. Skin conditions, including rashes, dermatitis, and acne, account for about 0.8% of terminations.

User Acceptance of Norplant

Overall, interview surveys throughout the world have indicated that women perceive sustained-release methods, Norplant in particular, as highly acceptable methods of contraception.[40,50–52] The most popular feature of Norplant is the ease of use. About 20% of U.S.

patients report that friends and relatives notice their implants. This may be a greater problem in warmer climates with less encompassing clothing. Only 25% of the women who report that the implants were noticed were bothered by this attention.[5]

In the U.S., the primary motivations for Norplant use have been problems with previous contraceptive methods and ease of Norplant use. Although fear of pain during Norplant insertion is a prominent source of anxiety for many women, the actual pain experienced does not match the expectations. The level of satisfaction has been high in users who were self-motivated and well-informed about Norplant. Teenagers provide an example of well-documented success. Their one-year pregnancy rates are much lower and continuation rates much higher that that with oral contraceptives.[53–56]

Studies of women's attitudes toward sustained-release contraceptives indicate that the great majority of women find them highly acceptable and perceive them as desirable alternatives to conventional contraceptives, although not everyone finds Norplant preferable.[57,58] Around the world, women who have used Norplant say they have recommended Norplant to friends and would like to use it again.[5,40,50,52,59]

Counseling Women

Frank information about negative factors such as irregular bleeding and possible weight changes will avoid surprise and disappointment, and encourage women to continue use long enough to enjoy the positive attributes such as convenience, safety, and efficacy. Open discussion of side effects will lead to public and media awareness of the disadvantages as well as the advantages of these methods. Helping women decide if they are good candidates for use of Norplant, for example, before they invest too much time and money in this long-acting contraceptive, is a very important objective of good counseling.

Common patient questions regarding Norplant are as follows;

- Is it effective?
- How is it inserted and removed; how long do these procedures take; does it hurt; and will it leave scars?
- Will the implants be visible under the skin?
- Will the implants be uncomfortable or restrict movement of the arm?

- Will the implants move in the body?
- Will the implants be damaged if they are touched or bumped?
- Will this contraceptive change sexual drive and enjoyment?
- What are the short- and long-term side effects?
- Are there any effects on future fertility?
- What do the implants look and feel like?
- What happens if pregnancy occurs during use?
- How long will it take for the method to be effective after insertion?
- Can a partner tell if this method is being used?

General Advantages

One of the major advantages of sustained-release methods is the high degree of efficacy, nearly equivalent to the theoretical effectiveness. In couples for whom elective abortion is unacceptable in the event of an unplanned pregnancy, the high efficacy rate is especially important. There are no forgotten pills, broken condoms, or lost diaphragms. For women who are at high risk of medical complications should they become pregnant, these methods present a significant safety advantage. Users should be reassured that Norplant use has not been associated with changes in carbohydrate or lipid metabolism, coagulation, liver or kidney function, or immunoglobulin levels. Since many women wanting Norplant will have had negative experiences with other contraceptives, it is important that the differences between this method and previous methods be explained.

Norplant is a good method for breastfeeding women. There are no effects on breast milk quality or quantity, and infants grow normally.[60,61] If new nursing mothers will not have a later opportunity (within 3 months), Norplant can be inserted immediately postpartum.

Another advantage of Norplant is that it allows women to plan their pregnancies precisely; return of fertility after removal is prompt, in contrast to the 18 month delay in ovulation that can follow Depo-Provera injections.[13,62] In addition, anemia is less likely in Norplant users.[21]

General Disadvantages

The cost of implants plus fees for insertion total an amount that seems high to many patients unless they compare it to the total cost of using other methods for up to 5 years.[59] Nevertheless, short-term use is expensive compared with the relatively low initial costs of other reversible methods, and most women cannot be expected to use long-acting methods for their full duration of action.

Sustained-release, progestin-only methods do not increase the risk of developing STDs, but it is not known whether they provide any protection. Women who have multiple partners, or whose partners do, should use condoms as well. All users must be aware of the possible menstrual changes. It is important to stress that all of the menstrual changes are expected, that they do not cause or represent illness, and that most women revert back to a more normal pattern with increasing duration of use.

Cultural factors can influence the acceptability of menstrual changes. Hispanic users of Norplant, for example, are very accepting of irregular or prolonged bleeding.[5] Some cultures restrict a woman from participating in religious activity, household activities, or sexual intercourse while menstruating.

Insertion and removal of implants will be a new experience for most women. As with any new experience, women will approach it with varying degrees of apprehension and anxiety. In reality, most patients are able to watch in comfort as implants are inserted or removed. Women should be told that the incisions used for the procedures are very small and heal quickly, leaving small scars which are usually difficult to see because of their location and size.

Prospective users should be allowed to see and touch implants. Women should be reassured that the implants will not be damaged or move if the skin above them is accidentally injured. Normal activity cannot damage or displace the implants. Most women become unaware of their presence.

A few women report sensing the implants if they have been touched or manipulated for a prolonged period of time, or after vigorous exercise. The implants can be visible in slender women with good muscle tone. Darker-skinned users may notice further darkening of the skin directly over the implants; this resolves after removal.

167

Finally, a small minority of women cannot use implants because of their need to take other medications, such as rifampin or the antiepileptics (phenobarbitol, phenytoin, carbamazepine) that reduce Norplant's efficacy.[63]

New Developments in Implant Contraception

The two implant system, "Norplant II," uses levonorgestrel suspended in a Silastic matrix and covered with a Silastic membrane. Like the 6 capsule Norplant and the single capsule, Implanon, Norplant II should be removed when serum levonorgestrel levels are too low for contraception, at least 3 years after insertion, but possibly as long as 5 years. Bleeding, pregnancy, and continuation rates are like those of the 6 capsule system, but insertion and removal are easier.[13]

The newer progestins (desogestrel, gestodene, nestorone, nomegestrol, and norgestimate) are less androgenic than levonorgestrel and could prove useful in contraceptive implants. An example is "Implanon," a single implant 4 cm long, that contains 60 mg of 3-keto desogestrel in a core of ethinyl vinyl acetate wrapped with a membrane of the same material. The hormone is released at a rate of about 60 µg per day. Implanon is designed to provide contraception for 2–3 years after which the implant should be removed. Efficacy and side effects appear to be similar to those with Norplant.[64,65] Another single implant contraceptive is "Uniplant," containing 38 mg nomegestrol acetate in a 4 cm Silastic tube with a 100 µg per day release rate. It provides contraception for one year.[66–68]

Biodegradable implants deliver sustained levels of progestin for variable periods of time from a vehicle that dissolves in body tissues. The utility of implant contraception would be improved by the elimination of the need for surgical removal. Two types are under evaluation: Capronor and norethindrone pellets.

Capronor is a single capsule, biodegradable, levonorgestrel-releasing subdermal implant composed of the polymer E-caprolactone. Implants measure 0.24 cm in diameter and either 2.5 or 4 cm in length, providing contraception for one year. The shorter capsule contains 16 mg levonorgestrel, and the longer contains 26 mg. Levonorgestrel escapes from caprolactone at a rate 10 times faster than from Silastic. The shorter implant maintains circulating levels of levonorgestrel of 0.2–0.3 ng/mL, while the longer implant maintains higher levels equivalent to those found in Norplant users. The longer capsule suppresses ovulation in a higher proportion (about 50%) of cycles than reported with Norplant, but the shorter implant allows ovulation in most users. The higher release rate allows the use of a smaller implant. Experience is still too limited to report pregnancy rates, but the longer implant should provide contraception comparable to Norplant.

When exposed to tissue fluids, E-caprolactone slowly breaks down into E-hydroxycaproic acid, then finally to carbon dioxide and water. The capsule remains intact during the first 12 months of use, allowing easy removal. After 12 months, the capsule begins to disappear.

Capronor shares the advantages of Norplant with convenience of use and few metabolic effects. There is no adverse impact on the lipoprotein profile. Removal is easier and quicker. The disadvantages are also similar to Norplant: changes in menstrual patterns and the other side effects typical of low-dose, continuous progestin systems. Biodegradable implants could continue to release small, noncontracpetive amounts of hormone after their period of use as a contraceptive has expired. Although it is unlikely that such low serum levels of progestin would be harmful to users or to their pregnancies, this question needs to be resolved. The degrading implants can be removed in the event of pregnancy.[69]

Biodegradable subdermal norethindrone pellets are expected to maintain circulating concentrations of this progestin at contraceptive levels for 12–18 months, and to completely disappear within 24 months. The pellets are composed of 10% pure cholesterol and 90% norethindrone, and are about the size of a grain of rice. This method is currently under development to determine the correct size and number of pellets and the cholesterol/hormone ratio necessary to obtain the release rates that provide contraception. Preliminary trials of 2, 3, and 4 pellets have demonstrated that bleeding patterns are disrupted during the first few months of use, then return to normal patterns. Users of 4 pellets are more likely to be amenorrheic and anovulatory.[70]

References

1. **Segal SJ,** A new delivery system for contraceptive steroids, Am J Obstet Gynecol 157:1090, 1987.

2. **Sivin I,** International experience with Norplant and Norplant-2 contraceptives, Stud Fam Plann 19:81, 1988.

3. **Roy S, Mishell DR Jr, Robertson D, Krauss RM, Lacarra M, Duda MJ,** Long-term reversible contraception with levonorgestrel-releasing Silastic rods, Am J Obstet Gynecol 148:1006, 1984.

4. **Trussell J, Hatcher RA, Cates W Jr, Stewart FH, Kost K,** Contraceptive failure in the United States: an update, Stud Fam Plann 21:51, 1990.

5. **Darney PD, Elizazbeth A, Tanner S, MacPherson S, Hellerstein S, Alvardo A,** Acceptance and perceptions of Norplant among users in San Francisco, USA, Stud Fam Plann 21:152, 1990.

6. **Brache V, Faundes A, Johansson E, Alvarez F,** Anovulation, inadequate luteal phase, and poor sperm penetration in cervical mucus during prolonged use of Norplant implants, Contraception 31:261, 1985.

7. **Brache V, Alvarez-Sanchez F, Faundes A, Tejada AS, Cochon L,** Ovarian endocrine function through five years of continuous treatment with Norplant subdermal contraceptive implants, Contraception 41:169, 1990.

8. **Affandi B, Cekan S, Boonkasemanti R, Samil RS, Dicsfalusy E,** The interaction between sex hormone binding globulin and levonorgestrel released from Norplant, an implantable contraceptive, Contraception 35:135, 1987.

9. **Alvarez F, Brache V, Tejada AS, Faundes A,** Abnormal endocrine profile among women with confirmed or presumed ovulation during long-term Norplant use, Contraception 33:111, 1986.

10. **Croxatto HB, Diaz S, Salvatierra AM, Morales P, Ebensperger C, Brandeis A,** Treatment with Norplant subdermal implants inhibits sperm penetration through cervical mucus in vitro, Contraception 36:193, 1987.

11. **Segal SJ, Alvarez-Sanchez F, Brache V, Faundes A, Vilja P, Tuohimaa P,** Norplant implants: the mechanism of contraceptive action, Fertil Steril 56:273, 1991.

12. **Dunson TR, Amatya RN, Krueger SL,** Complications and risk factors associated with the removal of Norplant implants, Obstet Gynecol 85:543, 1995.

13. **Sivin I, Stern J, Diaz S, Pavez M, Alvarez F, Brache V, Mishell DR Jr, Lacarra M, McCarthy T, Holma P, Darney P, Klaisle C, Olsson S-E, Odlind V,** Rates and outcomes of planned pregnancy after use of Norplant capsules, Norplant II rods, or levonorgestrel-releasing or copper TCu 380Ag intrauterine contraceptive devices, Am J Obstet Gynecol 166:1208, 1992.

14. Darney PD, Klaisle CM, Tanner ST, Alvarado AM, Sustained release contraceptives, Curr Prob Obstet Gynecol Fertil 13:87, 1990.

15. Centers for Disease Control and Prevention, Ectopic pregnancy in the United States, 1970–1988, CDC Surveillance Summaries, MMWR 38:1, 1989.

16. Franks AL, Beral V, Cates W Jr, Hogue CJ, Contraception and ectopic pregnancy risk, Am J Obstet Gynecol 163:1120, 1990.

17. Sivin I, Alvarez-Sanchez F, Diaz S, Holma P, Coutinho E, McDonald O, Robertson DN, Stern J, Three-year experience with Norplant subdermal contraception, Fertil Steril 39:799, 1983.

18. Shoupe D, Mishell DR Jr, Bopp B, Fiedling M, The significance of bleeding patterns in Norplant implant users, Obstet Gynecol 77:256, 1991.

19. Sivin I, Diaz S, Holma P, Alvarez-Sanchez F, Robertson DN, A four-year clinical study of Norplant implants, Stud Fam Plann 14:184, 1983.

20. Nilsson C, Holma P, Menstrual blood loss with contraceptive subdermal levonorgestrel implants, Fertil Steril 35:304, 1981.

21. Fakeye O, Balogh S, Effect of Norplant contraceptive use on hemoglobin, packed cell volume, and menstrual bleeding patterns, Contraception 39:265, 1989.

22. Diaz S, Croxatto HB, Pavez M, Belhadj H, Stern J, Sivin I, Clinical assessment of treatments for prolonged bleeding in users of Norplant implants, Contraception 42:97, 1990.

23. Croxatto HB, Diaz S, Robertson D, Pavez M, Clinical chemistries in women treated with levonorgestrel implant (Norplant) or a TCu 200 IUD, Contraception 27:281, 1983.

24. Konje JC, Otolorin EO, Ladipo OA, Changes in carbohydrate metabolism during 30 months on Norplant, Contraception 44:163, 1991.

25. Shaaban MM, Elwan SI, El-Sharkawy MM, Farghaly AS, Effect of subdermal lenonorgestrel contraceptive implants, Norplant, on liver functions, Contraception 30:407, 1984.

26. Singh K, Viegas OAC, Liew D, Singh P, Ratnam SS, Two-year follow-up of changes in clinical chemistry in Singaporean Norplant acceptors: metabolic changes, Contraception 39:129, 1989.

27. Shaaban MM, Elwan SI, El-Kabsh MY, Farghaly SA, Thabet N, Effect of levonorgestrel contraceptive implants, Norplant, on bleeding and coagulation, Contraception 30:421, 1984.

28. Singh K, Viegas OAC, Koh SCL, Ratnam SS, Effect of long-term use of Norplant implants on haemostatic function, Contraception 45:203, 1992.

29. Abdulla K, Elwan SI, Salem HS, Shaaban MM, Effect of early postpartum use of the contraceptive implants, Norplant, on the serum levels of immunoglobulin of the mothers and their breastfed infants, Contraception 32:261, 1985.

30. Bayad M, Ibrahim I, Fayad M, et al, Serum cortisol in women users of subdermal levonorgestrel implants, Contracept Deliv Syst 4:133, 1983.

31. Shaaban MM, Elwan SI, Abdalla SA, Dawish HA, Effect of subdermal levonorgestrel contraceptive implants, Norplant, on serum lipids, Contraception 30:413, 1984.

32. Otubu JAM, Towobola OA, Aisien AO, Ogunkeye OO, Effects of Norplant contraceptive subdermal implants on serum lipids and lipoproteins, Contraception 47:149, 1993.

33. Koopersmith TB, Lobo RA, Insulin sensitivity is unaltered by the use of the Norplant subdermal implant contraceptive, Contraception 51:197, 1995.

34. Gu S, Du M, Zhang L, Liu YL, Wang SH, Sivin I, A 5-year evaluation of Norplant contraceptive implants in China, Obstet Gynecol 83:673, 1994.

35. Wysowski DK, Green L, Serious adverse events in Norplant users reported to the Food and Drug Administration's MedWatch Spontaneous Reporting System, Obstet Gynecol 85:538, 1995.

36. Pasquale SA, Knuppel RA, Owens AG, Bachmann GA, Irregular bleeding, body mass index and coital frequency in Norplant contraceptive users, Contraception 50:109, 1994.

37. Faundes A, Brache V, Tejada AS, Cochon L, Alvarez-Sanchez F, Ovulatory dysfunction during continuous administration of low-dose levonorgestrel by subdermal implants, Fertil Steril 56:27, 1991.

38. Darney PD, Taylor RN, Klaisle C, Bottles K, Zaloudek C, Serum concentrations of estradiol, progesterone, and levonorgestrel are not determinants of endometrial histology or abnormal bleeding in long-term Norplant implant users, Contraception, Vol 38, 1996.

39. Phemister DA, Lauarent S, Harrison FNH Jr, Use of Norplant contraceptive implants in the immediate postpartum period: safety and tolerance, Am J Obstet Gynecol 172:175, 1995.

40. Zimmerman M, Haffey J, Crane E, Szumowski D, Alvarez F, Bhiromrut P, Brache V, Lubis F, Salah M, Shaaban MM, Shawly B, Sidiip S, Assessing the acceptability of Norplant implants in four countries: findings from focus group research, Stud Fam Plann 21:92, 1990.

41. Bromham DR, Davey A, Gaffikin L, Ajello CA, Materials, methods and results of the Norplant training program, Br J Fam Plann 10:256, 1995.

42. Nelson AL, Neutralizing pH of lidocaine reduces pain during Norplant system insertion procedures, Contraception 51:299, 1995.

43. **Klavon SL, Grubb G,** Insertion site complications during the first year of Norplant use, Contraception 41:27, 1990.

44. **Darney PD, Klaisle CM, Walker DM,** The pop-out method of Norplant removal, Adv Contraception 8:188, 1992.

45. **Glauser SJ, Scharling ES, Stovall TG, Zagoria RJ,** Ultrasonography: usefulness in localization of the Norplant contraceptive implant system, J Ultrasound Med 14:411, 1995.

46. **Letterie GS, Garnaas M** Localization of "lost" Norplant capsules using compression film screen mammography, Obstet Gynecol 85:886, 1995.

47. **Praptohardjo U, Wibowo S,** The "U" technique: a new method for Norplant implants removal, Contraception 48:526, 1993.

48. **Frank ML, Ditmore JR, Llegbodu AE, Bateman L, Poindexter AN III,** Characteristics and experiences of American women electing for early removal of contraceptive implants, Contraception 52:159, 1995.

49. **Gu S, Sivin I, Du M, Zhang L, Ying-Lin L, Meng F, Wu S, Wang P, Gao Y, He X, Qi L, Chen C, Liu Y, Wang D,** Effectiveness of Norplant implants through seven years: a large-scale study in China, Contraception 52:99, 1995.

50. **Salah M, Ahmed A, Abo-Eloyoun M, Shaaban MM,** Five-year experience with Norplant implants in Assiut, Egypt, Contraception 35:543, 1987.

51. **Bashayake S, Thapa S, Balogh A,** Evaluation of safety, efficacy, and acceptability of Norplant implants in Sri Lanka, Stud Fam Plann 19:39, 1988.

52. **Dugoff L, Jones OW III, Allen-Davis J, Hurst BS, Schlaff WD,** Assessing the acceptability of Norplant contraceptive in four patient populations, Contraception 52:45, 1995.

53. **Cromer BA, Smith RD, Blair JM, Dwyer J, Brown RT,** A prospective study of adolescents who choose among levonorgestrel implant (Norplant), medroxyprogesterone acetate (Depo-Provera), or the combined oral contraceptive pill as contraception, Pediatrics 94:687, 1994.

54. **Cullins VE, Remsburg RE, Blumenthal PD, Huggins GR,** Comparison of adolescent and adult experience with Norplant levonorgestrel contraceptive implants, Obstet Gynecol 83:1026, 1994.

55. **Polaneczky M, Slap G, Forke C, Rappaport A, Sondheimer S,** The use of levonorgestrel implants (Norplant) for contraception in adolescent mothers, New Engl J Med 331:1201, 1994.

56. **Berenson AB, Wiemann CM,** Use of levonorgestrel implants versus oral contraceptives in adolescence: a case-control study, Am J Obstet Gynecol 172:1128, 1995.

173

57. **Gao J, Wang SL, Wu SC, Sun BL, Allonen H, Luukkainen T,** Comparison of the clinical performance, contraceptive efficacy and acceptability of levonorgestrel-releasing IUD and Norplant implants in China, Contraception 41:485, 1990.

58. **Sihvo S, Ollila E, Hemminki E,** Who uses Norplant: a study from Finland, Acta Obstet Gynecol Scand 73:476, 1994.

59. **Trussell J, Leveque JA, Koenig JD, London R, Borden S, Henneberry J, LaGuardia KD, Stewart F, Wilson G, Wysocki S, Strauss M,** The economic value of contraception: a comparison of 15 methods, Am J Public Health 85:494, 1995.

60. **Shaaban MM, Salem HT, Abdullah KA,** Influence of levonorgestrel contraceptive implants, Norplant, initiated early postpartum, upon lactation and infant growth, Contraception 32:623, 1985.

61. **Diaz S, Herreros C, Juez G, Casado ME, Salvatierra AM, Miranda P, Peralta O, Croxatto HB,** Fertility regulation in nursing women: influence of Norplant levonorgestrel implants upon lactation and infant growth, Contraception 32:53, 1985.

62. **Diaz S, Pavez M, Cardenas H, Croxatto HB,** Recovery of fertility and outcome of planned pregnancies after the removal of Norplant subdermal implants or copper-T IUDs, Contraception 35:569, 1987.

63. **Haukkamaa M,** Contraception by Norplant subdermal capsules is not reliable in epileptic patients on anticonvulsant treatment, Contraception 33:559, 1986.

64. **Olsson S-E, Odlind V, Johansson E,** Clinical results with subcutaneous implants containing 3-keto desogestrel, Contraception 42:1, 1990.

65. **Diaz S, Pavez M, Moo-Young AJ, Bardin CW, Croxatto HB,** Clinical trial with 3-keto-desogestrel subdermal implants, Contraception 44:393, 1991.

66. **Coutinho EM,** One year contraception with a single subdermal implant containing nomegestrel acetate (Uniplant), Contraception 47:94, 1993.

67. **Haukkamaa M, Laurikka-Routti M, Heikinheimo O, Moo-Young A,** Contraception with subdermal implants releasing the progestin ST-1435: a dose-finding study, Contraception 45:49, 1992.

68. **Diaz S, Schiappacasse V, Pavez M, Zepeda A, Moo-Young AJ, Brandeis A, Lahteenmaki P, Croxatto HB,** Clinical trial with Nestorone subdermal contraceptive implants, Contraception 51:33, 1995.

69. **Darney PD, Klaisle CM, Monroe SE, Cook CE, Phillips N, Schindler A,** Evaluation of a 1-year levonorgestrel-releasing contraceptive implant: side effects, release rates, and biodegradability, Fertil Steril 58:137, 1992.

70. **Singh M, Saxena BB, Landesman R, Ledger WJ,** Contraceptive efficacy of bioabsorbable pellets of norethindrone (NET) as subcutaneous implants: Phase II clinical study, Adv Contraception 1:131, 1985.

174

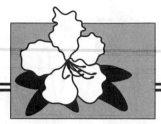

5

Injectable Contraception: Depo-Provera

DEPO-PROVERA (medroxyprogesterone acetate) is the most thoroughly studied progestin-only contraceptive. Although its approval for contraception in the U.S. is recent (1992), it has been available in some countries since the mid 1960s. Much of our knowledge of the safety, efficacy, and acceptability of long-acting hormonal contraception comes from Thailand and Mexico where Depo-Provera has been used and studied for decades. The long-delayed approval as a contraceptive in the U.S. was based on political and economic considerations, not scientific ones.[1]

Depo-Provera comes as microcrystals, suspended in an aqueous solution. The correct dose for contraceptive purposes is 150 mg intramuscularly (gluteal or deltoid) every 3 months. A comparative trial established that the 100 mg dose is significantly less effective.[2] The contraceptive level is maintained for at least 14 weeks, providing a safety margin for one of the most effective contraceptives available, about 1 pregnancy per 100 women after 5 years of consistent use.[2,3]

Depo-Provera is not a "sustained release" system, but relies on higher peaks of progestin to inhibit ovulation and thicken cervical mucus. The difference between serum levels of progestins in a sustained release system like Norplant and a depot system like Depo-Provera is illustrated in the following diagram.

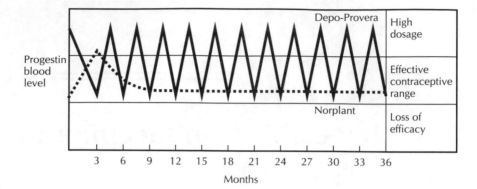

Several injectable contraceptives are in use around the world, but only Depo-Provera is available in the U.S. Other widely-used injectables are norethindrone enanthate (NET-EN), 200 mg every 2 months, and the monthly injectables, Cyclofem (25 mg medroxyprogesterone acetate and 5 mg estradiol cypionate) and Mesigyna (50 mg norethindrone enanthate and 5 mg estradiol valerate).

Mechanism of Action

The mechanism of action with Depo-Provera is different than the other lower-dose, progestin-only methods because, in addition to thickening of the cervical mucus and alteration of the endometrium, the circulating level of the progestin is high enough to effectively block the LH surge, and therefore, ovulation does not occur. Suppression of FSH is not as intense as with the combination oral contraceptive, therefore follicular growth is maintained sufficiently to produce estrogen levels comparable to those in the early follicular phase of a normal menstrual cycle.[4] Symptoms of estrogen deficiency, such as vaginal atrophy or a decrease in breast size, do not occur.

The injection should be given within the first 5 days of the current menstrual cycle, otherwise a back-up method is necessary for 2 weeks. The duration of action can be shortened if attention is not paid to proper administration. The injection must be given deeply in muscle by the Z-track technique and not massaged. It is prudent to avoid locations at risk for massage by daily activities.

Efficacy

The efficacy of this method is equal to that of sterilization. and better than that of all the other temporary methods.[5] Because serum concentrations are relatively high, efficacy is not influenced by weight or by the use of medications that stimulate hepatic enzymes. On the contrary, Depo-Provera is an excellent contraceptive choice for women taking antiepileptic drugs because the high progestin levels raise the seizure threshold.[6]

Advantages

Like other sustained release forms of contraception, this method is not associated with compliance problems and is not related to the coital event. Depo-Provera is useful for women whose ability to remember contraceptive requirements is limited. It should be considered for women who lead disorganized lives or who are mentally retarded.

The freedom from the side effects of estrogen allows Depo-Provera to be considered for patients with congenital heart disease, sickle cell anemia, patients with a previous history of thromboembolism, and women over 30 who smoke or have other risk factors. The absolute safety in regard to thrombosis is mainly theoretical; it has not been proven in a controlled study. However, an increased risk of thrombosis has not been observed in epidemiologic evaluation of Depo-Provera users.[3]

A further advantage in patients with sickle-cell disease is evidence indicating an inhibition of in vivo sickling with hematologic improvement during treatment.[7]

Another advantage is the finding that Depo-Provera increases the quantity of milk in nursing mothers, a direct contrast to the effect seen with combination oral contraception. The concentration of the drug in the breast milk is very small, and no effects of the drug on infant growth and development have been observed.[8–10]

As noted, Depo-Provera should be considered in patients with seizure disorders; an improvement in seizure control can be achieved probably because of the sedative properties of progestins.[6]

Other benefits associated with Depo-Provera use include a decreased risk of endometrial cancer,[11] and probably the same benefits associated with the progestin impact of oral contraceptives: reduced menstrual flow and anemia, less PID, less endometriosis, fewer uterine fibroids, and fewer ectopic pregnancies. A failure to document a reduced risk of ovarian cancer by the World Health Organization probably reflects the study's low statistical power and the high parity in the Depo-Provera users.[12]

Depo-Provera, like oral contraception, may reduce the risk of pelvic inflammatory disease; however, the only study was hampered by small numbers.[13] Suppression of ovulation means that ectopic pregnancies are abolished and ovarian cysts are rare.

Summary of Advantages

1. Easy to use, no daily or coital action required.
2. Safe, no serious health effects.
3. Very effective, as effective as sterilization and intrauterine and implant contraception.
4. Free from estrogen-related problems.
5. Private, use not detectable.
6. Enhances lactation.
7. Has noncontraceptive benefits.

Problems with Depo-Provera

Major problems with Depo-Provera are irregular menstrual bleeding, breast tenderness, weight gain, and depression.[2,3] By far the most common problem is the change in menstrual bleeding. Up to 25% of patients discontinue in the first year because of irregular bleeding.[14] The bleeding is rarely heavy; in fact, hemoglobin values rise in Depo-Provera users. The incidence of irregular bleeding is 70% in the first year, and 10% thereafter. Bleeding and spotting decrease progressively with each re-injection so that after 5 years, 80% of users are amenorrheic (compared to 10% of Norplant users).[15]

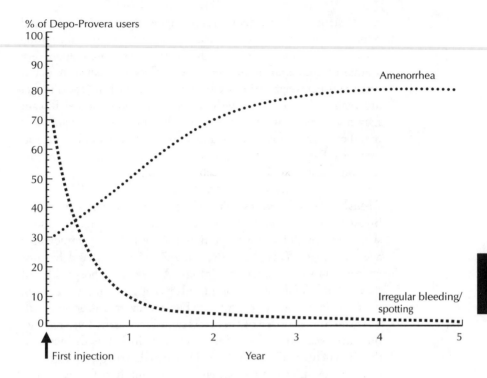

% of Depo-Provera users

Amenorrhea

Irregular bleeding/
spotting

First injection

Year

179

If necessary, the bleeding can be treated with exogenous estrogen, 1.25 mg conjugated estrogens, or 2 mg estradiol, given daily for 7 days. A nonsteroidal anti-inflammatory product given for a week is also effective. Giving the Depo-Provera injection earlier (more frequently) does not change the bleeding pattern.[16] Most women can wait for amenorrhea without treatment if they know what to expect with time.

About half of women who discontinue Depo-Provera can expect normal menses to return in 6 months after the last injection, but 25% will wait a year before resumption of a normal pattern.[15]

In a large international study, the most common medical reasons for discontinuing Depo-Provera during the first two years of use were:[3]

1. Headaches   —   2.3%
2. Weight gain   —   2.1%
3. Dizziness   —   1.2%
4. Abdominal pain   —   1.1%
5. Anxiety   —   0.7%

In Western societies, depression, fatigue, decreased libido, and hypertension are also encountered. Whether medroxyprogesterone acetate causes these side effects is difficult to know since they are very common complaints in nonusers as well.[17] Even attempts to document a greater weight gain specifically associated with Depo-Provera are unable to do so.[18,19] As with oral contraception, the weight gain may not be hormone-induced, but reflect lifestyle and aging. Remember if symptoms are truly due to the progestin, unlike pills and implants, Depo-Provera takes 6–8 months to be gone after the last injection. Clearance is slower in heavier women.

Breast Cancer. This progestin, in large continuous doses, produced breast tumors in beagle dogs (perhaps because in dogs progestins stimulate growth hormone secretion, known to be a mammotropic agent in dogs). This is an effect unique with dogs, and has not appeared in women after years of use. A very large, hospital-based case-control WHO study conducted over 9 years in 3 developing countries indicated that exposure to Depo-Provera is associated with a very slightly increased risk in breast cancer in the first 4 years of use, but there was no evidence for an increase in risk with increased duration of use.[20] The results were interpreted to suggest that growth of already existing tumors is enhanced. The number of cases was not large, and the confidence intervals reflected this.

Two earlier population-based case-control studies indicated a possible association between breast cancer and Depo-Provera. One, from Costa Rica, was based on only 19 cases.[21] The other, from New Zealand, did not find an increased relative risk in ever-users but did find an indication of increased risk shortly after initiating use at an early age, less than age 25.[22] A pooled analysis of the WHO and New Zealand data indicated that the highest risk was in women who had received a single injection.[23] The risk, if real, is very slight, and it is equally possible that the suggestions of increased risk based on a small number of cases have not been free of confounding variables. Because recent use appears to be the key factor, it is appropriate to emphasize that these studies did not find evidence for an overall increased risk of breast cancer, and the risk did not increase with duration of use. However, clinicians should consider informing patients that Depo-Provera might accelerate the growth of an already present occult cancer.

Other Cancers. An increased risk of cervical dysplasia cannot be documented even with long-term use (4 or more years).[24] The WHO study has not detected an increased risk of invasive squamous cell cancer of the cervix in Depo-Provera users; however, the risk of cervical carcinoma *in situ* was slightly elevated in the WHO case-control study, and it is not certain whether this is a real finding or a consequence of unrecognized biases.[25,26] In New Zealand, a modest increase in the risk of cervical dysplasia among users of Depo-Provera could be attributed to an increased prevalence of known risk factors for dysplasia among women who choose this method of contraception.[24] Nevertheless, it is prudent to insist on annual Pap smear surveillance in all users of contraception, no matter what method. Women at higher risk because of their sexual behavior (multiple partners, history of STDs) should have Pap smears every 6 months.

As noted, Depo-Provera is associated with a reduction in the risk of endometrial cancer, and there is probably a modest reduction in the risk of ovarian cancer.

There is no evidence that liver cancer risk is changed by the use of Depo-Provera.[27]

Metabolic Effects. The impact of Depo-Provera on the lipoprotein profile is uncertain. While some fail to detect an adverse impact, and claim that this is due to the avoidance of a first pass through effect in the liver,[28] others have demonstrated a decrease in HDL-cholesterol and increases in total cholesterol and LDL-cholesterol.[29,30] In a multicenter clinical trial by the World Health Organization, a transient adverse impact was present only in the few weeks after injection when blood levels were high.[31] The clinical impact of these changes, if any, have yet to be reported. It seems prudent to monitor the lipid profile annually in women using Depo-Provera for long durations. The emergence of significant adverse changes in LDL-cholesterol and HDL-cholesterol warrant reconsideration of contraceptive choice.

There are no clinically significant changes in carbohydrate metabolism or in coagulation factors.[29,32]

There is some concern that the blood levels of estrogen with this method of contraception are relatively lower over a period of time compared to a normal menstrual cycle, and therefore patients can lose bone to some degree.[33] Another possible mechanism is displacement of cortisol by the progestin from its binding globulin in the circulation, resulting in elevated levels of free cortisol. It is unlikely that this bone loss is sufficient to raise the risk of osteoporosis later in life. Furthermore, bone density measurements in women who stopped using Depo-Provera indicated that the loss is regained even after long-term use.[34] This concern will require on-going surveillance, especially of past users, but at the present time, this should not be a reason to avoid this method of contraception.

Effect on Future Fertility

The delay in becoming pregnant after ceasing use of Depo-Provera is a problem unique to injectable contraception; all the other temporary methods allow a more prompt return to fertility.[35] However, medroxyprogesterone acetate does not permanently suppress ovarian function, and the concern that infertility with suppressed menstrual function may be caused by Depo-Provera has not been supported by epidemiologic data. The pregnancy rate in women discontinuing the injections because of a desire to become pregnant is normal.[36] By 18 months after the last injection, 90% of Depo-Provera users have become pregnant, the same proportion as for other methods.[37] The delay to conception is about 9 months after the last injection, and the delay does not increase with increasing duration of use. Because of this delay, women who want to conceive promptly after discontinuing their contraceptive should not use Depo-Provera. Suppressed menstrual function persisting beyond 12 months after the last injection is not due to the drug and deserves evaluation.

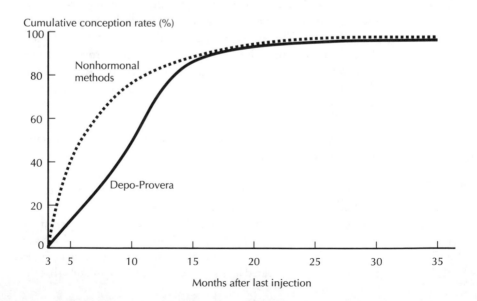

Accidental pregnancies occurring at the time of the initial injection of Depo-Provera have been reported to be associated with higher neonatal and infant mortality rates, probably due to an increased risk of intrauterine growth retardation.[38,39] The timing of the first injection is, therefore, very important. To ensure effective contraception, the first injection should be administered within the first 5 days of the menstrual cycle (before a dominant follicle emerges), or a back-up method is necessary for 2 weeks.

Summary of Disadvantages

1. Menstrual irregularities.
2. Weight gain, mood changes.
3. Can't be removed.
4. Return to fertility is delayed.
5. Regular injections required.
6. No STD or HIV protection.

Counseling Women About Depo-Provera

The greater the number of choices women have, the more likely they are to find a contraceptive that works well for them. For some women the primary advantages of Depo-Provera are privacy and ease of use. No one but the user need know about the injection, and the 3-month schedule can be easy to maintain for women who don't mind injections. In some societies injections are respected as efficacious; in these situations, Depo-Provera is the most popular contraceptive despite bleeding changes and other side effects.

Indications

1. At least one year of birth spacing desired.
2. Highly effective long-acting contraception not linked to coitus.
3. Estrogen-free contraception needed.
4. Breastfeeding.
5. Sickle cell disease.
6. Seizure disorder.
7. Private, coitally-independent method desired.

Absolute Contraindications

1. Pregnancy.
2. Unexplained genital bleeding.

Relative Contraindications

1. Liver disease.
2. Breast cancer.
3. Severe cardiovascular disease.
4. Rapid return to fertility desired.
5. Difficulty with injections.
6. Severe depression.

Norethindrone Enanthate

Norethindrone enanthate is given in a dose of 200 mg intramuscularly every 2 months. This progestin acts in the same way as Depo-Provera, and has the same problems.[3] A combination (Mesigyna) of norethindrone enanthate (50 mg) with estradiol valerate (5 mg) given monthly provides effective contraception with good cycle control.[40] Compared to Cyclofem (25 mg medroxyprogesterone acetate and 5 mg estradiol cypionate), Mesigyna has less bleeding problems.[41]

New Developments in Injectable Contraception

It is unlikely that the other depot injectables in use in other countries will become available in the U.S. More probable is the eventual introduction of sustained release injectables that provide lower, more stable levels of contraceptive progestins than Depo-Provera.

Microspheres or microcapsules have been studied for several years.[42,43] They consist of a biodegradable copolymer and one or more hormones. Like other injectable contraceptives, they are easy to administer and are highly effective. Unlike implants, injectables do not require surgical skills of the clinician and can be discontinued by the patient simply by declining to have another injection. Unlike implants, the microspheres cannot be removed once they are injected. If a woman experiences side effects or becomes pregnant, the hormone will remain in the body until completely metabolized. For this reason, the duration of action of the norethindrone capsules has been limited to a few months.

The carrier of the microsphere is composed of a polymer commonly used in biodegradable suture, poly-dl-lactide-co-glycolide. The size of the microspheres varies from 0.06 to 0.1 mm in diameter, and each is composed of about 50% norethindrone dispersed within the polymer. The release of norethindrone occurs initially by diffusion and later by degradation of the carrier. The size of the microspheres, the amount of hormone contained within the carrier, and the quantity of microspheres delivered by injection determine the daily dose of norethindrone delivered. Injections currently under evaluation contain a total dose of either 65 mg or 100 mg norethindrone, and the amount released daily is approximately the same as that delivered by low-dose oral contraception, but circulating levels are more stable.

The microspheres come preloaded in a syringe and are put into suspension with the addition of 2.5 mL of dextran diluent and vigorously agitated. The mixture must be shaken until all of the microspheres are in suspension, and again immediately prior to injection. The microspheres are deposited in the gluteal muscle using a 21-gauge needle and Z-track intramuscular injection technique.

As with other progestin-only methods of contraception, menstrual changes occur and are the most common cause of discontinuation during the first year of use. Users may experience amenorrhea or persistent or irregular spotting or bleeding. In contrast to Depo-Provera, hormone levels decline rapidly after the microspheres have degraded, so that contraceptive effectiveness ends promptly at the predicted time. Most users will resume ovulatory cycles within 2–3 months after the predicted duration of the injection. If pregnancy occurs shortly after expiration of the norethindrone microspheres, the fetus will not be exposed to significant levels of norethindrone.

Microsphere preparations containing norethindrone combined with ethinyl estradiol are also under development. It is hoped that the addition of estrogen at a low dose will lead to fewer menstrual irregularities.

References

1. **Rosenfield A, Maine D, Rochat R, Shelton J, Hatcher RA,** The Food and Drug Administration and medroxyprogesterone acetate: what are the issues? JAMA 249:2922, 1983.

2. **WHO,** A multicentered phase III comparative clinical trial of depot-medroxyprogesterone acetate given three-monthly at doses of 100 mg or 150 mg: I. Contraceptive efficacy and side effects, Contraception 34:223, 1986.

3. **WHO,** Multinational comparative clinical evaluation of two long-acting injectable contraceptive steroids: norethisterone enanthate and medroxyprogesterone acetate. Final report, Contraception 28:1, 1983.

4. **Fraser IS, Weisberg EA,** A comprehensive review of injectable contaception with special emphasis on depot medroxyprogesterone acetate, Med J Aust 1(Suppl):3, 1981.

5. **Harlap S, Kost K, Forrest DJ,** *Preventing Pregnancy, Protecting Health: A New Look at Birth Control Choices in the United States,* The Alan Guttmacher Institute, New York, New York, 1991.

6. **Mattson RH, Cramer JA, Caldwell BV, Siconolfi BC,** Treatment of seizures with medroxyprogesterone acetate: preliminary report, Neurology 34:1255, 1984.

7. **DeCeular K, Gruber C, Hayes R, Serjeant GR,** Medroxyprogesterone acetate and homozygous sickle-cell disease, Lancet 2:229, 1982.

8. **Jimenez J, Ochoa M, Soler MP, Portales P,** Long-term follow-up of children breast-fed by mothers receiving depot-medroxyprogesterone acetate, Contraception 30:523, 1984.

9. **Zacharias S, Aguilena J, Assanzo JR, Zanatu J,** Effects of hormonal and non-hormonal contracepters on lactation and incidence of pregnancy, Contraception 33:203, 1986.

10. **Pardthaisong T, Yenchit C, Gray R,** The long-term growth and development of children exposed to Depo-Provera during pregnancy or lactation, Contraception 45:313, 1992.

11. **WHO, Collaborative Study of Neoplasia and Steroid Contraceptives,** Depot-medroxyprogesterone acetate (DMPA) and risk of endometrial cancer, Int J Cancer 49:186, 1991.

12. **WHO, Collaborative Study of Neoplasia and Steroid Contraceptives,** Depot-medroxyprogesterone acetate (DMPA) and risk of epithelial ovarian cancer, Int J Cancer 49:191, 1991.

13. **Gray RH,** Reduced risk of pelvic inflammatory disease with injectable contraceptives, Lancet 1:1046, 1985.

14. **Cromer BA, Smith RD, Blair JM, Dwyer J, Brown R,** A prospective study of adolescents who choose among levonorgestrel implant (Norplant), medroxyprogesteorne acetate (Depo-Provera), or the combined oral contraceptive pill as contraception, Pediatrics 94:687, 1994.

15. **Gardner JM, Mishell DR Jr,** Analysis of bleeding patterns and resumption of fertility following discontinuation of a long-acting injectable contraceptive, Fertil Steril 21:286, 1970.

16. **Harel Z, Biro FM, Kollar LM,** Depo-Provera in adolescents: effects of early second injection or prior oral contraception, J Adolesc Health 16:379, 1995.

17. **Westhoff C, Wieland D, Tiezzi L,** Depression in users of depo-medroxyprogesterone acetate, Contraception 51:351, 1995.

18. **Moore LL, Valuck R, McDougall C, Fink W,** A comparative study of one-year weight gain among users of medroxyprogesterone acetate, levonorgestrel implants, and oral contraceptives, Contraception 52:215, 1995.

19. **Mainwaring R, Hales HA, Stevenson K, Hatasaka HH, Poulson AM, Jones KP, Peterson CM,** Metabolic parameters, bleeding, and weight changes in U.S. women using progestin only contraceptives, Contraception 51:149, 1995.

20. **WHO Collaborative Study of Neoplasia and Steroid Contraceptives,** Breast cancer and depot-medroxyprogesterone acetate: a multinational study, Lancet 338:833, 1991.

21. **Lee NC, Rosero-Bixby L, Oberle MW, Grimaldo C, Whatley AS, Rovira EZ,** A case-control study of breast cancer and hormonal contraception in Costa Rica, J Natl Cancer Inst 79:1247, 1987.

22. **Paul C, Skegg DCG, Spears GFS,** Depot medroxyprogesterone (Depo-Provera) and risk of breast cancer, Br Med J 299:759, 1989.

23. **Skegg DCG, Noonan EA, Paul C, Spears GFS, Meirik O, Thomas DB,** Depot medroxyprogesterone acetate and breast cancer: a pooled analysis of the World Health Organization and New Zealand studies, JAMA 273:799, 1995.

24. **The New Zealand Contraception and Health Study Group,** History of long-term use of depot-medroxyprogesterone acetate in patients with cervical dysplasia; case-control analysis nested in a cohort study, Contraception 50:443, 1994.

25. **WHO Collaborative Study of Neopolasia and Steroid Contraception,** Depot-medroxyprogesterone acetate (DMPA) and risk of invasive squamous cell cervical cancer, Contraception 45:299, 1992.

26. **Thomas DB, Ye Z, Ray RM, and the WHO Collaborative Study of Neoplasia and Steroid Contraception,** Cervical carcinoma *in situ* and use of depot-medroxyprogesterone aceate (DMPA), Contraception 51:25, 1995.

187

27. **WHO,** Depo-medroxyprogesterone acetate (DMPA) and cancer; memorandum from a WHO meeting, Bull World Health Organization 64:375, 1986.

28. **Garza-Flores J, De la Cruz DL, Valles de Bourges V, Sanchez-Nuncio R, Martinez M, Fuziwara JL, Perez-Palacios G,** Long-term effects of depot-medroxyprogesterone acetate on lipoprotein metabolism, Contraception 44:61, 1991.

29. **Fahmy K, Khairy M, Allam G, Gobran F, Allush M,** Effect of depo-medroxyprogesterone acetate on coagulation factors and serum lipids in Egyptian women, Contraception 44:431, 1991.

30. **Enk L, Landgren BM, Lindberg U-B, Silverstolpe G, Crona N,** A prospective, one-year study on the effects of two long acting injectable contraceptives (depot-medroxyprogesterone acetate and norethisterone enanthate) on serum and lipoprotein lipids, Horm Metab Res 24:85, 1992.

31. **WHO,** A multicentre comparative study of serum lipids and apolipoproteins in long-term users of DMPA and a control group of IUD users, Contraception 47:177, 1993.

32. **Fahmy K, Abdel-Razik M, Shaaraway M, Al-Kholy G, Saad S, Wagdi A, Al-Azzony M,** Effect of long-acting progestagen-only injectable contraceptives on carbohydrate metabolism and its hormonal profile, Contraception 44:419, 1991.

33. **Cundy T, Evans M, Roberts H, Wattie D, Ames R, Reid IR,** Bone density in women receiving depot medroxyprogesterone acetate for contraception, Br Med J 303:13, 1991.

34. **Cundy T, Cornish J, Evans MC, Roberts H, Reid IR,** Recovery of bone density in women who stop using medroxyprogesterone acetate, Br Med J 308:247, 1994.

35. **Garza-Flores J, Cardenas S, Rodriguez V, Cravioto MC, Diaz-Sanchez V, Perez-Palacios G,** Return to ovulation following the use of long-acting injectable contraceptives: a comparative study, Contraception 31:361, 1985.

36. **Pardthaisong T,** Return of fertility after use of the injectable contraceptive Depo Provera: up-dated analysis, J Biosoc Sci 16:23, 1984.

37. **Schwallie P, Assenze J,** The effect of depo medroxyprogesterone acetate on pituitary and ovarian function, and the return of fertility following its discontinuation. A review, Contraception 10:181, 1974.

38. **Pardthaisong T, Gray RH,** In utero exposure to steroid contraceptives and outcome of pregnancy, Am J Epidemiol 134:795, 1991.

39. **Gray RH, Pardthaisong T,** In utero exposure to steroid contraceptives and survival during infancy, Am J Epidemiol 134:804, 1991.

40. **Kesseru Ev, Aydinlik S, Etchepareborda JJ,** Multicentered, phase III clinical trial of norethisteone enanthate 50 mg plus estradiol valerate 5 mg as a monthly injectable contraceptive; final three-year report, Contraception 50:329, 1994.

41. **Sang GW, Shao QX, Ge RS, Chen JK, Song S, Fang KJ, He ML, Luo SY, Chen SF, Chen XB, Li MX, Wu SC, Sun GL, Zhou HE, Zhang SF, Zhu LL, Ye BL, Zhang JH, Ma FL, Jiang BY, Zhou ZQ, Dong QH, Shenm HC, Liu YX, Shao JY, Wang SX, Ming HD, Zhu ZR, Cheng HZ, Chen SH, Yu HY, Zhang ZY, Qing YN, Wang XY, Hall PE, d'Arcangues C, Snow RC,** A multicentred phase III comparative clinical trial of Mesigyna, Cyclofem, and injectable no. 1 given monthly by intramuscular injection to Chinese women. I. Contraceptive efficacy and side effects, Contraception 51:167, 1995. II. The comparison of bleeding patterns, Contraception 51:185, 1995.

42. **Beck L, Pope V,** Long-acting injectable norethindrone contraceptive system: review of clinical studies, Res Front Fertil Reg 3:1, 1984.

43. **Grubb GS, Welch JD, Cole L, Goldsmith A, Rivera R,** A comparative evaluation of the safety and contraceptive effectiveness of 65 mg and 100 mg of 90-day norethindrone (NET) injectable microspheres: a multicenter study, Fertil Steril 51:803, 1989.

6

Intrauterine Contraception (The IUD)

INTRAUTERINE CONTRACEPTIVES are used by nearly 100 million women worldwide, but fewer than 1 million of these are American. The growing need for reversible contraception in the United States would be well served by increasing utilization of intrauterine contraception with the intrauterine device (the IUD). The efficacy of modern IUDs in actual use is superior to that of oral contraception. Problems with IUD use can be minimized to a very low rate of minor side effects with careful screening and technique. We hope that American clinicians and patients will "rediscover" this excellent method of contraception.

History

A frequently told, but not well-documented story, assigns the first use of IUDs to caravan drivers who allegedly used intrauterine stones to prevent pregnancies in their camels during long journeys.

The forerunners of the modern IUD were small stem pessaries used in the 1800s, small button-like structures which covered the opening of the cervix and which were attached to stems extending into the cervical canal.[1] It is not certain these pessaries were used for contraception, but this seems to have been intended. In 1902, a pessary which extended into the uterus was developed by Hollweg in Germany and used for contraception. This pessary was sold for self-insertion, but the hazard of infection was great, earning the condemnation of the medical community.

191

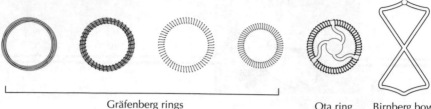

Gräfenberg rings   Ota ring   Birnberg bow

In 1909, Richter in Germany, reported success with a silkworm catgut ring having a nickle and bronze wire protruding through the cervix.[2] Shortly after, Pust combined Richter's ring with the old button-type pessary, and replaced the wire with a catgut thread.[3] This IUD was used during World War I in Germany, although the German literature was quick to report infections with its insertion and use. In the 1920s, Gräfenberg removed the tail and pessary because he believed this was the cause of infection. He reported his experience in 1930, using rings made of coiled silver and gold, then steel.[4]

The Gräfenberg ring was short-lived, falling victim to Nazi political philosophy which was bitterly opposed to contraception. The non-Aryan Gräfenberg was finally sent to jail, but he managed to flee Germany, dying in New York City in 1955. He never received the recognition which was his just due.

The Gräfenberg ring was associated with a high rate of expulsion. This was solved by Ota in Japan who added a supportive structure to the center of his gold or silver plated ring in 1934.[5] Ota also fell victim to World War II politics, being sent into exile, but his ring continued to be used.

The Gräfenberg and Ota rings were essentially forgotten by the rest of the world throughout the World War II period. An awareness of the explosion in population and its impact began to grow in the first two decades after World War II. In 1959, reports from Japan and Israel by Ishihama and Oppenheimer once again stirred interest in the rings.[6,7] The Oppenheimer report was in the American Journal of Obstetrics and Gynecology, and several American gynecologists were stimulated to use rings of silver or silk, and others to develop their own devices.

In the 1960s and 1970s, the IUD thrived. Techniques were modified and a plethora of types introduced. The various devices developed in the 1960s were made of plastic (polyethylene) impregnated with barium sulfate so that they would be visible on an x-ray. The Margulies Coil, developed by Lazer Margulies, in 1960, at Mt. Sinai Hospital in New York City, was the first plastic device with a memory, allowing the use of an inserter and reconfiguration of the shape when it was expelled into the uterus. The Coil was a large device (sure to cause cramping and bleeding) and its hard plastic tail proved risky for the male partner.

In 1962, the Population Council, at the suggestion of Alan Guttmacher, who that year became president of the Planned Parenthood Federation of America, organized the first international conference on IUDs in New York City. It was at this conference that Jack Lippes of Buffalo presented experience with his device, which fortunately as we will see, had a single filament thread as a tail. The Margulies Coil was rapidly replaced by the Lippes Loop, which quickly became the most widely prescribed IUD in the United States in the 1970s.

The 1962 conference also led to the organization of a program established by the Population Council, under the direction of Christopher Tietze, to evaluate IUDs, the Cooperative Statistical Program. The Ninth Progress Report in 1970 was a landmark comparison of efficacy and problems with the various IUDs being used.[8]

Many other devices came along, but with the exception of the four sizes of Lippes Loops and the two Saf-T-Coils, they had limited use. Stainless steel devices incorporating springs were designed to compress for easy insertion, but the movement of these devices allowed them to embed in the uterus, making them too difficult to remove. The Majzlin Spring is a memorable example.

The Dalkon Shield was introduced in 1970. Within 3 years, a high incidence of pelvic infection was recognized. There is no doubt that the problems with the Dalkon Shield were due to defective construction, pointed out as early as 1975 by Tatum.[9] The multifilamented tail (hundreds of fibers enclosed in a plastic sheath) of the Dalkon Shield provided a pathway for bacteria to ascend protected from the barrier of cervical mucus.

Although sales were discontinued in 1975, a call for removal of all Dalkon Shields was not issued until the early 1980s. The large number of women with pelvic infections led to many lawsuits against the pharmaceutical company, ultimately causing its bankruptcy. Unfortunately, the Dalkon Shield problem tainted all IUDs and ever since, media and the public have inappropriately regarded all IUDs in a single, generic fashion.

About the time of the introduction of the Dalkon Shield, the U.S. Senate conducted hearings on the safety of oral contraception. Young women who were discouraged from using oral contraceptives following these hearings turned to IUDs, principally the Dalkon Shield which was promoted as suitable for nulliparous women. Changes in sexual behavior in the 1960s and 1970s, and failure to use protective contraception (condoms and oral contraceptives), led to an epidemic of sexually transmitted diseases (STDs) and pelvic inflammatory disease (PID) for which IUDs were held partially responsible.[10]

The first epidemiologic studies of the relationship between IUDs and PID used as controls women who depended on oral contraception or barrier methods, and who were, therefore, at reduced risk of PID compared to non-contraceptors and IUD users.[11,12] In addition these first studies failed to control for the characteristics of sexual behavior which are now accepted as risk factors for PID (multiple partners, early age at first intercourse, and increased frequency of intercourse).[13] The Dalkon Shield magnified the risk attributed to IUDs because its high failure rate in young women who were already at risk of STDs led to septic spontaneous abortions and, in some cases, death.[14] Reports of these events led the American public to regard all IUDs as dangerous, including those which, unlike the Dalkon Shield, had undergone extensive clinical trials and post-marketing surveillance.

The 1980s saw the decline of IUD use in the United States as manufacturers discontinued marketing in response to the burden of litigation. Despite the fact that most of the lawsuits against the copper devices were won by the manufacturer, the cost of the defense combined with declining use affected the financial return. It should be emphasized that this action was the result of corporate business decisions related to concerns for profit and liability, not for medical or scientific reasons. The number of women using the IUD in the U.S. decreased by two-thirds from 1981 to 1988, from 2.2 million to 0.7 million (7.1% to 2% of married couples).[15] Nevertheless, in the rest of the world, the IUD is the most widely used method of reversible contraception; currently, about 100 million women use the IUD.

Use of the IUD in the U.S. and the World in 1988 [15, 16]

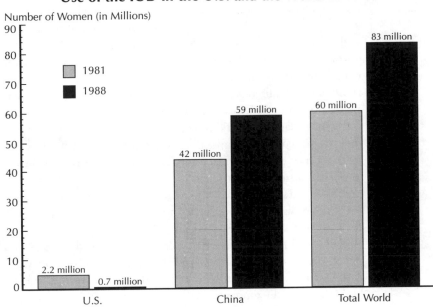

The reason for the decline in the U.S. is the consumer fear of IUD-related pelvic infection. The final blow to the IUD in the U.S. came in 1985 with the publication of two reports indicating that the use of IUDs was associated with tubal infertility.[17,18] Later, better controlled studies identified the Dalkon Shield as a high risk device, and failed to demonstrate an association between PID and other IUDs, except during the period shortly after insertion. Efforts to point out that the situation was different for the copper IUDs, and that in fact, pelvic inflammatory disease was not increased in women with a single sexual partner,[19] failed to prevent the withdrawal of IUDs from the American market and the negative reaction to IUDs by the American public.

Ironically, the IUD declined in the country which developed the modern IUD. It is time for a revival!

The Modern IUD

The addition of copper to the IUD was suggested by Jaime Zipper of Chile, whose experiments with metals indicated that copper acted locally on the endometrium.[20] Howard Tatum combined Zipper's suggestion with the development of the T-shape to diminish the uterine reaction to the structural frame, and produced the copper-T. The first copper IUD had copper wire wound around the straight shaft of the T, the TCu-200 (200 mm^2 of exposed copper wire), also known as the Tatum-T.[21] Tatum's reasoning was that the T-shape would conform to the shape of the uterus in contrast to the other IUDs which required the uterus to conform to their shape. Furthermore, the copper IUDs could be much smaller than those of simple, inert plastic devices and still provide effective contraception. Studies indicate that copper exerts its effect before implantation of a fertilized ovum; it may be spermicidal, or it may diminish sperm motility or fertilizing capacity. The addition of copper to the IUD and reduction in the size and structure of the frame improved tolerance, resulting in fewer removals for pain and bleeding.

The Cu-7 with a copper wound stem was developed in 1971 and quickly became the most popular device in the U.S. Both the Cu-7 and the Tatum-T were withdrawn from the U.S. market in 1986 by G. D. Searle and Company.

IUD development continued, however. More copper was added by Population Council investigators, leading to the TCu-380A (380 mm^2 of exposed copper surface area — copper wound around the stem plus a copper sleeve on each horizontal arm).[22] The "A" in TCu-380A is for arms, indicating the importance of the copper sleeves. Making the copper solid and tubular increased effectiveness and the lifespan of the IUD. It has been in use in more than 30 countries since 1982, and in 1988, it was marketed in the U.S. as the "ParaGard."

The "Progestasert" was developed by the Alza Corporation at the same time that the copper IUDs were developed. This T-shaped device releases 65 µg of progesterone per day for at least one year. The progesterone diminishes the amount of cramping and the amount of blood loss, thus it is especially useful for women who have heavy periods and cramping. The short lifespan can be and has been solved by using a more potent progestin, such as levonorgestrel.

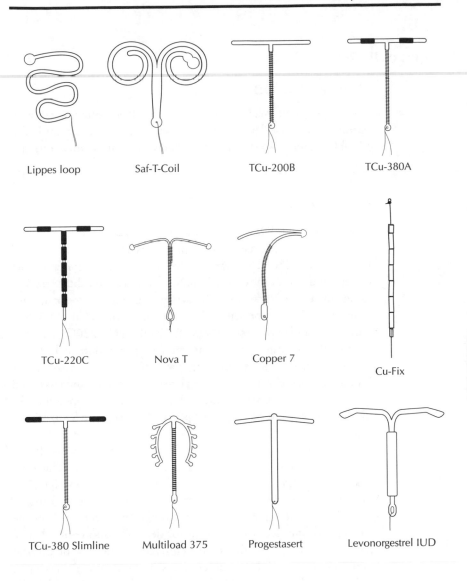

| Lippes loop | Saf-T-Coil | TCu-200B | TCu-380A |

| TCu-220C | Nova T | Copper 7 | Cu-Fix |

| TCu-380 Slimline | Multiload 375 | Progestasert | Levonorgestrel IUD |

197

Efforts continue to develop IUDs which address the main problems of bleeding and cramping. The IUDs of the future will possibly be medicated and frameless.

Types of IUDs

Unmedicated IUDs

The Lippes Loop, made of plastic (polyethylene) impregnated with barium sulfate, is still used throughout the world (except in the U.S.). Flexible stainless steel rings are widely used in China, but not elsewhere.[23]

Copper IUDs

The first copper IUDs were wound with 200 to 250 mm² of wire, and two of these are still available (except in the U.S.), the TCu-200 and the Multiload-250. The more modern copper IUDs contain more copper, and part of the copper is in the form of solid tubular sleeves, rather than wire, increasing efficacy and extending lifespan. This group of IUDs is represented in the U.S. by the TCu-380A (the ParaGard), and in the rest of the world, by the TCu-220C, the Nova T, and the Multiload-375. The modern generation of IUDs in China includes a stainless steel ring with copper wire that also releases indomethacin (very effective with a low expulsion rate and less blood loss), a V-shaped copper IUD, and a copper IUD shaped like the uterine cavity.[23] The Sof-T is a copper IUD used only in Switzerland.

The TCu-380A is a T-shaped device with a polyethylene frame holding 380 mm² of exposed surface area of copper. The pure electrolytic copper wire wound around the 36 mm stem weighs 176 mg, and copper sleeves on the horizontal arms weigh 66.5 mg. A polyethylene monofilament is tied through the 3 mm ball on the stem, providing two white threads for detection and removal. The ball at the bottom of the stem helps reduce the risk of cervical perforation. The IUD frame contains barium sulfate, making it radiopaque. The TCu-380Ag is identical to the TCu-380A, but the copper wire on the stem has a silver core to prevent fragmentation and extend the lifespan of the copper. The TCu-380 Slimline has the copper sleeves flush at the ends of the horizontal arms to facilitate easier loading and insertion. The performance of the TCu-380Ag and the TCu-380 Slimline is equal to that of the TCu-380A.[24,25]

The Multiload-375 has 375 mm² of copper wire wound around its stem. The flexible arms were designed to minimize expulsions. This is a popular device in many parts of the world. The Multiload-375 and the TCu-380A are similar in their efficacy and performance.[26]

The Nova T is similar to the TCu-200, containing 200 mm² of copper; however, the Nova T has a silver core to the copper wire, flexible arms, and a large, flexible loop at the bottom to avoid injury to cervical tissue. There is some concern that the efficacy of the Nova T decreased after 3 years in WHO data; however, results from Finland and Scandinavia indicate low and stable pregnancy rates over 5 years of use.[26]

Hormone-Releasing IUDs

The only hormone-releasing device marketed in the U.S. (since 1976) is the Progestasert. The Progestasert is a T-shaped IUD made of ethylene/vinyl acetate copolymer containing titanium dioxide. The vertical stem contains a reservoir of 38 mg progesterone together with barium sulfate dispersed in silicone fluid. The horizontal arms are solid and made of the same copolymer. Two blue-black, monofiliment strings are attached at a hole in the base of the stem. Progesterone is released at a rate of 65 µg per day.

The LNG-20, manufactured by Leiras in Finland, releases *in vitro* 20 µg of levonorgestrel per day. It has been marketed in Europe.[27] This T-shaped device has a collar attached to the vertical arm, which contains 52 mg levonorgestrel dispersed in polydimethylsiloxane and released at a rate of 15 µg per day *in vivo*. The levonorgestrel IUD lasts up to 10 years and reduces menstrual blood loss and pelvic infection rates.[28-30]

Future IUDs

Modifications of the copper IUD are being studied throughout the world. The Ombrelle-250 and Ombrelle-380, designed to be more flexible in order to reduce expulsion and side effects, have been marketed in France. A frameless IUD, the FlexiGard (also known as the Cu-Fix), consists of 6 copper sleeves (330 mm² of copper) strung on a surgical nylon (polypropylene) thread which is knotted at one end. The knot is pushed into the myometrium during insertion with a notched needle which works like a miniature harpoon. Because it is frameless, it is expected to have low rates of removal for bleeding or pain, but because insertion is more difficult, there is a higher expulsion rate.[31]

Mechanism of Action

The contraceptive action of all IUDs is mainly in the uterine cavity. Ovulation is not affected, nor is the IUD an abortifacient.[32,33] It is currently believed that the mechanism of action for IUDs is the production of an intrauterine environment that is spermicidal.

Nonmedicated IUDs depend for contraception upon the general reaction of the uterus to a foreign body. It is believed that this reaction, a sterile inflammatory response, produces tissue injury of a minor degree, but sufficient enough to be spermicidal. Very few, if any, sperm reach the ovum in the fallopian tube. Normally cleaving, fertilized ova cannot be obtained by tubal flushing in women with IUDs in contrast to noncontraceptors, indicating the failure of sperm to reach the ovum, and thus fertilization does not occur.[34] If this action should fail, the inflammatory response would also prevent implantation. In women using copper IUDs, sensitive assays for human chorionic gonadotropin (HCG) do not find evidence of fertilization.[35,36] This is consistent with the fact that the copper IUD protects against both intrauterine and ectopic pregnancies (see below).

The copper IUD releases free copper and copper salts which have both a biochemical and morphological impact on the endometrium, and also produce alterations in cervical mucus and endometrial secretions. There is no measurable increase in the serum copper level. Copper has many specific actions, including the enhancement of prostaglandin production and the inhibition of various endometrial enzymes. The copper IUD is associated with an enhanced inflammatory response, marked by production in the endometrium of cytokine peptides known to be cytotoxic.[37] An additional spermicidal effect probably takes place in the cervical mucus.

The progestin-releasing IUDs add the endometrial action of the progestin to the foreign body reaction. The endometrium becomes decidualized with atrophy of the glands. The progesterone IUD (serum progesterone levels are not increased) probably has two mechanisms of action: inhibition of implantation and inhibition of sperm capacitation and survival. The levonorgestrel IUD produces serum concentrations of the progestin about half those of Norplant so that ovarian follicular development and ovulation are only partially inhibited. Finally, the progestin IUDs thicken the cervical mucus, creating a barrier to sperm penetration. The progestin IUDs decrease menstrual blood loss (about 40–50%) and dysmenorrhea; with the levonorgestrel IUD, bleeding can be reduced by 90% one year after insertion.[38] Average hemoglobin and iron levels increase over time compared to preinsertion values.

Following removal of IUDs, the normal intrauterine environment is rapidly restored. In large studies, there is no delay, regardless of duration of use, in achieving pregnancy at normal rates, which belies the assertion that IUD use is associated with infection leading to infertility.[39–42] There has been no significant difference in cumulative pregnancy rates between parous and nulliparous or nulligravid women.[41,42]

Efficacy of IUDs

Intrauterine Pregnancy

The TCu-380A is approved for use in the United States for 10 years. The TCu-200 is approved for 4 years and the Nova T for 5 years. The progesterone-releasing IUD must be replaced every year because the reservoir of progesterone is depleted in 12–18 months. The levonorgestrel IUD can be used for at least 7 years, and probably 10.[26] The progesterone IUD has a slightly higher failure rate, but the levonorgestrel device that releases 15–20 μg levonorgestrel per day is as effective as the new copper IUDs.[24,28,43,44]

The nonmedicated IUDs never have to be replaced. The deposition of calcium salts on the IUD can produce a structure which is irritating to the endometrium. If bleeding increases after a nonmedicated IUD has been in place for some time, it is worth replacing it. Some clinicians (as do we) recommend replacing all older IUDs with the new, more effective copper IUDs.

First Year Clinical Trial Experience in Parous Women [45]

Device	Pregnancy Rate	Expulsion Rate	Removal Rate
Lippes Loop	3%	12–20%	12–15%
Cu–7	2–3	6	11
TCu–200	3	8	11
TCu–380A	0.5–0.8	5	14
Progesterone IUD	1.3–1.6	2.7	9.3
Levonorgestrel IUD	0.2	6	17

Considering all IUDS together, the actual use failure rate in the first year is approximately 3%, with a 10% expulsion rate, and a 15% rate of removal, mainly for bleeding and pain. With increasing duration of use and increasing age, the failure rate decreases, as do removals for pain and bleeding. The performance of the TCu-380A in recent years, however, has proved to be superior.

Ten-Year Experience with ParaGard, TCu-380A
Rate per 100 users per year

| | \multicolumn{10}{c}{Year} | | | | | | | | | |
	1	2	3	4	5	6	7	8	9	10
Pregnancy	0.7	0.3	0.6	0.2	0.3	0.2	0.0	0.4	0.0	0.0
Expulsion	5.7	2.5	1.6	1.2	0.3	0.0	0.6	1.7	0.2	0.4
Bleeding/ Pain removal	11.9	9.8	7.0	3.5	3.7	2.7	3.0	2.5	2.2	3.7
Medical removals	2.5	2.1	1.6	1.7	0.1	0.3	1.0	0.4	0.7	0.3
Continuation	76.8	78.3	81.2	86.2	89.0	91.9	87.9	88.1	92.0	91.8
Number starting each year	4932	3149	2018	1121	872	621	563	483	423	325

Data from Population Council (n = 3536) and WHO (n = 1396) trials.

203

In careful studies, with attention to technique and participation by motivated patients, the failure rate with the TCu-380A and the other newer copper IUDs is less than one per 100 women per year.[26,45,46] The cumulative net pregnancy rate after 7 years of use is 1.5 per 100 woman-years.[47] In developing countries, the failure rate with IUDs is less than that with oral contraception.[48] Failure rates are slightly higher in younger (less than age 25), more fertile women.

Women use IUDs longer than other reversible methods of contraception. The IUD continuation rate is higher than that with oral contraception, condoms, or diaphragms. This may reflect the circumstances surrounding the choice of an IUD (older, parous women).

Expulsion

Approximately 5% of patients spontaneously expel the TCu-380A within the first year. This event can be associated with cramping, vaginal discharge, or uterine bleeding. However, in some cases, the only observable change is lengthening or absence of the IUD strings. Patients should be cautioned to request immediate attention if expulsion is suspected. A partially expelled IUD should be removed.

If pregnancy or infection is not present, a new IUD can be inserted immediately (in this instance, antibiotic prophylaxis is recommended).

Ectopic Pregnancy

The previous use of an IUD does not increase the risk of a subsequent ectopic pregnancy.[41,49,50] The current use of an IUD, other than the progesterone-releasing device, offers some protection against ectopic pregnancy.[49-54] The largest study, a WHO multicenter study, concluded that IUD users were 50% less likely to have an ectopic pregnancy when compared to women using no contraception.[49] This protection is not as great as that achieved by inhibition of ovulation with oral contraception. Therefore, when an IUD user becomes pregnant, the pregnancy is more likely to be ectopic. However, the actual occurrence of an ectopic pregnancy in an IUD user is a rare event.

The lowest ectopic pregnancy rates are seen with the most effective IUDs, like the TCu-380A (90% less likely compared to noncontraceptors).[54] The rate is about one-tenth the ectopic pregnancy rate associated with the Lippes Loop or with devices with less copper such as the TCu-200.[54] The progesterone-releasing IUD has a higher rate, probably because its action is limited to a local effect on the endometrium,[52] while very few ectopic pregnancies have been reported with the levonorgestrel IUD, presumably because it is associated with a partial suppression of gonadotropins with subsequent disruption of normal follicular growth and development, and in a significant number of cycles (20–30%), inhibition of ovulation.[24,43,44,55,56]

The risk of ectopic pregnancy does not increase with increasing duration of use with the TCu-380A or the levonorgestrel IUD.[24,47] In a 7-year prospective study, not a single ectopic pregnancy was encountered with the levonorgestrel IUD.[24] In 8,000 woman-years of experience in randomized multicenter trials, there has been only a single ectopic pregnancy reported with the TCu-380A (which is one tenth the rate with the Lippes Loop or TCu-200).[24]

The protection against ectopic pregnancy provided by the TCu-380A and the levonorgestrel IUD makes these IUDs acceptable choices for contraception in women with previous ectopic pregnancies.

Ectopic Pregnancy Rates per 1,000 Woman-Years [54,57]

Non-contraceptive users	3.00–4.50
Progesterone IUD (based on small numbers, thus probably the same as non-contraceptive users)	6.80
Levonorgestrel IUD	0.20
TCu-380A IUD	0.20

Side Effects

With effective patient screening and good insertion technique, the copper and medicated IUDs are not associated with an increase risk of infertility after their removal. Even if IUDs are removed for problems, subsequent fertility rates are normal.[41,42,44]

The symptoms most often responsible for IUD discontinuation are increased uterine bleeding and increased menstrual pain. Within one year, 5–15% of women discontinue IUD use because of these problems. Smaller copper and progestin IUDs have reduced the incidence of pain and bleeding considerably, but a careful menstrual history is still important in helping a woman consider an IUD. Women with prolonged, heavy menstrual bleeding or significant dysmenorrhea may not be able to tolerate copper IUDs but may benefit from a progestin IUD.[38] Because bleeding and cramping are most severe in the first few months after IUD insertion, treatment with a nonsteroidal anti-inflammatory (NSAID) agent (an inhibitor of prostaglandin synthesis) during the first several menstrual periods can reduce bleeding and cramping and help a patient through this difficult time. Even persistent heavy menses can be effectively treated with NSAIDs.[58] NSAID treatment should begin at the onset of menses and be maintained for 3 days. It is not unusual to have a few days of intermenstrual spotting or light bleeding. Although aggravating, this does not cause significant blood loss. Such bleeding deserves the usual evaluation for cervical or endometrial pathology. These changes can be objectionable for women who are prevented from having intercourse while bleeding.

Following insertion of a modern copper IUD, menstrual blood loss increases by about 55%, and this level of bleeding continues for the duration of IUD use.[59] This is associated with a slight (1–2 day) prolongation of menstruation. Over a year's time, this amount of blood loss does not result in changes (e.g., serum ferritin) indicative of iron deficiency. Assessment for iron depletion and anemia should be considered, however, in long-term users and in women susceptible to iron deficiency anemia.

Because of a decidualizing, atrophic impact on the endometrium, amenorrhea can develop over time with the progestin-containing IUDs. With the levonorgestrel IUD, 70% of patients are oligomenorrheic and 30% amenorrheic within 2 years.[24] For some women, the lack of periods is so disconcerting that they request removal. On the other hand, this effect on menstruation is manifested by an increase in blood hemoglobin levels.[24,45] Sufficient progestin reaches the systemic circulation from the levonorgestrel-containing IUD so that androgenic side effects can occur such as acne and hirsutism. More extensive clinical studies are needed to assess the impact of this IUD on the lipoprotein profile; however, it is unlikely that the low dose of levonorgestrel has an important effect on cardiovascular risk.

Some women report an increased vaginal discharge while wearing an IUD. This complaint deserves examination for the presence of vaginal or cervical infection. Treatment can be provided with the IUD remaining in place.

Long-term use of the IUD is associated with impressive safety and lack of side effects. In a 7-year prospective study, the use of either the copper IUD or the levonorgestrel IUD beyond 5 years led to no increase in pelvic infection, no increase in ectopic pregnancy rates, no increase in anemia, and no increase in abnormal Pap smears.[24] Duration of use does not affect pregnancy rates or outcome.

The presence of copper may yield some benefits. There are epidemiologic data indicating that the copper IUD reduces the risks of endometrial cancer and invasive cervical cancer.[60–62] Presumably this protective effect is due to copper-induced biochemical alterations that affect cellular responses.

Infections

IUD-related bacterial infection is now believed to be due to contamination of the endometrial cavity at the time of insertion. Mishell's classic study indicated that the uterus is routinely contaminated by bacteria at insertion.[63] Infections that occur 3–4 months after insertion are believed to be due to acquired STDs, not the direct result of the IUD. The early, insertion-related infections, therefore, are polymicrobial, derived from the endogenous cervicovaginal flora, with a predominance of anaerobes.

A review of the World Health Organization data base derived from all of the WHO IUD clinical trials concluded that the risk of pelvic inflammatory disease was 6 times higher during the 20 days after the insertion compared to later times during follow-up, but, most importantly, PID was extremely rare beyond the first 20 days after insertion.[64] In nearly 23,000 insertions, however, only 81 cases of PID were diagnosed, and a scarcity of PID was observed in those situations where STDs are rare. There was no statistically significant difference comparing the copper IUD to the inert Lippes Loop or progestin-containing IUDs. These data confirm earlier studies that the risk of infection is highest immediately after insertion and that PID risk does not increase with long-term use.[14,19] The problem of infection can be minimized with careful screening and the use of aseptic technique. Even women with insulin-dependent diabetes mellitus do not have an increased risk for infection.[65,66]

Doxycycline (200 mg) or azithromycin (500 mg) administered orally one hour prior to insertion can provide protection against insertion-associated pelvic infection, but prophylactic antibiotics are probably of little benefit for women at low risk for STDs.

Compared with oral contraception, barrier methods, and hormonal IUDs, there is no reason to think that nonmedicated or copper IUDs can confer protection against STDs.[67] However, the levonorgestrel-releasing IUD has been reported to be associated with a protective effect against pelvic infection, and the copper IUD is associated with lower titers of anti-chlamydial antibody.[68,69] In vitro, copper inhibits chlamydial growth in endometrial cells.[70] Thus, the association between IUD use and pelvic infection (and infertility) is now seriously questioned.[71] Women who use IUDs must be counseled to employ condoms along with the IUD whenever they have intercourse with a partner who could be an STD carrier. Because sexual behavior is the most important modifier of the risk of infection, clinicians should ask prospective IUD users about numbers of partners, their partner's sexual practices, the frequency and age of onset of intercourse, and history of STDs.[72] Women at low risk are unlikely to have pelvic infections while using IUDs.[19]

It is not certain that the IUD is inappropriate for women who are at increased risk of bacterial endocarditis (previous endocarditis, rheumatic heart disease, or the presence of prosthetic heart valves). The bacteriologic contamination of the uterine cavity at insertion is short-lived.[63] Three studies have attempted to document bacteremia during IUD insertion or removal.[73-75] Only one of the three could find blood culture evidence of bacteremia, and it was present transiently in only a few patients.[75] In our view, the IUD is acceptable for patients at risk of bacterial endocarditis, *but antibiotic prophylaxis (amoxicillin 2 g) should be provided one hour before insertion or removal.*

Asymptomatic IUD users whose cervical cultures show gonorrheal or chlamydia infection should be treated with the recommended drugs without removal of the IUD. If, however, there is evidence that an infection has ascended to the endometrium or fallopian tubes, treatment must be instituted and the IUD removed promptly. Vaginal bacteriosis should be treated (metronidazole, 500 mg bid for 7 days), but the IUD need not be removed unless pelvic inflammation is present.

For simple endometritis, in which uterine tenderness is the only physical finding, doxycycline (100 mg bid for 14 days) is adequate. If tubal infection is present, as evidenced by cervical motion tenderness, abdominal rebound tenderness, adnexal tenderness or masses, or elevated white blood count and sedimentation rate, parenteral treatment is indicated with removal of the IUD as soon as antibiotic serum levels are adequate. The previous presence of an IUD does not alter the treatment of PID. IUD-associated pelvic infection is more likely to be caused by non-STD organisms.[76]

Appropriate outpatient management of less severe infections:

> Cefoxitin (2 g IM) plus probenecid (1 g orally), or
> Ceftriaxone (250 mg IM) plus doxycycline (100 mg bid orally), for 14 days.

Severe infections require hospitalization and treatment with:

Cefoxitin (2 g IV q 6 h), or
Cefotetan (2 g IV q 12 h)
Plus doxycycline (100 mg bid orally or IV)
Followed by 14 days of an oral regimen of antibiotics.

The following is an alternative regimen:

Clindamycin (900 mg IV q 8 h), plus
Gentamicin (2 mg/kg IV or IM followed by 1.5 mg/kg
    q 8 h).

There is a suggestion that IUD use increases the risk of HIV transmission from man to woman, especially when the IUD is inserted or removed during exposure to the infected man.[77,78] However, this is not a strong suggestion, because the risk with IUD use was ascertained compared to other contraceptive methods (which can protect against transmission) and the many and various influencing factors are difficult to adjust and control.

Actinomyces

The significance of actinomycosis infection in IUD users is unclear. There are several reports of IUD users with unilateral pelvic abscesses containing *Actinomyces*.[79,80] However, *Actinomyces* are found in Pap smears of up to 30% of plastic IUD wearers when cytologists take special care to look for the organisms. The rate is much lower (less than 1%) with copper devices and varies with duration of use.[79–82] Furthermore, *Actinomyces* are commonly present in the normal vagina.[83] The clinician must decide whether to remove the IUD and treat the patient, treat with the IUD in place, or simply remove the IUD. These patients are almost always asymptomatic and without clinical signs of infection. If uterine tenderness or a pelvic mass is present, the IUD should always be removed after the initiation of treatment with oral penicillin G, 500 mg qid that should continue for a month. If *Actinomyces* are present on the Pap smear of an asymptomatic well woman, in our view it is not necessary to administer antibiotic treatment or to remove the IUD. Although it has been recommended that the IUD should be removed in this instance and replaced when a repeat Pap smear is negative, there is no evidence to support this recommendation. Another anaerobic, gram-positive rod, *Eubacterium nodatum*, resembles *Actinomyces* and has also been reported to be associated with colonization of an IUD.[84] *E. nodatum* can be mistaken for *Actinomyces* on Pap smears. Our recommendations can be applied to both *E. nodatum* and *Actinomyces.*

Pregnancy with an IUD in situ

Spontaneous Abortion. Spontaneous abortion occurs more frequently among women who become pregnant with IUDs in place, a rate of approximately 40–50%. Because of this high rate of spontaneous abortion, IUDs should always be removed if pregnancy is diagnosed and the string is visible. Use of instruments inside the uterus should be avoided if the pregnancy is desired, unless sonographic guidance can help avoid rupture of the membranes.[85] After removal of an IUD with visible strings, the spontaneous abortion rate is approximately 30%.[86,87] Combining ultrasonography guidance with carbon dioxide hysteroscopy, an IUD with a missing tail can be identified and removed during early pregnancy.[88] *If the IUD is easily removed without trauma or expelled during the first trimester, the risk of spontaneous abortion is not increased.*[89,90]

Septic Abortion. In the past, if the IUD could not be easily removed, the patient was offered therapeutic abortion because it was believed that the risk of life-threatening septic, spontaneous abortion in the second trimester was increased 20-fold if the pregnancy continued with the IUD in utero. However, this belief was derived from experiences with the Dalkon Shield. There is no evidence that there is an increased risk of septic abortion if pregnancy occurs with an IUD in place other than the Shield.[90,91] There have been no deaths in the United States since 1977 among women pregnant with an IUD.[92]

If a patient plans to terminate a pregnancy which has occurred with an IUD in place, the IUD should be removed immediately. If there is no evidence of infection, the IUD can safely be removed in a clinic or office.

If an IUD is in an infected, pregnant uterus, removal of the device should be undertaken only after antibiotic therapy has been initiated, and equipment for cardiovascular support and resuscitation is immediately available. These precautions are necessary because removal of an IUD from an infected, pregnant uterus can lead to septic shock.

Congenital Anomalies. There is no evidence that exposure of a fetus to medicated IUDs is harmful. The risk of congenital anomalies is not increased among infants born to women who become pregnant with an IUD in place.[90,93] A case-control study did not find an increased incidence of IUD use in pregnancies resulting in limb reduction deformities.[94]

Preterm Labor and Birth. The incidence of preterm labor and delivery is increased approximately 4-fold when an IUD is left in place during pregnancy.[87,90,95–97]

Other Complications. Obstetrical complications at delivery (such as hemorrhage, stillbirth, and difficulties wth placenta removal) have been reported only with the Dalkon Shield *in situ.*

IUD Insertion

Patient Selection

Patient selection for successful IUD use requires attention to menstrual history and the risk for STDs. Age and parity are not the critical factors in selection; the risk factors for STDs are the most important consideration. Women who have multiple sexual partners, whose partners have multiple partners, who are drug or alcohol dependent, and who are not in a stable sexual relationship are at greater risk of pelvic infection at the time of IUD insertion and at greater risk of acquiring a sexually transmitted disease after IUD insertion.[17–19] It would be appropriate for these women to use condoms for STD protection and an IUD for effective contraception. Current, recent,or recurrent PID is a contraindication for IUD use. Hormonal and barrier methods are better choices for these women. Nulliparous and nulligravid women can safely use the IUD if both sexual partners are monogamous. In a national U.S. survey, only 13% of adults had more than one sexual partner in the previous year.[98] Most women are good candidates for the IUD.

Patients with heavy menstrual periods should be cautioned regarding the increase in menstrual bleeding associated with the copper IUD. Women who are anticoagulated or have a bleeding disorder are obviously not good candidates for the copper IUD, but might benefit from a progestin IUD.

There are other conditions which can compromise success. Women who have abnormalities of uterine anatomy (bicornuate uterus, submucous myoma, cervical stenosis) may not accommodate an IUD. The IUD is not a good choice when the uterine cavity is distorted by leiomyomata. According to conventional wisdom, the few individuals who have allergies to copper or have Wilson's disease (a prevalence of about 1 in 200,000) should not use copper IUDs; however, no cases of difficulty have ever been recorded and it is doubtful, considering the low exposure to copper, that there would be a problem. The amount of copper released into the circulation per day is less than that consumed in a normal diet.[99]

Immunosuppressed patients should not use IUDs. Patients at risk for endocarditis should be treated with prophylactic antibiotics at insertion and removal. In our view, cervical dysplasia does not preclude IUD insertion or continued use.

Because many older women have diabetes mellitus, it is worth emphasizing that no increase in adverse events has been observed with copper IUD use in women with either insulin-dependent or non-insulin-dependent diabetes.[65,66,100] Indeed, the IUD can be an ideal choice for a woman with diabetes, especially if vascular disease is present.

The IUD should not be dismissed just because the patient is an adolescent. Although the clinical performance of the IUD in a study of parous adolescents was not as good as in older women, it was still similar or slightly better than other reversible methods used by adolescents.[101] Given appropriate screening, counseling, and care, the IUD can provide long-term effective contraception for adolescents.

A careful speculum and bimanual examination is essential prior to IUD insertion. It is important to know the position of the uterus; undetected extreme posterior uterine position is the most common reason for perforation at the time of IUD insertion. However, perforation is rare; the incidence is estimated to be less than 1 per 3,000 insertions.[102] A very small or large uterus, determined by examination and sounding, can preclude insertion. For successful IUD use, the uterus should preferably not sound less than 6 cm or more than 9 cm.

Preferably, the absence of cervical or vaginal infection should be established before insertion. If this is not feasible, insertion should definitely be delayed if a mucopurulent discharge of the cervix or a significant vaginitis (including vaginal bacteriosis) is present.

Key Points in Patient Counseling

Prospective IUD users should be aware of the following important points:

1. Protection against unwanted pregnancy begins immediately after insertion.
2. Menses can be longer and heavier (except with hormonal IUDs); tampons can be used.
3. There is a slightly increased risk of pelvic infection in the first few months after insertion.
4. Protection against infections transmitted through the vaginal mucosa requires the use of condoms.
5. Ectopic pregnancies can still occur.
6. The IUD can be spontaneously expelled; monthly palpation of the IUD strings is important to avoid unwanted pregnancies. If the strings are not felt or something hard is palpable (suggestive of the IUD frame), a clinician should be notified as soon as possible. Backup contraception should be provided until the patient can be examined.

Summary: IUD Use and Medical Conditions

1. A woman with a previous ectopic pregnancy can use a copper IUD or the levonorgestrel IUD.
2. Women with heavy menses and dysmenorrhea, including women who have a bleeding disorder or are anticoagulated, should consider a progestin-releasing IUD.
3. Women at risk for bacterial endocarditis should receive prophylactic antibiotics at insertion and removal.
4. Current, recent, or recurrent PID is a contraindication for IUD use.
5. Women with diabetes mellitus, either insulin-dependent or non-insulin-dependent, can use IUDs.
6. IUD insertion is relatively easier in breastfeeding women, and the rates of expulsion and uterine perforation are not increased.

Timing

An IUD can be safely inserted at any time after delivery, abortion, or during the menstrual cycle. Expulsion rates were higher when the older, large plastic IUDs were inserted sooner than 8 weeks postpartum, however studies indicate that the copper IUDs can be inserted between 4 and 8 weeks postpartum without an increase in pregnancy rates, expulsion, uterine perforation, or removals for bleeding and/or pain.[103,104] Insertion can even occur immediately after a vaginal delivery; it is not associated with an increased risk of infection, uterine perforation, postpartum bleeding, or uterine subinvolution.[105] This is not recommended if intrauterine infection is present, and a slightly higher expulsion rate is to be expected compared to insertion 4–8 weeks postpartum. The IUD can also be inserted at cesarean section; the expulsion rate is slightly lower than that with insertion immediately after vaginal delivery.[106]

Insertion of an IUD in breastfeeding women is relatively easier, and is associated with a lower removal rate for bleeding or pain.[105] An early suggestion that uterine perforation is more common in lactating women has not been substantiated.[105,107]

An IUD can be inserted immediately after a first trimester abortion, but after a second trimester abortion, it is recommended to wait until uterine involution occurs.[108,109]

Insertions can be more difficult if the cervix is closed between menses. The advantages of insertion during or shortly after a menstrual period include a more open cervical canal, the masking of insertion-related bleeding, and the knowledge that the patient is not pregnant. These relative advantages may be outweighed by the risk of unintended pregnancy if insertion is delayed to await menstrual bleeding. In addition, there is evidence that the expulsion rate and termination rates for pain, bleeding, and pregnancy are lower if insertions are done after day 11 of the menstrual cycle, and the infection rate may be lower with insertions after the 17th cycle day.[110]

Technique for the TCu-380A and the Progestasert

Inserting an IUD requires only a few minutes, has few complications, and is rarely painful, but preoperative examination, medication, and the right equipment will insure a good experience for your patient. After introducing a vaginal spectrum, the cervix is cleaned with

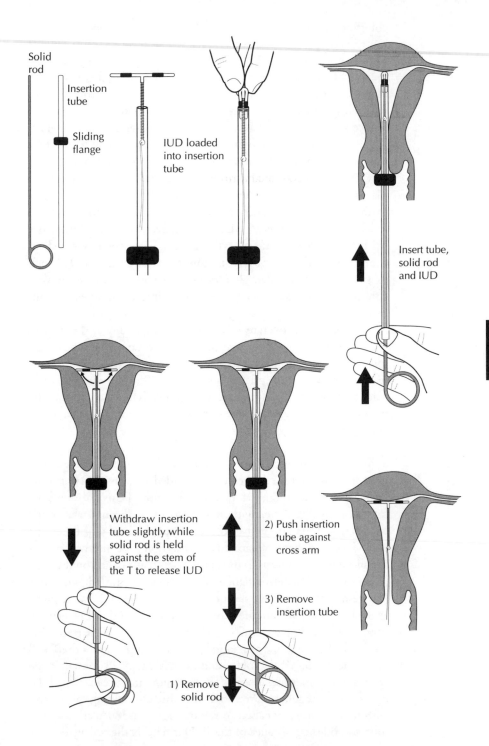

Solid rod

Insertion tube

Sliding flange

IUD loaded into insertion tube

Insert tube, solid rod and IUD

Withdraw insertion tube slightly while solid rod is held against the stem of the T to release IUD

2) Push insertion tube against cross arm

3) Remove insertion tube

1) Remove solid rod

215

chlorhexadine or povidone-iodine. Leave the antiseptic-soaked cotton-tipped applicator in the cervical canal during the procedures prior to insertion of the IUD. Place a paracervical block by injecting one mL of local anesthetic (1% chloroprocaine) into the cervical lip (anterior if the uterus is anterior in the pelvis and posterior if it lies posteriorly). Inclusion of atropine, 0.4 mg, in the anesthetic will reduce the incidence of vasovagal reactions. After one minute grasp the cervical lip with the tenaculum ratcheting it only to the first position in a slow, deliberate fashion. Use the tenaculum to move the cervix to the patient's right, revealing the left lateral vaginal fornix. Place the needle tip in the cervical mucosa at 3 o'clock, 1–2 cm lateral to the cervical os, advance it about 1.5 inches (4 cm) under the mucosa and inject about 4 mL of anesthetic, leaving an additional 1 mL behind under the mucosa as the needle is withdrawn. Now deflect the cervix to the patient's left and inject local anesthetic at 9 o'clock in similar fashion. *Wait 2–3 minutes before proceeding.* A very common mistake is to not allow sufficient time for anesthetic action.

Many women can tolerate IUD insertion, especially at the time of menses, without a paracervical block. For some women, however, insertion is less painful with local anesthetic and with administration of a nonsteroidal anti-inflammatory agent 30 minutes to one hour prior to the procedure. If a paracervical block is not used, having the patient cough just as the tenaculum is applied reduces pain and the chance of a vasovagal reaction.

Sound and measure the depth of the uterus (the insertion tube can be used for this purpose). The IUD is loaded into its insertion tube immediately prior to insertion. The arms of the TCu-380A must be folded manually, either with sterile gloves or through the sterile wrapper, and maneuvered into the end of the insertion tube, just enough to hold them in place during insertion. The insertion tube is advanced into the uterus to the correct depth as marked on the tube either by a sliding plastic flange (TCu-380A) or printed gradations (Progestasert). The flange should be twisted to be in the same plane as the horizontal arms. When the insertion tube and IUD reach the fundus, withdraw a few mm. Check to make sure that the transverse arm of the IUD is in the horizontal plane so that the tips of the T will rest in the cornual regions of the endometrial cavity. Placement in the vertical plane increases the risk of expulsion and pregnancy.[111] To release the Progestasert, remove the thread-retaining plug, and withdraw the insertor tube. To release the TCu-380A, advance the solid rod till the resistance of the IUD is felt, fix the rod against the tenaculum which is held in traction, and withdraw the insertion tube while the solid insertion rod is held against the stem of the T, releasing the transverse arms into high fundal position. Remove the solid rod and finally the inserter tube taking care not to pull on the strings. You can ensure that the TCu-380A is in a high fundal position if, after removing the solid rod, you push the insertor tube up against the cross arm of the T prior to withdrawing it completely from the cavity. Trim the strings to about 4 cm from the external os, and record their length in the chart. Shorter strings can cause unpleasant bristle-like sensations. With the Progestasert, the shorter string verifies correct placement, the longer thread should be trimmed.

Patients with newly inserted IUDs should attempt to feel the strings before they leave the examining room. Giving them the cut ends of the strings as a sample of what to feel is helpful. Palpation should be performed monthly by the patient to verify continuing presence of the IUD after each menstrual flow. Patients should return within 3 months, preferably after the first menses, to confirm the presence of the IUD and to provide support, because bleeding changes and expulsion are most likely to occur during this time. Caution the patient that the first 2 menses are typically heavier. As with all office procedures, patients should be provided a 24-hour phone number for urgent questions or concerns, and especially to report unusual pain, bleeding, or vaginal discharge.

Prophylactic Antibiotics

Doxycycline (200 mg) administered orally one hour prior to insertion can provide protection against insertion-associated pelvic infection, but two double-blind randomized studies conducted in Africa found no significant advantage in the treated groups.[112,113] Azithromycin in a dose of 500 mg has also been used prophylactically, presumably offering more protection because of a longer half-life.[114] In women at low risk for STDs, the incidence of infection is so low that there is little benefit to be expected with prophylactic antibiotics.

IUD Removal

Removal of an IUD can usually be accomplished by grasping the string with a ring forcep or uterine dressing forceps and exerting firm traction. If strings cannot be seen, they can often be extracted from the cervical canal by rotating two cotton-tipped applicators or a Pap smear cytobrush in the endocervical canal. If further maneuvers are required, a paracervical block should be administered. Oral administration of a nonsteroidal anti-inflammatory drug beforehand will reduce uterine cramping.

If IUD strings cannot be identified or extracted from the endocervical canal, a light plastic uterine sound should be passed into the endometrial cavity after administration of a paracervical block. A standard metal sound is too heavy and insensitive for this purpose. The IUD can frequently be felt with the sound and localized against the anterior or posterior wall of the uterus. The device can then be removed using a Facit polyp or alligator type forceps directed to where the device was felt, taking care to open the forceps widely immediately on passing it through the internal cervical os so that the IUD can be caught between the jaws. If removal is not easily accomplished using this forceps, direct visualization of the IUD with sonography or hysteroscopy can facilitate removal. Sonography is less painful and more convenient, and should be tried first.

Fertility returns promptly and pregnancies after removal of an IUD occur at a normal rate, sooner than after oral contraception.[39-44] Pregnancy outcome after IUD removal is assocated with a normal incidence of spontaneous abortion and ectopic pregnancy.[44]

If a patient wishes to continue use of an IUD, a new device can be placed immediately after removal of the old one. In this case, antibiotic prophylaxis is advised.

Embedded IUDs

If removal is not easily accomplished, direct visualization of the IUD with sonography or hysteroscopy can be helpful. Sonography is safer and less expensive.[85,115] Transvaginal ultrasonography provides the best image to confirm the location of the IUD, but there is little room for the removal procedure. A better approach is to fill the bladder and use an abdominal sector transducer to image the uterine cavity as the forceps are introduced. Open the forceps widely and see if the IUD moves when the forceps close upon it. If it moves, close the forceps tightly and extract the IUD. If unsuccessful, re-introduce the forceps in a different plane, keeping one jaw of the open forceps firmly against first the anterior than the posterior uterine wall. If this approach is not successful, hysteroscopy is indicated.

Finding a Displaced IUD

When an IUD cannot be found, besides expulsion, one has to consider perforation of the uterus into the abdominal cavity (a very rare event) or embedment into the myometrium. All IUDs are radiopaque, but localizing them radiographically requires 2–3 views, is time-consuming and expensive, and does not allow intrauterine direction of instruments. A quick, real-time sonographic scan in the office is the best method to locate a lost IUD, whether or not removal is desired. If the IUD cannot be visualized with ultrasonography, abdominal x-rays are necessary because the IUD can be high and hidden.

If the IUD is identified perforating the myometrium or in the abdominal cavity, it should be removed using operative laparoscopy, usually under general anesthesia. If the IUD is in the uterine cavity, but cannot be grasped with a forceps under sonographic guidance, hysteroscopy is the best approach. Both routes may be helpful if an IUD is partially perforated.

Copper in the abdominal cavity can lead to adhesion formation, making laparoscopic removal difficult.[116] Although inert perforated devices without closed loops were previously allowed to remain in the abdominal cavity, current practice is to remove any perforated IUD. Because IUD perforations usually occur at the time of insertion, it is important to check for correct position by identifying the string within a few weeks after insertion. Uterine perforation itself is unlikely to cause more than transient pain and bleeding, and can go undetected at the time of IUD insertion. If you believe perforation has occurred, prompt sonography is indicated so that the device can be removed before adhesion formation can occur.

This problem should be put into perspective. With the new generation of IUDs (copper and medicated), adhesion formation appears to be an immediate reaction which does not progress, and rarely leads to serious complications.[117] In appropriate situations (where the risk of surgery is considerable), clinician and patient may elect not to remove the translocated IUD. However, a case has been reported of sigmoid perforation occurring 5 years after insertion, and the general consensus continues to favor removal of a perforated IUD immediately upon diagnosis.[118]

IUD Myths

We hope the information in this chapter will lay to rest 4 specific myths associated with IUDs. For emphasis, the following sentences provide the correct responses to what we believe are common misconceptions among clinicians:

1. IUDs are *NOT* abortifacients.
2. An increased risk of infection with the modern IUD is related *ONLY* to the insertion.
3. The modern IUD *HAS NOT* exposed clinicians to litigation.
4. IUDs *DO NOT* increase the risk of ectopic pregnancy.

References

1. **Huber SC, Piotrow PT, Orlans B, Dommer G,** Intrauterine devices, Pop Reports, Series B, No.2, 1975.

2. **Richter R,** Ein mittel zur verhutung der konzeption, Deutsche Med Wochenschrift 35:1525, 1909.

3. **Pust K,** Ein brauchbarer frauenschutz, Deutsche Med Wochenschrift 49:952, 1923.

4. **Gräfenberg E,** An intrauterine contraceptive method, in Sanger M, Stone HM, editors, *The Practice of Contraception: Proceedings of the 7th International Birth Control Conference, Zurich, Switzerland,* Williams & Wilkins, Baltimore, Maryland, 1930, pp 33–47.

5. **Ota T,** A study on birth control with an intra-uterine instrument, Jap J Obstet Gynecol 17:210, 1934.

6. **Ishihama A,** Clinical studies on intrauterine rings, especially the present state of contraception in Japan and the experiences in the use of intra-uterine rings, Yokohama Med Bull 10:89, 1959.

7. **Oppenheimer W,** Prevention of pregnancy by the Graefenberg ring method: A re-evaluation after 28 years' experience, Am J Obstet Gynecol 78:446, 1959.

8. **Tietze C,** Evaluation of intrauterine devices. Ninth progress report of the cooperative statistical program, Stud Fam Plann 1:1, 1970.

9. **Tatum HJ, Schmidt FH, Phillips DM, McCarty M, O'Leary WM,** The Dalkon shield controversy, structural and bacteriologic studies of IUD tails, JAMA 231:711, 1975.

10. **Kessel E,** Pelvic inflammatory disease with intrauterine device use: A reassessment, Fertil Steril 51:1, 1989.

11. **Eschenbach DA, Harnisch JP, Holmes KK,** Pathogenesis of acute pelvic inflammatory disease: Role of contraception and other risk factors, Am J Obstet Gynecol 128:838, 1977.

12. **Kaufman DW, Shapiro S, Rosenberg L, Monson RR, et al,** Intrauterine contraceptive device use and pelvic inflammatory disease, Am J Obstet Gynecol 136:159, 1980.

13. **Kaufman DW, Watson J, Rosenberg L, Helmrich SP, et al,** The effect of different types of intrauterine devices on the risk of pelvic inflammatory disease, JAMA 250:759, 1983.

14. **Lee NC, Rubin GL, Ory HW, Burkman RT,** Type of intrauterine device and the risk of pelvic inflammatory disease, Obstet Gynecol 62:1, 1983.

15. **Mosher WD, Pratt WF,** Contraceptive use in the United States, 1973–1988, Advance data from vital and health statistics; No. 182, National Center for Health Statistics, Hyattsville, Maryland, 1990.

16. **Population Crisis Committee,** Access to birth control: A world assessment, Population Briefing Paper No. 19, Washington, D.C., 1986.

17. **Daling JR, Weiss NS, Metch BJ, Chow WH, Soderstrom RM, Moore DE, Spadoni LR, Stadel BV,** Primary tubal infertility in relation to the use of an intrauterine device, New Engl J Med 312:937, 1985.

18. **Cramer DW, Schiff I, Schoenbaum SC, Gibson M, Belisle S, Albrecht B, Stillman RJ, Berger MJ, Wilson E, Stadel BV, Seible M,** Tubal infertility and the intrauterine device, New Engl J Med 312:941, 1985.

19. **Lee NC, Rubin GL, Borucki R,** The intrauterine device and pelvic inflammatory disease revisited: new results from the Women' Health Study, Obstet Gynecol 72:1, 1988.

20. **Zipper JA, Medel M, Prager R,** Suppression of fertility by intrauterine copper and zinc in rabbits: A new approach to intrauterine contraception, Am J Obstet Gynecol 105:529, 1969.

21. **Tatum HJ,** Milestones in intrauterine device development, Fertil Steril 39:141, 1983.

22. **Sivin I, Tatum HJ,** Four years of experience with the TCu 380A intrauterine contraceptive device, Fertil Steril 36:159, 1981.

23. **Sujuan G, Liuqu Z, Yuhao W, Feng L,** Chinese IUDs, in Bardin CW, Mishell DR Jr, editors, *Proceedings from the Fourth International Conference on IUDs,* Butterworth-Heinemann, Boston, 1994, pp 308–318,

24. **Sivin I, Stern J, International Committee for Contraception Research,** Health during prolonged use of levonorgestrel 20 μg/d and the copper TCu 380 Ag intrauterine contraceptive devices: a multicenter study, Fertil Steril 61:70, 1994.

25. **Sivin I, Diaz S, Pavez M, Alvarez F, Brasche V, Diaz J, Odlind V, Olsson S-E, Stern J,** Two-year comparative trial of the gyne T 380 slimline and gyne T 380 intrauterine copper devices, Contraception 44:481, 1991.

26. **Chi I-c,** The TCu-380A (AG), MLCu375, and Nova-T IUDs and the IUD daily releasing 20 μg levonorgestrel-four pillars of IUD contraception for the nineties and beyond? Contraception 47:325, 1993.

27. **Luukkainen T, Allonen H, Haukkamaa M, Lahteenmake P, Nilsson CG, Toivonen J,** Five years' experience with levonorgestrel-releasing IUDs, Contraception 33:139, 1986.

28. **Sivin I, Stern J, Coutinho E, Mattos CER, El Mahgoub S, Diaz S, Pavez M, Alvarez F, Brache V, Thevinin F, Diaz J, Faundes A, Diaz MM, McCarthy T, Mishell DR Jr, Shoupe D,** Prolonged intrauterine contraception: A seven-year randomized study of the levonorgestrel 20 mcg/day (LNg 20) and the copper T380 Ag IUDs, Contraception 44:473, 1991.

29. **Toivonen J, Luukkainen T, Alloven H,** Protective effect of intrauterine release of levonorgestrel on pelvic infections: three years' comparative experience of levonorgestrel with copper-releasing intrauterine devices, Obstet Gynecol 77:261, 1991.

30. Bilian X, Liying Z, Xuling Z, Mengchun J, Luukkainen T, Allonen H, Pharmacokinetic and pharmacodynamic studies of levonorgestrel-releasing intrauterine device, Contraception 41:353, 1990.

31. UNDP, UNFPA, and WHO Special Programme of Research, Development and Research Training in Human Reproduction, World Bank: IUD Research Group, The TCu-380A IUD and the frameless IUD "the Flexigard:" interim three-year data from an international multicenter trial, Contraception 52: 77, 1995.

32. Sivin I, IUDs are contraceptives, not abortifacients: A comment on research and belief, Stud Fam Plann 20:355, 1989.

33. Ortiz ME, Croxatto HB, The mode of action of IUDs, Contraception 36:37, 1987.

34. Alvarez F, Guiloff E, Brache V, Hess R, Fernandez E, Salvatierra AM, Guerrero B, Zacharias S, New insights on the mode of action of intrauterine contraceptive devices in women, Fertil Steril 49:768, 1988.

35. Segal SJ, Alvarez-Sanchez F, Adejuwon CA, Brache De Mejla V, Leon P, Faundes A, Absence of chorionic gonadotropin in sera of women who use intrauterine devices, Fertil Steril 44:214, 1985.

36. Wilcox AJ, Weinberg CR, Armstrong EG, Canfield RE, Urinary human chorionic gonadotropin among intrauterine device users: Detection with a highly specific and sensitive assay, Fertil Steril 47:265, 1987.

37. Ämmälä M, Nyman T, Strengell L, Rutanen, E-M, Effect of intrauterine contraceptive devices on cytokine messenger ribonucleic acid expression in the human endometrium, Fertil Steril 63:773, 1995.

38. Andersson J, Rybo G, Levonorgestrel-releasing intrauterine device in the treatment of menorrhagia, Br J Obstet Gynecol 97:697, 1990.

39. Vessey MP, Lawless M, McPherson K, Yeates D, Fertility after stoppping use of intrauterine contraceptive device, Br Med J 283:106, 1983.

40. Belhadj H, Sivin I, Diaz S, Pavez M, Tejada A-S, Brache V, Alvarez F, Shoupe D, Breaux H, Mishell DR Jr, McCarthy T, Yo V, Recovery of fertility after use of the levonorgestrel 20 mcg/day or copper T 380Ag intrauterine device, Contraception 34:261, 1986.

41. Wilson JC, A prospective New Zealand study of fertility after removal of copper intrauterine devices for conception and because of complications: A four-year study, Am J Obstet Gynecol 160:391, 1989.

42. Skjeldestadt FE, Bratt H, Fertility after complicated and non-complicated use of IUDs. A controlled prospective study, Adv Contracept 4:179, 1988.

43. Sivin I, Stern J, Diaz J, Diaz MM, Faundes A, Mahgoub SE, Diaz S, Pavéz M, Coutinho E, Mattos CER, McCarthy T, Mishell DR Jr, Shoupe D, Alvarez F, Brache V, Jimenez E, Two years of intrauterine contraception with levonorgestrel and with copper: A randomized comparison of the TCu 380Ag and levonorgestrel 20 mcg/day devices, Contraception 35:245, 1987.

223

44. **Sivin I, Stern J, Diaz S, Pavéz M, Alvarez F, Brache V, Mishell DR Jr, Lacarra M, McCarthy T, Holma P, Darney P, Klaisle C, Olsson S-E, Odlind V,** Rates and outcomes of planned pregnancy after use of Norplant capsules, Norplant II rods, or levonorgestrel-releasing or copper TCu 380Ag intrauterine contraceptive devices, Am J Obstet Gynecol 166:1208, 1992.

45. **Sivin I, Schmidt F,** Effectiveness of IUDs: A review, Contraception 36:55, 1987.

46. **Petta CA, Amatya R, Farr G,** Clinical evaluation of the Tcu 380A IUD at six Latin American centers, Contraception 50:17, 1994.

47. **WHO Special Programme of Research, Development and Research Training in Human Reproduction. Task Force on the Safety and Efficacy of Fertility Regulating Methods,** The TCu 380A, TCu 220C, Multiload 250, and Nova T IUDs at 3, 5, and 7 years of use, Contraception 42:141, 1990.

48. **Farr G, Amatya R,** Contraceptive efficacy of the copper T 380A and copper T 200 intrauterine devices: results from a comparative clinical trial in six developing countries, Contraception 49:231, 1994.

49. **WHO Special Programme of Research, Development and Research Training in Human Reproduction. Task Force on Intrauterine Devices for Fertility Regulation,** A multinational case-control study of ectopic pregnancy, Clin Reprod Fertil 3:131, 1985.

50. **Marchbanks PA, Annegers JE, Coulam CB, Strathy JH, Kurland LT,** Risk factors for ectopic pregnancy. A population based study, JAMA 259:1823, 1988.

51. **Ory HW,** Ectopic pregnancy and intrauterine contraceptive devices: New perspectives, Obstet Gynecol 57:2, 1981.

52. **Edelman DA, Porter CW,** The intrauterine device and ectopic pregnancy, Contraception 36:85, 1987.

53. **Makinen JI, Erkkola RU, Laippala PJ,** Causes of the increase in incidence of ectopic pregnancy — a study on 1017 patients from 1966 to 1985 in Turku, Finland, Am J Obstet Gynecol 160:642, 1989.

54. **Sivin I,** Dose- and age-dependent ectopic pregnancy risks with intrauterine contraception, Obstet Gynecol 78:291, 1991.

55. **Barbosa I, Bakos O, Olsson S-E, Odlind V, Johansson EDB,** Ovarian function during use of a levonorgestrel-releasing IUD, Contraception 42:51, 1990.

56. **Bilian X, Liying Z, Xuling Z, Mengchun J, Luukkainen T, Allonen H,** Pharmacokinetic and pharmacodynamic studies of levonorgestrel-releasing intrauterine device, Contraception 41:353, 1990.

57. **Franks AL, Beral V, Cates W Jr, Hogue CJ,** Contraception and ectopic pregnancy risk, Am J Obstet Gynecol 163:1120, 1990.

58. Cameron IT, Haining R, Lumsden M-A, Thomas VR, Smith SK, The effects of mefenamic acid and norethisterone on measured menstrual blood loss, Obstet Gynecol 76:85, 1990.

59. Milsom I, Andersson K, Jonasson K, Lindstedt G, Rybo G, The influence of the Gyne-T 380S IUD on menstrual blood loss and iron status, Contraception 52:175, 1995.

60. Castellsague X, Thompson WD, Dubrow R, Intra-uterine contraception and the risk of endometrial cancer, Internatl J Cancer 54:911, 1993.

61. Lassise DL, Savitz DA, Hamman RF, Baron AE, Brinton LA, Levines RS, Invasive cervical cancer and intrauterine device use, Internatl J Epidemiol 20:865, 1991.

62. Parazzini F, La Vecchia C, Negri E, Use of intrauterine device and risk of invasive cervical cancer, Internatl J Epidemiol 21:1030, 1992.

63. Mishell DR Jr, Bell JH, Good RG, Moyer DL, The intrauterine device: a bacteriologic study of the endometrial cavity, Am J Obstet Gynecol 96:119, 1966.

64. Farley MM, Rosenberg MJ, Rowe PJ, Chen J-H, Meirik O, Intrauterine devices and pelvic inflammatory disease: an international perspective, Lancet 339:785, 1992.

65. Skouby SO, Molsted-Pedersen L, Kosonen A, Consequences of intrauterine contraception in diabetic women, Fertil Steril 42:568, 1984.

66. Kimmerle R, Weiss R, Berger M, Kurz K, Effectiveness, safety, and acceptability of a copper intrauterine deivce (Cu Safe 300) in type I diabetic women, Diabetes Care 16:1227, 1993.

67. Buchan H, Villard-Mackintosh L, Vessey M, Yeates D, McPherson K, Epidemiology of pelvic inflammatory disease in parous women with special reference to intrauterine device use, Br J Obstet Gynaecol 97:780, 1990.

68. Toivonen J, Luukkainen T, Alloven H, Protective effect of intrauterine release of levonorgestrel on pelvic infection: three years' comparative experience of levonorgestrel and copper-releasing intrauterine devices, Obstet Gynecol 77:261, 1991.

69. Mehanna MTR, Rizk MA, Ramadan M, Schachter J, Chlamydial serologic characteristics among intrauterine contraceptive device users: Does copper inhibit chlamydial infection int he female genital tract? Am J Obstet Gynecol 171:691, 1994.

70. Kleinman D, Insler V, Sarov I, Inhibition of *Chlamydia trachomatis* growth in endometrial cells by copper: possible relavance for the use of copper IUDs, Contraception 39:665, 1989.

71. Kronmal RA, Whitney CW, Mumford SD, The intrauterine device and pelvic inflammatory disease; the Women's Health Study reanalyzed, J Clin Epidemiol 44:109, 1991.

225

72. Lee NC, Rubin GL, Grimes DA, Measures of sexual behavior and the risk of pelvic inflammatory disease, Obstet Gynecol 77:425, 1991.

73. Everett ED, Reller LB, Droegemueller W, Greer BE, Absence of bacteremia after insertion or removal of intrauterine device, Obstet Gynecol 47:207, 1976.

74. Hall SM, Jamieson JR, Witcomb MA, Bacteraemia after insertion of intrauterine devices, S Afr Med J 50:1232l, 1976.

75. Murray S, Hickey JB, Houang E, Significant bacteremia associated with replacement of intrauterine contraceptive device, Am J Obstet Gynecol 156:698, 1987.

76. Jossens MOR, Schachter J, Sweet RL, Risk factors associated with pelvic inflammatory disease of differing microbial etiologies, Obstet Gynecol 83:989, 1994.

77. European Study Group, Risk factors for male to female transmission of HIV, Br Med J 298:411, 1989.

78. Musicco M, Nicolosi A, Saracco A, Lazzarin A, IUD use and man to woman sexual transmission of HIV-1, in Bardin CW, Mishell DR Jr, editors, *Proceedings from the Fourth International Conference on IUDs*, Butterworth-Heinemann, Boston, 1994, pp 179–188.

79. Chapin DS, Sullinger JC, A 43-year old woman with left buttock pain and a presacral mass, New Engl J Med 323:183, 1990.

80. Keebler C, Chatwani A, Schwartz R, Actinomycosis infection associated with intrauterine contraceptive devices, Am J Obstet Gynecol 145:596, 1983.

81. Duguid HLD, Actinomycosis and IUDs, Int Plann Parenthood Fed Med Bull 17:3, 1983.

82. Petitti DB, Yamamoto D, Morgenstern N, Factors associated with actinomyces-like organisms on Papanicolaou smear in users of IUDs, Am J Obstet Gynecol 145:338, 1983.

83. Persson E, Holmberg K, Dahlgren S, Nielsson L, Actinomyces Israelii in genital tract of women with and without intrauterine contraception devices, Acta Obstet Gynecol Scand 62:563, 1983.

84. Hill GB, *Eubacterium nodatum* mimics *Actinomyces* in intrauterine device-associated infections and other settings within the female genital tract, Obstet Gynecol 79:534, 1992.

85. Stubblefield P, Fuller A, Foster S, Ultrasound-guided intrauterine removal of intrauterine contraceptive devices in pregnancy, Obstet Gynecol 72:961, 1988.

86. Lewit S, Outcome of pregnancy with intrauterine device, Contraception 2:47, 1970.

87. Alvior GT Jr, Pregnancy outcome with removal of intrauterine device, Obstet Gynecol 41:894, 1973.

88. Assaf A, Gohar M, Saad S, El-Nashar A, Abdel Aziz A, Removal of intrauterine devices with missing tails during early pregnancy, Contraception 45:541, 1992.

89. Foreman H, Stadel VB, Schlesselman S, Intrauterine device usage and fetal loss, Obstet Gynecol 58:669, 1981.

90. United Kingdom Family Planning Research Network, Pregnancy outcome associated with the use of IUDs, Br J Fam Plann 15:7, 1989.

91. Williams P, Johnson B, Vessey M, Septic abortion in women using intrauterine devices, Br Med J iv:263, 1975.

92. Atrash HK, Frye A, Hogue CJR, Incidence of morbidity and mortality with IUD in situ in the 1980s and 1990s, in Bardin CW, Mishell DR Jr, editors, *Proceedings from the Fourth International Conference on IUDs,* Butterworth-Heinemann, Boston, 1994, pp 76–87.

93. Guillebaud J, IUD and congenital malformation, Br Med J I:1016, 1975.

94. Layde PM, Goldberg MF, Safra MJM, Oakley GP, Failed intrauterine device contraception and limb reduction deformities: a case-control study, Fertil Steril 31:18, 1979.

95. Tatum HJ, Schmidt FH, Jain AK, Management and outcome of pregnancies associatd with the copper-T intrauterine contraceptive device, Am J Obstet Gynecol 7:869, 1976.

96. Vessey MP, Doll R, Peto R, Johnson B, Wiggins P, A long term follow up of women using different methods of contraception. An interim report, J Biosoc Sci 8:373, 1976.

97. Chaim W, Mazor M, Pregnancy with an intrauterine device in situ and preterm delivery, Arch Gynecol Obstet 252:21, 1992.

98. Leigh BC, Temple MT, Trocki KF, The sexual behavior of US adults: results from a national survey, Am J Pub Health 83:1400, 1993.

99. Newton J, Tacchi D, Long-term use of copper intrauterine devices, Br J Fam Plann 16:116, 1990.

100. Kjos SL, Ballagh SA, La Cour M, Xiang A, Mishell DR Jr, The copper T380A intrauterine device in women with Type II diabetes mellitus, Obstet Gynecol 84:1006, 1994.

101. Diaz J, Pinto-Neto AM, Bahamondes L, Diaz M, Arce XE, Castro S, Performance of the copper T 200 in parous adolescents: are copper IUDs suitable for these women? Contraception 48:23, 1993.

102. Edelman D, Van Os W, Safety of intrauterine contraception, Adv Contracept 6:207, 1990.

103. Mishell DR Jr, Roy S, Copper intrauterine contraceptive device event rates following insertion 4 to 8 weeks post partum, Am J Obstet Gynecol 143:29, 1982.

104. **Zhuang L, Wang H, Yang P,** Observations of the clinical efficacies and side effects of six different timings of IUD insertions, Clin J Obstet Gynecol 22:350, 1987.

105. **Chi I-c, Farr G,** Postpartum IUD contraception — A review of an international experience, Adv Contracept 5:127, 1989.

106. **Zhou S, Chi I-c,** Immediate postpartum IUD insertions ina Chinese hospital — A two-year follow-up, Int J Gynaecol Obstet 35:157, 1991.

107. **Chi I-c, Potts M, Wilkens L, Champion C,** Performance of the TCu-380A device in breastfeeding and non-breastfeeding women, Contraception 39:603, 1989.

108. **Nielsen NC, Nygren K-G, Allonen H,** Three years of experience after post-abortal insertion of Nova-T and Copper-T-200, Acta Obstet Gynecol Scand 63:261, 1984.

109. **QueridoL, Ketting E, Haspels AA,** IUD insertion following induced abortion, Contraception 31:603, 1985.

110. **White MK, Ory HW, Rooks JB, Rochat RW,** Intrauterine device termination rates and the menstrual cycle day of insertion, Obstet Gynecol 55:220, 1980.

111. **Anteby E, Revel A, Ben-Chetrit A, Rosen B, Tadmor O, Yagel S,** Intrauterine device failure: relation to its location within the uterine cavity, Obstet Gynecol 81:112, 1993.

112. **Sinei SKA, Schulz KF, Laptey PR, Grimes D, Arnsi J, Rosenthal S, Rosenberg M, Rivon G, Njage P, Bhullar V, Ogendo H,** Preventing IUCD-related pelvic infection: The efficacy of prophylactic doxycycline at insertion, Br J Obstet Gynecol 97:412, 1990.

113. **Lapido OA, farr G, Otolorin E, Konje JC, Sturgen K, Cox P, Champion CB,** Prevention of IUD-related pelvic infection: the efficacy of prophylactic doxycycline at IUD insertion, Adv Contracept 7:43, 1991.

114. **Walsh TL, Bernstein GS, Grimes DA, Frezieres R, Bernstein L, Coulson AH, IUD Study Group,** Effect of prophylactic antibiotics on morbidity associated with IUD insertion: results of a pilot randomized controlled trial, Contraception 50:319, 1994.

115. **Sachs BP, Gregory K, McArdle C, Pinshaw A,** Removal of retained intrauterine contraceptive devices in pregnancy, Am J Perinatol 9:139, 1992.

116. **Gorsline J, Osborne N,** Management of the missing intrauterine contraceptive device: Report of a case, Am J Obstet Gynecol 153:228, 1985.

117. **Adoni A, Chetrit AB,** The management of intrauterine devices following uterine perforation, Contraception 43:77, 1991.

118. **Gronlund B, Blaabjerg J,** Serious intestinal complication five years after insertion of a Nova-T, Contraception 44:517, 1991.

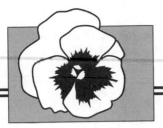

7

Barrier Methods

BARRIER METHODS of contraception have been the most widely used contraceptive technique throughout recorded history. These methods, the oldest of methods, are now being thrust into the forefront as we respond to the personal and social impact of sexually transmitted diseases (STDs). A new need for sexual safety has brought modern respect and new developments to the condom, while the other barrier methods continue to serve well for appropriate couples.

History

The use of vaginal contraceptives is probably as ancient as homo sapiens. References to sponges and plugs appear in the earliest of writings. Substances with either barrier or spermicidal properties (or both) have included honey, alum, spices, oils, tannic acids, lemon juice, and even crocodile dung. However, the diaphragm and the cervical cap were not invented until the late 1800s, the same time period which saw the beginning of investigations with spermicidal agents.

Intravaginal contraception was widespread in isolated cultures throughout the world. The Japanese used balls of bamboo paper; Islamic women used willow leaves; and the women in the Pacific Islands used seaweed. References can be found throughout ancient writings to sticky plugs, made of gumlike substances, to be placed in the vagina prior to intercourse. In preliterate societies, an effective method had to have been the result of trial and error, with some good luck thrown in.

How was contraceptive knowledge spread? Certainly, until modern times, individuals did not consult physicians for contraception. Contraceptive knowledge was folklore, undoubtedly perpetuated by the oral tradition. The social and technical circumstances of ancient times conspired to make communication of information very difficult. But even when knowledge was lacking, the desire to prevent conception was not. Hence, the widespread use of potions, body movements, and amulets; all of which can be best described as magic.

Egyptian papyri dating from 1850 B.C. refer to plugs of honey, gum, acacia, and crocodile dung. The descriptions of contraceptive techniques by Soranus are viewed as the best in history until modern times.[1] Soranus of Ephesus lived from 98 to 138, and has often been referred to as the greatest gynecologist of antiquity. He studied in Alexandria, and practiced in Rome. His great text was lost for centuries, and was not published until 1838.

Soranus gave explicit directions how to make concoctions which probably combined a barrier with spermicidal action. He favored making pulps from nuts and fruits (probably very acidic and spermicidal) and advocated the use of soft wool placed at the cervical os. He actually described up to 40 different combinations.

The earliest penis protectors were just that, intended to provide prophylaxis against infection. Gabriello Fallopius, one of the early authorities on syphilis, described, in 1564, a linen condom which covered the glans penis. The linen condom of Fallopius was followed by full covering with animal skins and intestines, but use for contraception cannot be dated to earlier than the 1700s.

There are many versions accounting for the origin of the word, "condom." Most attribute the word to a Dr. Condom, a physician in England in the 1600s. The most famous story declares that Dr. Condom invented the sheath in response to the annoyance displayed by Charles II at the number of his illegitimate children. All attempts to trace this physician have failed. This origin of the word can neither be proved or disproved.

By 1800, condoms were available at brothels throughout Europe, but nobody wanted to claim responsibility. The French called the condom the English cape; the English called condoms French letters.

Vulcanization of rubber dates to 1844, and by 1850 rubber condoms were available in the U.S. The vulcanization of rubber revolutionized transportation and contraception. The introduction of liquid latex and automatic machinery ultimately made reliable condoms both plentiful and affordable.

Diaphragms first appeared in publication in Germany in the 1880s. A practicing German gynecologist, C. Haase, wrote extensively about his diaphragm, using a pseudonym of Wilhelm P.J. Mensinga. The Mensinga diaphragm retained its original design with little change until modern times.

The cervical cap was available for use before the diaphragm. A New York gynecologist, E.B. Foote, wrote a pamphlet describing its use around 1860. By the 1930s, the cervical cap was the most widely prescribed method of contraception in Europe. Why was the cervical cap not accepted in the U.S.? The answer is not clear. Some blame the more prudish attitude towards sexuality as an explanation for why American women had difficulty learning self-insertion techniques.

Scientific experimentation with chemical inhibitors of sperm began in the 1800s. By the 1950s, more than 90 different spermicidal products were being marketed, and some of them were used in the first efforts to control fertility in India.[2] With the availability of the intrauterine device and the development of oral contraception, interest in spermicidal agents waned, and the number of products declined.

In the last decades of the 1800s, condoms, diaphragms, pessaries, and douching syringes were widely advertised; however, they were not widely utilized. It is only since 1900 that the knowledge and application of contraception have been democratized, encouraged, and promoted. And it is only since 1960, that contraception teaching and practice became part of the program in academic medicine, but not without difficulty.

In the 1960s, Duncan Reid, chair of obstetrics at Harvard Medical School, organized and cared for women in a clandestine clinic for contraception. Called "Dr. Reid's Clinic," women of Boston were able to receive contraceptives not available elsewhere in the city.

In 1961, C. Lee Buxton, chair of obstetrics and gynecology at Yale Medical School, and Estelle Griswold, the 61-year-old executive director of Connecticut Planned Parenthood, opened four Planned Parenthood clinics in New Haven, in a defiant move against the current Connecticut law. In an obvious test of the Connecticut law, Buxton and Griswold were arrested at the Orange Street clinic, in a prearranged scenario scripted by Buxton and Griswold at the invitation of the district attorney. Found guilty, and fined $100, imprisonment was deferred as the obvious goal was a decision by the United States Supreme Court. Buxton was forever rankled by the trivial amount of the fine. On June 7, 1965, the Supreme Court voted 7–2 to overturn the Connecticut law on the basis of a constitutional right of privacy. It was not until 1972 and 1973 that the last state laws prohibiting the distribution of contraceptives were overthrown.

Efficacy of Barrier Methods

Failure Rates During the First Year of Use, United States [3]

Method	Percent of Women with Pregnancy	
	Lowest Expected	Typical
No method	85.0%	85.0%
Spermicides	3.0	21.0
Cervical cap	6.0	18.0
Sponge		
Parous women	9.0	28.0
Nulliparous women	6.0	18.0
Diaphragm and spermicides	6.0	18.0
Condom	2.0	12.0

Risks and Benefits Common to All Barrier Methods

Barrier (condoms and diaphragms) and spermicide methods provide protection (about a 50% reduction) against STDs and pelvic inflammatory disease (PID).[4-8] This includes infections with chlamydia, gonorrhea, herpes simplex, cytomegalovirus, human papillomavirus, and human immunodeficiency virus (HIV); however, only the condom has been proven to prevent HIV infection. STD protection has a beneficial impact on the risk of tubal infertility and ectopic pregnancy.[6,9] There have been no significant clinical studies on STDs and cervical caps or the female condom, but these methods should be effective. Women who have never used barrier methods of contraception are almost twice as likely to develop cancer of the cervix.[9,10] The risk of toxic shock syndrome is increased with female barrier methods, but the actual incidence is so rare that this is not a significant clinical consideration.[11] Women who have had toxic shock syndrome, however, should be advised to avoid barrier methods.

Barrier Methods and Preeclampsia. An initial case-control study indicated that methods of contraception that prevented exposure to sperm were associated with an increased risk of preeclampsia.[12] This was not confirmed in a careful analysis of two large cohort prospective pregnancy studies.[13] This latter conclusion was more compelling in that it was derived from a large prospective cohort data base.

The Diaphragm

The first effective contraceptive method under a woman's control was the vaginal diaphragm. Distribution of diaphragms led to Margaret Sanger's arrest in New York City in 1918. This was still a contentious issue in 1965 when the Supreme Court's decision in Griswold v. Connecticut ended the ban on contraception in that state. By 1940, one-third of contracepting American couples were using the diaphragm. This decreased to 10% by 1965 after the introduction of oral contraceptives and intrauterine devices, and fell to about 3% by 1988 (Chapter 1).

Efficacy

Failure rates for diaphragm users vary from as low as 2% per year of use to a high of 23%. The typical use failure rate after one year of use is 18%.[3] Older, married women with longer use achieve the highest efficacy, but young women can use diaphragms very successfully if they are properly encouraged and counseled. There have been no adequate studies to determine whether efficacy is different with and without spermicides.[14]

Side Effects

The diaphragm is a safe method of contraception that rarely causes even minor side effects. Occasionally women report vaginal irritation due to the latex rubber or the spermicidal jelly or cream used with the diaphragm. Less than 1% discontinue diaphragm use for these reasons. Urinary tract infections are approximately twice as common among diaphragm users as among women using oral contraception.[15] Possibly the rim of the diaphragm presses against the urethra and causes irritation which is perceived as infectious in origin, or true infection may result from touching the perineal area or incomplete emptying of the bladder. It is more probable that spermicides used with the diaphragm can increase the risk of bacteriuria with *E coli*, perhaps due to an alteration in the normal vaginal flora.[16] Clinical experience suggests that voiding after sexual intercourse is helpful, and if necessary, a single postcoital dose of a prophylactic antibiotic can be recommended. Postcoital prophylaxis is effective, using trimethoprim-sulfamethoxazole (1 tablet postcoitus), nitrofurantoin (50 or 100 mg postcoitus), or cephalexin (250 mg postcoitus).

Improper fitting or prolonged retention (beyond 24 hours) can cause vaginal abrasion or mucosal irritation. There is no link between the normal use of diaphragms and the toxic shock syndrome.[17] It makes sense, however, to minimize the risk of toxic shock by removing the diaphragm after 24 hours and during menses.

Benefits

Diaphragm use reduces the incidence of cervical gonorrhea,[18] pelvic inflammatory disease,[19] and tubal infertility.[5, 9] This protection may be due in part to the simultaneous use of a spermicide. There are no data, as of yet, regarding the effect of diaphragm use on the transmission of the AIDS virus (HIV). An important advantage of the diaphragm is low cost. Diaphragms are durable, and with proper care, can last for several years.

Choice and Use of the Diaphragm

There are three types of diaphragms, and most manufacturers produce them in sizes ranging from 50 to 105 mm diameter, in increments of 2.5 to 5 mm. Most women use sizes between 65 and 80 mm.

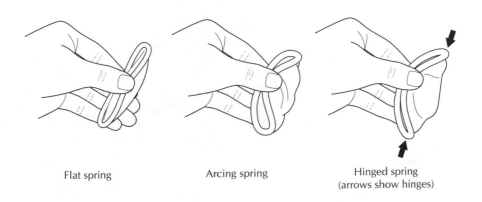

Flat spring   Arcing spring   Hinged spring
(arrows show hinges)

The diaphragm made with a *flat metal spring* or a *coil spring* remains in a straight line when pinched at the edges. This type is suitable for women with good vaginal muscle tone and an adequate recess behind the pubic arch. However, many women find it difficult to place the posterior edge of these flat diaphragms into the posterior cul-de-sac, and over the cervix.

Arcing diaphragms are easier to use for most women. They come in two types. The All-Flex type bends into an arc no matter where around the rim the edges are pinched together. The hinged type must be pinched between the hinges in order to form a symmetrical arc. The hinged type forms a narrower shape when pinched together, and thus may be easier for some women to insert. The arcing diaphragms allow the posterior edge of the diaphragm to slip more easily past the cervix and into the posterior cul-de-sac. Arcing diaphragms are used more successfully by women with poor vaginal muscle tone, cystocele, rectocele, a long cervix, or an anterior cervix of a retroverted uterus.

235

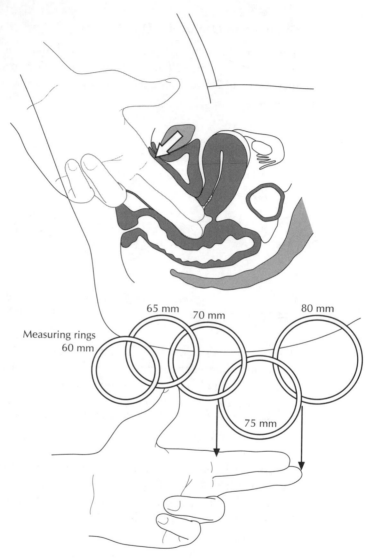

After S. Koperski from **Jackson, Berger, Keith**, *Vaginal Contraception*, G.K. Hall Publishers.

Fitting. Successful use of a diaphragm depends upon proper fitting. The clinician must have available aseptic fitting rings or diaphragms themselves in all diameters. These devices should be scrupulously disinfected by soaking in a bleach solution. At the time of the pelvic examination, the middle finger is placed against the vaginal wall and the posterior cul-de-sac, while the hand is lifted anteriorly until the pubic symphysis abuts the index finger. This point is marked with the examiner's thumb to approximate the diameter of the diaphragm.

The corresponding fitting ring or diaphragm is inserted, the fit to be assessed by both clinician and patient.

If the diaphragm is too tightly pressed against the pubic symphysis, a smaller size is selected. If the diaphragm is too loose (comes out with a cough or bearing down), the next larger size is selected. After a good fit is obtained, the diaphragm is removed by hooking the index finger under the rim behind the symphysis and pulling. It is important to instruct the patient in these procedures during and after the fitting. The patient should then insert the diaphragm, practice checking for proper placement, and attempt removal.

Timing. Diaphragm users need additional instruction about the timing of diaphragm use in relation to sexual intercourse and the use of spermicide. None of this advice has been rigorously assessed in clinical studies, therefore these recommendations represent the consensus of clinical experience.

The diaphragm should be inserted no longer than 6 hours prior to sexual intercourse. About a tablespoonful of spermicidal cream or jelly should be placed in the dome of the diaphragm prior to insertion, some of the spermicide should be spread around the rim with a finger. The diaphragm should be left in place for approximately 6 hours (but no more than 24 hours) after coitus. Additional spermicide should be placed in the vagina before each additional episode of sexual intercourse while the diaphragm is in place.

Reassessment. Weight loss, weight gain, vaginal delivery, and even sexual intercourse can change vaginal caliber. The fit of a diaphragm should be assessed every year at the time of the regular examination.

Care of the Diaphragm. After removal, the diaphragm should be washed with soap and water, rinsed, and dried. Powders of any sort need not and should not be applied to diaphragms. It is wise to use water to periodically check for leaks. Diaphragms should be stored in a cool and dark location.

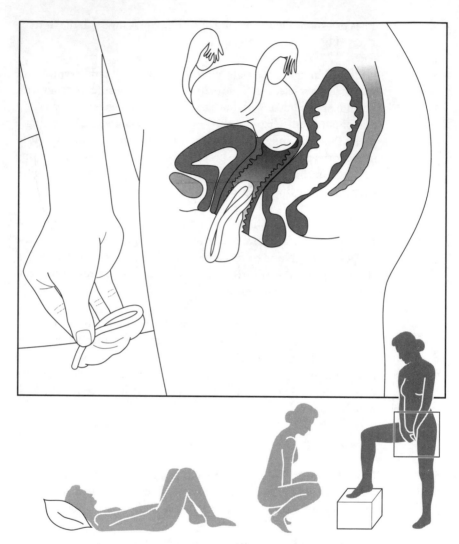

After S. Koperski from **Jackson, Berger, Keith**, *Vaginal Contraception*, G.K. Hall Publishers.

Diaphragm Insertion.

Above: Compression of the diaphragm with the cavity facing upward.

Below: Three commonly used positions for insertion.

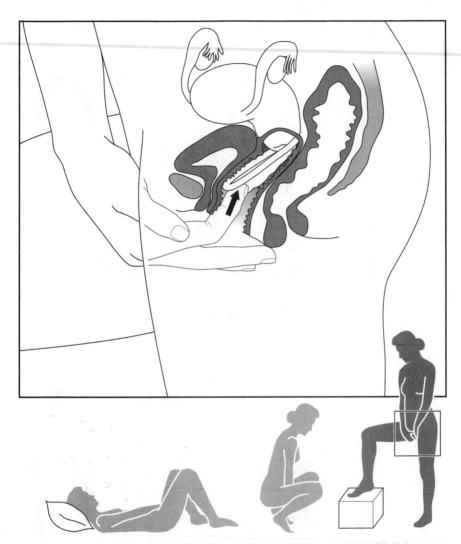

After S. Koperski from **Jackson, Berger, Keith**, *Vaginal Contraception*, G.K. Hall Publishers.

239

Diaphragm Insertion.

The diaphragm is pushed into the vagina as far as it will go. The leading edge is behind the cervix. The front edge is behind the symphysis pubis.

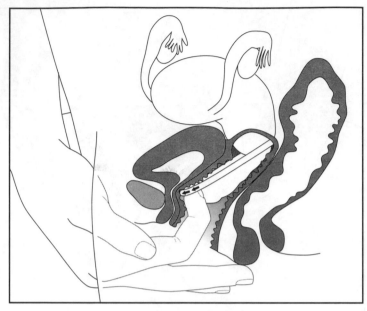

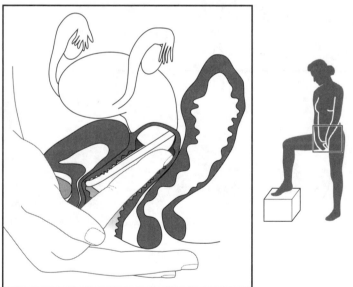

After S. Koperski from **Jackson, Berger, Keith**, *Vaginal Contraception*, G.K. Hall Publishers.

Checking Diaphragm Position.

Above: Checking for forward movement; it should be snug.

Below: Feeling the cervix to make sure it is covered. Move the finger back and forth to feel the rim, then find the bulge in the middle.

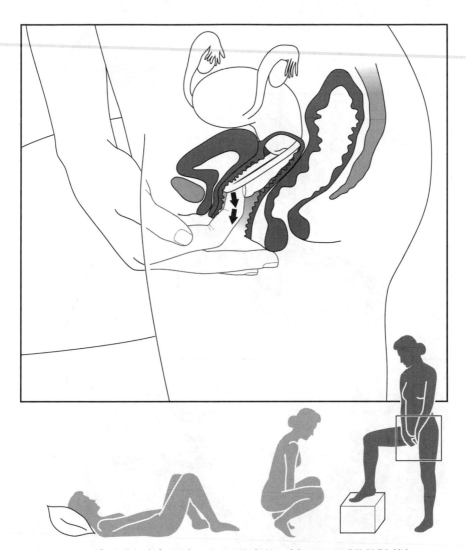

After S. Koperski from **Jackson, Berger, Keith**, *Vaginal Contraception*, G.K. Hall Publishers.

241

Diaphragm Removal.

Insert the index finger under the front rim and pull downward and outward. An alternative method is to approach the diaphragm with the palm down and insert the finger between the outer edge and the vagina.

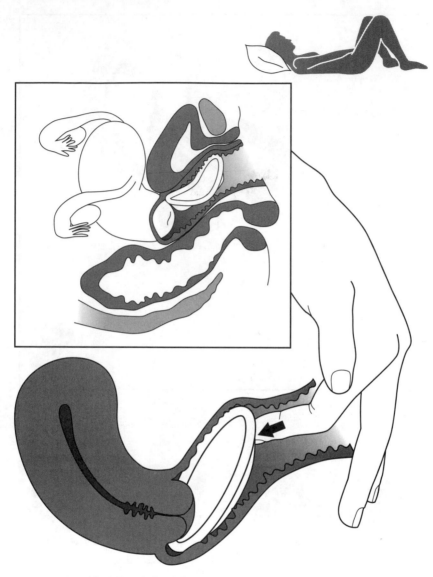

After S. Koperski from **Jackson, Berger, Keith,** *Vaginal Contraception,* G.K. Hall Publishers.

Incorrect Diaphragm Insertion.

Above: The outer rim is correct, but the leading rim is in front of the cervix.

Below: Incorrect placement can be repositioned with a downward push on the outer edge.

242

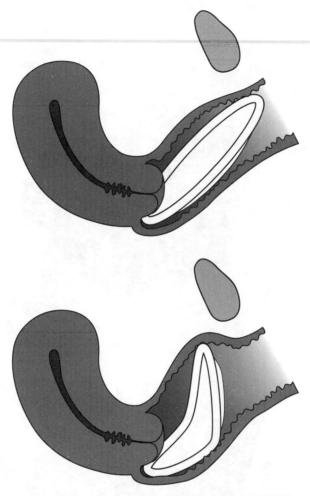

After S. Koperski from **Jackson, Berger, Keith**, *Vaginal Contraception*, G.K. Hall Publishers.

Incorrect Diaphragm Fit (Too Large).

Above: A diaphragm too large cannot fit behind the symphysis pubis.

Below: Forcing a diaphragm which is too large buckles the diaphragm and uncovers the cervix.

243

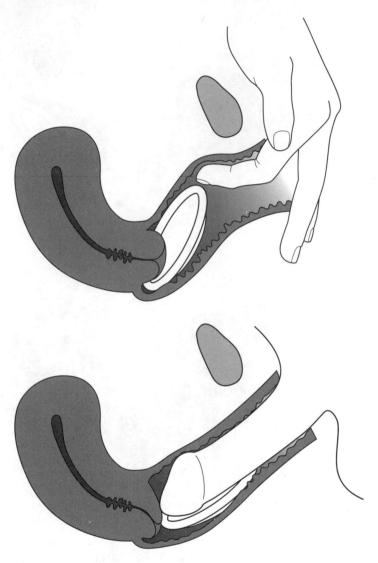

After S. Koperski from **Jackson, Berger, Keith**, *Vaginal Contraception*, G.K. Hall Publishers.

Incorrect Diaphragm Fit (Too Small).

Above: A diaphragm too small does not fit snugly behind the symphysis pubis.

Below: With a diaphragm too small, the penis displaces it and exposes the cervix.

The Cervical Cap

The cervical cap was popular in Europe long before its re-introduction into the United States. There are several types of cervical caps, but only the cavity rim (Prentif) cap is approved in the U.S. U.S. trials have demonstrated the cervical cap to be about as effective as the diaphragm, but somewhat harder to fit (it comes in only four sizes) and more difficult to insert (it must be placed precisely over the cervix).[20,21]

The cervical cap has several advantages over the diaphragm. It can be left in place for a longer time (up to 48 hours), and it need not be used with a spermicide. However, a tablespoonful of spermicide placed in the cap before application is reported to increase efficacy (to a 6% failure rate in the first year) and to prolong wearing time by decreasing the incidence of foul-smelling discharge (a common complaint after 24 hours).[21]

The size of the cervix varies considerably from woman to woman, and the cervix changes in individual women in response to pregnancy or surgery. Proper fitting can be accomplished in about 80% of women. Women with a cervix that is too long or too short, or with a cervix that is far forward in the vagina, may not be suited for cap use. However, women with vaginal wall or pelvic relaxation, who cannot retain a diaphragm, may be able to use the cap.

Those women who can be fitted with one of the 4 sizes must first learn how to identify the cervix, and then how to slide the cap into the vagina, up the posterior vaginal wall and onto the cervix. After insertion, and after each act of sexual intercourse, the cervix should be checked to make sure it is covered.

To remove the cap (at least 8 hours after coitus), pressure must be exerted with a finger tip to break the seal. The finger is hooked over the cap rim to pull it out of the vagina. Bearing down or squatting or both can help to bring the cervix within reach of the finger.

The cervical cap can be left in place for 2 days, but some women experience a foul-smelling discharge by 2 days. Like the diaphragm, it must be left in place for at least 8 hours after sexual intercourse in order to ensure that no motile sperm are left in the vagina.

The most common cause of failure is dislodgment of the cap from the cervix during sexual intercourse. There is no evidence that cervical caps cause toxic shock syndrome or dysplastic changes in the cervical mucosa.[22] It seems likely (although not yet documented) that cervical caps would provide the same protection from sexually transmitted diseases as the diaphragm.

The Fem Cap, made of nonallergic silicone rubber, is shaped like a sailor's hat, a design that allows a better fit over the cervix and in the vaginal fornices.[23] This cap may be easier to fit and use, and provides better efficacy.

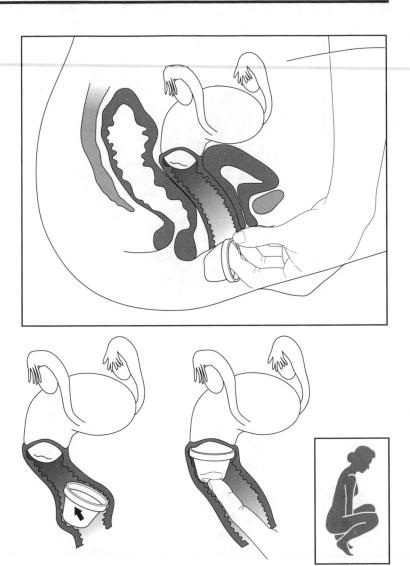

After S. Koperski from **Jackson, Berger, Keith**, *Vaginal Contraception*, G.K. Hall Publishers.

Insertion of the Cervical Cap.

Above: The cap is pushed into the vagina with the index
finger.

Below: The cap is pushed onto the cervix, and its position
is checked by feeling the cervix through the cap.

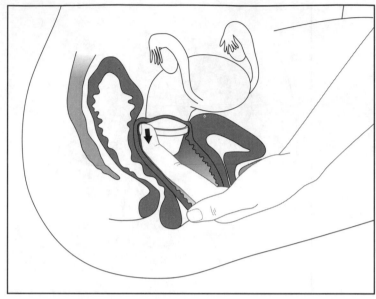

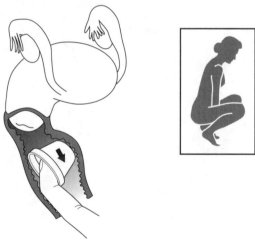

After S. Koperski from **Jackson, Berger, Keith,** *Vaginal Contraception,* G.K. Hall Publishers.

Removal of the Cervical Cap.

Above: The index finger is placed behind the rim, and the cap is dislodged with a downward motion.

Below: The cap is removed by inserting the finger into the cap.

The Contraceptive Sponge

The vaginal contraceptive sponge is a sustained release system for the spermicide, nonoxynol-9. The sponge also absorbs semen and blocks the entrance to the cervical canal. The "Today" sponge is a dimpled polyurethaned disc impregnated with one gram of nonoxynol-9. About 20% of the nonoxynol-9 is released over the 24 hours the sponge is left in the vagina. Production of the "Today" sponge in the U.S. ceased in 1995, and availability awaits a new manufacturer.

To insert, the sponge is moistened with water (squeezing out the excess) and placed firmly against the cervix. There should always be a lapse of at least 6 hours after sexual intercourse before removal, even if the sponge has been in place for 24 hours before intercourse (maximal wear time, therefore, is 30 hours). It can be inserted immediately before sexual intercourse or up to 24 hours beforehand. It is removed by hooking a finger through the ribbon attached to the back of the sponge. Obviously, the sponge is not a good choice for women with anatomical changes that make proper insertion and placement difficult.

In most studies, the effectiveness of the sponge exceeds that of foam, jellies, and tablets, but it is lower than that associated with diaphragm or condom use.[3,24] Some studies indicated higher failure rates (twice as high) in parous women, suggesting that one size may not fit all users.[25]

Discontinuation rates are generally higher among sponge users, compared to diaphragm and spermicide use. For some women, however, the sponge is preferred because it provides continuous protection for 24 hours regardless of the frequency of coitus. In addition, it is easier to use and less messy.

Side effects associated with the sponge include allergic reactions in about 4% of users. Another 8% complain of vaginal dryness, soreness, or itching. Some women find removal difficult. There is no risk of toxic shock syndrome, and in fact, the nonoxynol-9 retards staphylococcal replication and toxin production. There has been some concern that the sponge may damage the vaginal mucosa and enhance HIV transmission.[26]

Spermicides

Jellies, creams, foams, melting suppositories, foaming tablets, foaming suppositories, and soluble films are used as vehicles for chemical agents which inactivate sperm in the vagina before they can move into the upper genital tract. Some are used together with diaphragms, caps, and condoms, but even used alone, they can provide protection against pregnancy.

Various chemicals and a wide array of vehicles have been used vaginally as contraceptives for centuries. The first commercially available spermicidal pessaries were made in England in 1885 of cocoa butter and quinine sulfite. These or similar materials were used until the 1920s when effervescent tablets which released carbon dioxide and phenyl mercuric acetate were marketed. Modern spermicides, introduced in the 1950s, contain surface active agents which damage the sperm cell membranes (this same action occurs with bacteria and viruses, explaining the protection against STDs). The agents currently used are nonoxynol-9, octoxynol-9, and menfegol. Most preparations contain 60–100 mg of these agents in each vaginal application, with concentrations ranging from 2–12.5%.

Representative Products:

> **Vaginal Contraceptive Film — VCF**
> Foams　—　Delfen (nonoxynol-9, 12.5%)
> 　　　　　　Emko (nonoxynol-9, 8%)
> 　　　　　　Koromex (nonoxynol-9, 12.5%)
> **Jellies and Creams** —
> 　　　　　　Conceptrol (nonoxynol-9, 4%)
> 　　　　　　Delfen (nonoxynol-9, 12.5%)
> 　　　　　　Ortho Gynol (nonoxynol-9, 3%)
> 　　　　　　Ramses (nonoxynol-9, 5%)
> 　　　　　　Koromex Jelly (nonoxynol-9, 3%)
> Suppositories —
> 　　　　　　Encare (nonoxynol-9, 2.27%)
> 　　　　　　Koromex Inserts (nonoxynol-9, 125 mg)
> 　　　　　　Semicid (nonoxynol-9, 100 mg)

"Advantage 24" is a contraceptive gel that adheres to the vaginal mucosa and provides longer availability of nonoxynol-9; it is intended to be effective for 24 hours. Although available without prescription, adequate clinical trial data are not available.

Efficacy

Only periodic abstinence demonstrates as wide a range of efficacy in different studies as do the studies of spermicides. Efficacy seems to depend more on the population studied than the agent used. Efficacy ranges from less than 1% failure to nearly one-third in the first year of use. Failure rates of approximately 20% during a year's use are most typical.[3] There are no comparative studies to indicate which preparations, if any, are better or worse.

Spermicides require application 10–30 minutes prior to sexual intercourse. Jellies, creams, and foams remain effective for as long as 8 hours, but tablets and suppositories are good for less than one hour. If ejaculation does not occur within the period of effectiveness, the spermicide should be reapplied. Reapplication should definitely take place for each coital episode.

Vaginal douches are ineffective contraceptives even if they contain spermicidal agents. Postcoital douching is too late to prevent the rapid ascent of sperm (within seconds) to the fallopian tubes.

Advantages

Spermicides are relatively inexpensive and widely available in many retail outlets without prescription. This makes spermicides popular among adolescents and others who have infrequent or unpredictable sexual intercourse. In addition, spermicides are simple to use.

Spermicides provide protection against sexually transmitted diseases. In vitro studies have demonstrated that contraceptive spermicides kill or inactivate most STD pathogens, including HIV. Spermicides have been reported to prevent HIV seroconversion as well as to have no effect.[27–29] Clinical studies indicate reductions in the risk of gonorrhea,[30–32] pelvic infections,[33] and chlamydial infection.[30,32] There is little difference in the incidence of trichomoniasis, candidiasis, or bacterial vaginosis among spermicide users.[34]

Side Effects

No serious side effects or safety problems have arisen in all the years that spermicides have been used. The only serious question raised was that of a possible association between spermicide use and congenital abnormalities or spontaneous abortions. Epidemiologic analysis, including a meta-analysis, concluded that there is insufficient evidence to support these associations.[35–37] Spermicides are not absorbed through the vaginal mucosa in concentrations high enough to have systemic effects.[38] Vaginal and cervical mucosal damage has been observed with nonoxynol-9, and the overall impact on HIV transmission, although unknown, is of concern.[39,40]

The principal minor problem is allergy which occurs in 1–5% of users, related to either the vehicle or the spermicidal agent. Utilizing a different product often solves the problem.

Condoms

Six billion condoms were distributed world-wide in 1990. However, if condoms had been used in every sex act where they were needed, more than 12 billion would have been needed. Although awareness of condoms as an effective contraceptive method as well as protectors against STDs has increased tremendously in recent years, a great deal remains to be accomplished in order to reach the appropriate level of condom use. Contraceptive efficacy and STD prevention must be linked together and publicly promoted. The male condom is the only contraceptive proven to prevent HIV infection.

There are three specific goals: correct use, consistent use, and affordable, easy availability. If these goals are met, the year 2000 will see the annual manufacture of 20 billion condoms.

Various types of condoms are available. Most are made of latex; polyurethane and silicone rubber condoms are also now manufactured. "Natural skin" (lamb's intestine) condoms are still obtainable (about 1% of sales). Latex condoms are 0.3–0.8 mm thick. Sperm which are 0.003 mm in diameter cannot penetrate condoms. The organisms which cause STDs and AIDS also do not penetrate latex condoms, but they can penetrate condoms made from intestine.[41,42] Polyurethane condoms are expected to protect against STDs and HIV, based upon in vitro efficacy as a barrier to bacteria and viruses. Condom use (latex) also probably prevents transmission of human papillomavirus (HPV), the cause of condylomata acuminata. Because spermicides provide significant protection against STDs, condoms and spermicides used together offer more protection than either method used alone. The use of spermicides (or spermicide-coated condoms), however, increases the incidcence of *E. coli* bacteriuria because of the spermicide-induced alteration in vaginal fora.[16] Consistent use of condoms when one partner is HIV seropositive is highly effective in preventing HIV transmission (there was no seroconversion in 124 couples who used condoms consistently compared to 12.7% conversion after 24 months in couples with inconsistent use.[43] Women who are partners of condom users are less likely to be HIV positive.[44]

Condoms can be straight or tapered, smooth or ribbed, colored or clear, lubricated or nonlubricated. These are all marketing ventures aimed at attracting individual notions of pleasure and enjoyment.[45] Condoms which incorporate a spermicidal agent coating the inner and outer surfaces logically promise greater efficacy, but this remains to be determined. Some women are allergic to the spermicide, and it is a concern (not documented) that mucosal lesions can promote HIV transmission should a condom break.

An often repeated concern is the alleged reduction in penile glans sensitivity that accompanies condom use.[45] This has never been objectively studied, and it is likely that this complaint is perception (or excuse) not based on reality. A clinician can overcome this obstruction by advocating the use of thinner (and more esoteric) condoms, knowing that any difference is also more of perception than reality.

As is true for most contraceptive methods, older, married couples experienced in using condoms and strongly motivated to avoid another pregnancy are much more effective users than young, unmarried couples with little contraceptive experience. This does not mean that condoms are not useful contraceptives for adolescents, who are likely to have sex unexpectedly or infrequently. The recent decline in the teen pregnancy rate may reflect wider use of condoms by teens concerned about avoiding HIV infection.

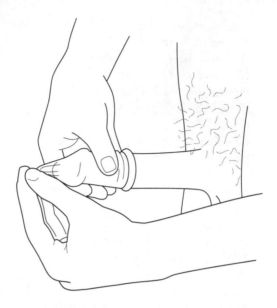

Prospective users need instructions if they are to avoid pregnancy and STDs. A condom must be placed on the penis before it touches a partner. Uncircumcised men must pull the foreskin back. Prior to unrolling the condom to the base of the penis, air should be squeezed out of the reservoir tip with a thumb and forefinger. The tip of the condom should extend beyond the end of the penis to provide a reservoir to collect the ejaculate (a half inch of pinched tip). If lubricants are used, they must be water based. Oil based lubricants (such as Vaseline) will weaken the latex. Couples should be concerned that any vaginal medication can compromise condom integrity. After intercourse, the condom should be held at the base as the still erect penis is withdrawn. Semen must not be allowed to spill or leak. The condom should be handled gently as finger nails and rings can penetrate the latex and cause leakage. If there is evidence of spill or leakage, a spermicidal agent should be quickly inserted into the vagina.

These instructions should be provided to new users of condoms who are likely to be reluctant to ask questions. Most condoms are acquired without medical supervision, and therefore, clinicians should use every opportunity to inform patients about their proper use.

Inconsistent use explains most condom failures. Incorrect use accounts for additional failures, and also, condoms sometimes break. Breakage rates range from 1–12 per 100 episodes of vaginal intercourse (and somewhat higher for anal intercourse). In a U.S. survey, one pregnancy resulted for every 3 condom breakages.[46] Concomitant use of spermicides lowers failure rates in case of breakage.

Breakage is a greater problem for couples at risk for STDs. An infected man transmits gonorrhea to a susceptible woman about two-thirds of the time.[47] If the woman is infected, transmission to the man occurs one-third of the time.[48] The chances of HIV infection after a single sexual exposure ranges from one in 1,000 to one in 10.[49,50]

Condom breakage rates depend upon sexual behavior and practices, experience with condom use, the condition of the condoms, and manufacturing quality. Condoms remain in good condition for up to 5 years unless exposed to ultraviolet light, excessive heat or humidity, ozone, or oils. Condom manufacturers regularly check samples of their products to make sure they meet national standards. These procedures limit the proportion of defects to less than 0.1% of all condoms distributed. Contraceptive failure is more likely to be due to nonuse or incorrect use.

When a condom breaks, or if there is reason to believe spillage or leakage occurred, a woman should contact a clinician within 72 hours. Emergency contraception, as discussed in Chapter 3, should be provided. Couples who rely upon condoms for contraception should be educated regarding emergency contraception and an appropriate supply of oral contraceptives should be kept available for self-medication (Chapter 3).

For the immediate future, prevention of STDs and control of the AIDS epidemic will require a great increase in the use of condoms. We must all be involved in the effort to promote condom use. Condom use must be portrayed in the positive light of STD prevention. The main motivation for condom use among women continues to be prevention of pregnancy, not prevention of STDs.[44,51] An important area of concentration is the teaching of the social skills required to ensure use by a reluctant partner. We believe that bans on condom advertising should be eliminated. Using scare tactics about STDs in order to encourage condom use is not sufficient. A more positive approach can yield better compliance. It is useful to emphasize that prevention of STDs will preserve future fertility.

We suggest that clinicians consider making free condoms available in their office. Manufacturers will sell condoms at a bulk rate, from $50–$100 per 1,000, depending upon style and lubrication.

U.S. Condom Manufacturers:
 Ansell Health Care (telephone: 800–327–8659)
 Carter Products (telephone: 609–655–6000)
 Meyer Laboratories (telephone: 800–426–6366)
 Okamoto USA (telephone: 800–283–7546)
 Schmid Laboratories (telephone: 800–829–0987)

The Female Condom

The female condom is a pouch made of polyurethane, which lines the vagina.[52] An internal ring in the closed end of the pouch covers the cervix and an external ring remains outside the vagina, partially covering the perineum. The female condom is prelubricated with silicone, and a spermicide need not be used. The female condom should be an effective barrier to STD infection;[53] however, high cost and acceptability are major problems. The devices are more cumbersome than condoms, and studies have indicated relatively high rates of problems such as slippage.[54] Women who have successfully used barrier methods and who are strongly motivated to avoid STDs are more likely to choose the female condom. With careful use, the efficacy rate should be similar to that of the diaphragm and the cervical cap.[55]

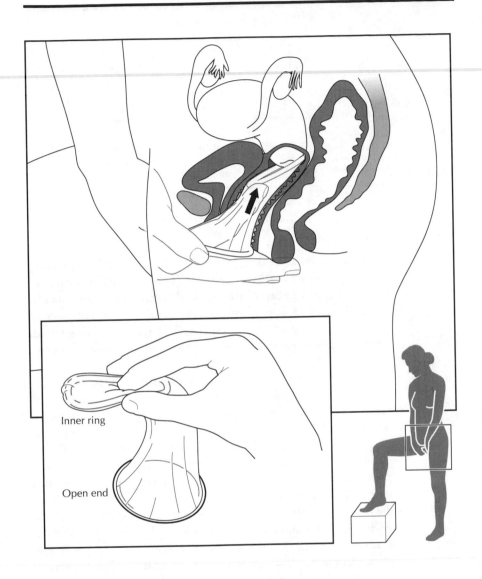

Inner ring

Open end

	Diaphragm	Cap	Sponge	Female Condom
Insertion before coitus, no longer than:	6 hrs	6 hrs	24 hrs	8 hrs
After coitus, should be left in place for:	6 hrs	8 hrs	6 hrs	6 hrs
Maximal wear time:	24 hrs	48 hrs	30 hrs	8 hrs

Future Developments

New barrier devices are being pursued, such as sponges incorporating several spermicides and cervical caps made of different materials. Chemical agents are being investigated that can combine spermicidal and antimicrobial actions, and vaginal spermicidal films of different materials and containing other spermicidal agents are being tested. Disposable diaphragms that release spermicide are in development.

Lea's Shield is a vaginal barrier contraceptive composed of silicone.[56,57] This soft, pliable device comes in one size and fits over the cervix, held in place by the pressure of the vaginal wall around it. There is a collapsible valve that communicates with a 9 mm opening in the bowl that fits over the cervix. This valve allows equalization of air pressure during insertion and drainage of cervical secretions and discharge, permitting a snug fit over the cervix. A thick U-shaped loop attached to the anterior side of the bowl is used to stabilize the device during insertion and for removal. The thicker part of the device is shaped to fill the posterior fornix, thus contributing to its placement and stability over the cervix. The addition of a spermicide, placed in the bowl, is recommended to enhance STD protection. Lea's Shield is designed to remain in place for 48 hours after intercourse. Clinical studies regarding efficacy and side effects are not yet available.

References

1. Himes NE, *Medical History of Contraception,* Williams & Wilkins Co., Baltimore, 1936.

2. Gamble CJ, Spermicidal times as aids to the clinician's choice of contraceptive materials, Fertil Steril 8:174, 1957.

3. Trussell J, Hatcher RA, Cates W Jr, Stewart FH, Kost K, Contraceptive failure in the United States: an update, Stud Fam Plann 21:51, 1990.

4. Grimes DA, Cates W Jr, Family planning and sexually transmitted diseases, in Holmes KK, Mardh P-A, Sparling PF, (editors), *Sexually Transmitted Diseases,* ed 2, McGraw-Hill, New York, 1990, pp 1087–1094.

5. Cramer DW, Goldman MB, Schiff I, Belisla S, Albrecht B, Stadel B, Gibson M, Wilson E, Stillman R, Thompson I, The relationship of tubal infertility to barrier method and oral contraceptive use, JAMA 257:2446, 1987.

6. Rosenberg MJ, Davidson AJ, Chen J-H, Judson FN, Douglas JM, Barrier contraceptives and sexually transmitted diseases in women: a comparison of female-dependent methods and condoms, Am J Pub Health 82:669, 1992.

7. Cates W, Stone K, Family planning, sexually transmitted diseases and contraceptive choice: a literature update: part I, Fam Plann Perspect 24:75, 1992.

8. Rowe PJ, You win some and you lose some — contraception and infections, Aust N Z Obstet Gynaecol 34:299, 1994.

9. Kost K, Forrest JD, Harlap S, Comparing the health risks and benefits of contraceptive choices, Fam Plann Perspect 23:54, 1991.

10. Coker AL, Hulka BS, McCann MF, Walton LA, Barrier methods of contraception and cervical intraepithelial neoplasia, Contraception 45:1, 1992.

11. Schwartz B, Gaventa S, Broome CV, Reingold AL, Hightower AW, Perlman JA, Wolf PH, Nonmenstrual toxic shock syndrome associated with barrier contraceptives: report of a case-control study, Rev Infect Dis 11(Suppl):S43, 1989.

12. Klonoff-Cohen HS, Savitz DA, Cefalo RC, McCann MF, An epidemiologic study of contraception and preeclampsia, JAMA 62:3143, 1989.

13. Mills JL, Klebanoff MA, Graubard BI, Carey JC, Berendes HW, Barrier contraceptive methods and preeclampsia, JAMA 265:70, 1991.

14. Craig S, Hepburn S, The effectiveness of barrier methods of contraception with and without spermicide, Contraception 26:347, 1982.

15. **Fihn SD, Latham RH, Roberts P, Running K, Stamm WE,** Association between diaphragm use and urinary tract infection, JAMA 254:240, 1985.

16. **Hooton TM, Hillier S, Johnson C, Roberts P, Stamm WE,** *Escherichia coli* bacteriuria and contraceptive method, JAMA 265:64, 1991.

17. **Centers for Disease Control,** Toxic shock syndrome, United States, 1970–1982, MMWR 31:201, 1982.

18. **Keith L, Berger G, Moss W,** Prevalence of gonorrhea among women using various methods of contraception, Br J Venereal Dis 51:307, 1975.

19. **Kelaghan J, Rubin GL, Ory HW, Layde PM,** Barrier method contraceptives and pelvic inflammatory disease, JAMA 248:184, 1982.

20. **Bernstein G, Kilzer LH, Coulson AH, Nakamara RM, Smith GC, Bernstein R, Frezieres R, Clark VA, Coan C,** Studies of cervical caps, Contraception 26:443, 1982.

21. **Richwald GA, Greenland S, Gerber MM, Potik R, Kersey L, Comas MA,** Effectiveness of the cavity-rim cervical cap: results of a large clinical study, Obstet Gynecol 74:143, 1989.

22. **Gollub EL, Sivin I,** The Prentif cervical cap and pap smear results: a critical appraisal, Contraception 40:343, 1989.

23. **Shihata AA, Trussell J,** New female intravaginal barrier contraceptive device, Contraception 44:11, 1991.

24. **Edelman DA, McIntyre SL, Harper J,** A comparative trial of the Today contraceptive sponge and diaphragm: a preliminary report, Am J Obstet Gynecol 150:869, 1984.

25. **McIntyre SL, Higgins JE,** Parity and use-effectiveness with the contraceptive sponge, Am J Obstet Gynecol 155:796, 1986.

26. **Costello Daly C, Helling-Giese GE, Mati JK, Hunter DJ,** Contraceptive methods and the transmission of HIV: implications for family planning, Genitourin Med 70:110, 1994.

27. **Hicks DR, Martin LS, Getchell JP, Heath JL, Francis DP, McDougal JS, Curran JW, Voeller B,** Inactivation of HTLV-III/LAV-infected cultures of normal human lymphocytes by nonoxynol-9 in vitro, Lancet 2:1422, 1985.

28. **Kreiss J, Ngugi E, Holmes K, Ndinya-Achola J, Waiyaki P, Roberts PL, Ruminjo I, Sajabi R, Kimata J, Fleming TR, Anzala A, Holton D, Plummer F,** Efficacy of nonoxynol-9 contraceptive sponge use in preventing heterosexual acquisition of HIV in Nairobi prostitutes, JAMA 268:477, 1992.

29. **Zekeng L, Feldblum PJ, Oliver RM, Kaptue L,** Barrier contraceptive use and HIV infection among high risk women in Cameroon, AIDS 7:725, 1993.

30. Louv WC, Austin H, Alexander WJ, Stagno S, Cheeks J, A clinical trial of nonoxynol-9 as a prophylaxis for cervical Neisseria gonorrhoeae and Chlamydia trachomatis infections, J Infect Dis 158:518, 1988.

31. Austin H, Louv WC, Alexander WJ, A case-control study of spermicides and gonorrhea, JAMA 251:2822, 1984.

32. Niruthisard S, Roddy RE, Chutivongse S, Use of nonoxynol-9 and reduction in rate of gonococcal and chlamydial cervical infections, Lancet 339:1371, 1992.

33. Kelaghan J, Rubin GL, Ory HW, Layde PM, Barrier-method contraceptives and pelvic inflammatory disease, JAMA 248:184, 1982.

34. Barbone F, Austin H, Louv WC, Alexander WJ, A follow-up study of methods of contraception, sexual activity, and rates of trichomoniasis, candidiasis, and bacterial vaginosis, Am J Obstet Gynecol 163:510, 1990.

35. Louik C, Mitchell AA, Werler MM, Hanson JW, Shapiro S, Maternal exposure to spermicides in relation to certain birth defects, New Engl J Med 317:474, 1987.

36. Bracken MB, Vita K, Frequency of non-hormonal contraception around conception and association with congenital malformations in offspring, Am J Epidemiol 117:281, 1983.

37. Einarson TR, Koren G, Mattice D, Schechter-Tsafriri O, Maternal spermicide use and adverse reproductive outcome: a meta-analysis, Am J Obstet Gynecol 162:655, 1990.

38. Malyk B, Preliminary results: serum chemistry values before and after the intravaginal administration of 5% nonoxynol-9 cream, Fertil Steril 35:647, 1981.

39. Niruthisard S, Roddy RE, Chutivonge S, The effects of frequent nonoxynol-9 use on vaginal and cervical mucosa, STD 268:521, 1991.

40. Roddy RE, Cordero M, Cordero C, Fortney JA, A dosing study of nonoxynol-9 and genital irritation, AIDS 4:165, 1993.

41. Stone KM, Grimes DA, Magder LS, Primary prevention of sexually transmitted diseases. A primer for clinicians, JAMA 255:1763, 1986.

42. Van de Perre P, Jacobs D, Sprecher-Goldberger S, The latex condom, an efficient barrier against sexual transmission of AIDS-related viruses, AIDS 1:49, 1987

43. DeVincenzi I, for the European Study Group on Heterosexual Transmission of HIV, A longitudinal study of human immunodeficiency virus transmission by heterosexual partners, New Engl J Med 331:341, 1994.

44. Diaz T, Schable B, Chu SY, and the Supplement to HIV and AIDS Surveillance Project Group, Relationship between use of condoms and other forms of contraception among human immunodeficiency virus-infected women, Obstet Gynecol 86:277, 1995.

45. Grady WR, Klepinger DH, Billy JOG, Tanfer K, Condom characteristics: the perceptions and preferences of men in the United States, Fam Plann Perspect 25:67, 1993.

46. **Population Infomation Program,** Condoms, now more than ever, Population Reports, H-81, The Johns Hopkins University, 1990, p 11.

47. **Platt R, Rice PA, McCormack WM,** Risk of acquiring gonorrhea and prevalence of abnormal adnexal findings among women recently exposed to gonorrhea, JAMA 250:3205, 1983.

48. **Hooper RR, Reynolds GM, Jones OG, Zaidi A, Wiesner RJ, Latimer KP, Lester A, Campbell AF, Harrison WO, Karney WW, Holmes KK,** Cohort study of venereal disease. I. The risk of gonorrhea transmission from infected women to men, Am J Epidemiol 108:136, 1978.

49. **Anderson RM, Medley GF,** Epidemiology of HIV infection and AIDS: incubation and infectious periods, survival and vertical transmissions, AIDS 2 (Suppl 1):557, 1988.

50. **Cameron DW, Simonsen JN, D'Costa LJ, et al,** Female to male transmission of human immunodeficiency virus type 1: risk factors for seroconverison in men, Lancet 2:403, 1989.

51. **Fleisher JM, Senie RT, Minkoff H, Jaccard J,** Condom use relative to knowledge of sexually transmitted disease prevention, method of birth control, and past or present infection, J Comm Health 19:395, 1994.

52. **Soper DE, Brockwell NJ, Dalton JP,** Evaluation of the effects of a female condom on the female lower genital tract, Contraception 44:21, 1991.

53. **Drew WL, Blair M, Miner RC, Conant M,** Evaluation of the virus permeability of a new condom for women, STD 17:110, 1990.

54. **Bounds W, Guillebaud J, Newman GB,** Female condom (Femidom). A clinical study of its use-effectiveness and patient acceptability, Br J Fam Plann 18:36, 1992.

55. **Trussell J, Sturgen K, Strickler J, Dominik R,** Comparative contraceptive efficacy of the female condom and other barrier methods, Fam Plann Perspect 26:66, 1994.

56. **Hunt WL, Gabbay L, Potts M,** Lea's Shield®, a new barrier contraceptive; preliminary clinical evaluations, three-day tolerance study, Contraception 50:551, 1994.

57. **Archer DF, Mauck CK, Viniegra-Sibal A, Anderson FD,** Lea's Shield®: a phase I postcoital study of a new contraceptive barrier device, Contraception 52:167, 1995.

8

Periodic Abstinence

PERIODIC ABSTINENCE as a method of contraception is keyed to the observation of naturally occurring signs and symptoms of the fertile phase of the menstrual cycle. This method must take into account the viability of sperm in the female reproductive tract (2 to 7 days) and the lifespan of the ovum (1–3 days). The variability in the timing of ovulation is the reason why the period of abstinence must be relatively lengthy unless barrier methods are used during the fertile days.

The period of maximal fertility begins 5 days before the day of ovulation and ends on the day of ovulation.[1] The probability of conception is abruptly lost the day after ovulation; however, conception occasionally occurs more than 6 days before ovulation or immediately following ovulation.[2] The likelihood of pregnancy steadily increases during this period of fertility and is highest the day of ovulation and the preceding 2 days.[1,2] Ovulation occurs at the following median times (note the relatively wide ranges):[3]

- 16 hours after the LH peak (range 8–40 hours).
- 24 hours after the estradiol peak (range 17–32 hours).
- 8 hours after the rise in progesterone (range 12.5 hours before to 16 hours after).

Approximately 1% of reproductive age women in the United States utilized some method of fertility timing in 1988.[4] This represented

263

a dramatic decline since the 1960s.[5] This method requires commitment from both partners; it is a way of life. Unsuccessful use can be predicted in couples who are unable to part with sexual spontaneity, women with irregular menses, disorganized people who cannot keep good records, and women with chronic problems of vaginitis or cervicitis. The advantage of periodic abstinence as a method of contraception is the availability of this method irregardless of economic status or the accessibility of other methods. Users of this method also avoid religious proscription and the need to use "unnatural" substances.

Methods

Although there are several specific methods, most teachers of periodic abstinence advocate the incorporation of features from more than one method.[6] The sophistication of these methods was made possible by the tremendous increase in the scientific knowledge of the events in the human menstrual cycle. The time of ovulation (the fertile period) was identified in the 1930s, but it wasn't until the 1960s with the advent of the radioimmunoassay, that relatively precise timing of the various events became possible.

The Rhythm or Calendar Method

This method of periodic abstinence was based on the assumption that menstrual cycles were relatively constant, and therefore, the fertile period of the subsequent month could be predicted by the timing of the past cycle.

The general rule is to record the length of 6 cycles, then estimate the beginning of the fertile period by subtracting 18 days from the length of the shortest cycle, and to estimate the end of the fertile period by subtracting 11 days from the length of the longest cycle. Thus a woman with cycles varying from 26–32 days will practice periodic abstinence from the 8th day until the 21st day, a formidable requirement of 14 days of abstinence per cycle. Indeed, because of the normal variation in menstrual cycles, the average couple would practice periodic abstinence 16 days each month.

This method is useful only for women who have relatively regular and consistant menstrual cycles. This method has a pregnancy rate of about 40 per 100 woman-years, and therefore, it is not advocated without combining it with other techniques. However, the utilization of programmed electronic devices to record temperatures, keep track of cycles, and provide a signal to the patient to use a barrier method during the fertile period can reduce pregnancy rates to approximately 10 per 100 woman-years.[7]

The Cervical Mucus Method

The effectiveness of periodic abstinence has been improved by the development of methods that allow decisions to be made within each cycle. The cervical mucus method is also called the ovulation method, or the Billings method.[8] This method requires sensing or observing the cervical mucus changes over time. A woman successfully practicing this method must become aware of the estrogen-induced changes in cervical mucus which occur at midcycle: an increase in the amount of clear, thin, stringy mucus. Practitioners of this method describe these changes as wet, sticky (but slippery), and moist. The day of ovulation corresponds closely to the day of peak mucus. This method requires the maintenance of a daily record, at least in the beginning.

The rules for intercourse are as follows:

- Not on consecutive days during the postmenstrual preovulatory period so that seminal fluid will not obscure observation of cervical mucus changes.
- Abstinence when the mucus becomes sticky and moist.
- Intercourse is permitted beginning on the 4th day after the last day of sticky, wet mucus.

The Symptothermal Method

This method utilizes at least two indicators to identify the fertile period, usually combining the cervical mucus method with the basal body temperature (BBT). The BBT is recorded with any thermometer before getting out of bed. Prior to ovulation the temperature is usually below the normal body temperature. It rises about 0.2–0.4° C or 0.4–0.8° F in response to the increasing levels of progesterone after ovulation. The BBT method is so variable that, if practiced alone, it requires abstinence until the night of the 3rd day of a shift in temperature.

Combining the BBT with the mucus method, abstinence begins when the mucus becomes sticky and moist. Intercourse resumes the night of either the 3rd day of a temperature shift or the 4th day after

265

the last day of sticky, wet mucus, whichever is later. Although this method is more complicated, the efficacy is slightly better, even approaching only 2 failures per 100 woman-years when practiced by experienced couples who follow all the rules.[9]

Individual women can be taught to incorporate other signals into their periodic abstinence method. For many women these additional signs and symptoms can add accuracy. These signals include mittleschmerz, breast tenderness, and changes in cervical position and texture.

Resources

It is too much to expect the average clinician to provide the necessary instruction and support for these methods. Referral to a local resource is both appropriate and recommended. The local affiliate of the Planned Parenthood Federation of America can direct a clinician to a community program. A directory of all methods and related resources in the U.S., including support groups, is available:

> Cooper SA, *Fertility Awareness and Natural Family Planning Resource Directory,* Small World Publications, Corvallis, Oregon, 1988.

Most teachers of this method utilize detailed charts for recording changes and signals. The following resources can be contacted for advice, charts, and teaching plans:

> Los Angeles Regional Family Planning Council
> 3600 Wilshire Boulevard
> Los Angeles, California 90010

> The Couple to Couple League Foundation
> PO Box 111184
> Cincinnati, Ohio 45211

> Natural Family Planning Program
> Center for Life
> 498 O'Connor Drive
> San Jose, California 95128

Efficacy

The World Health Organization completed a remarkable clinical trial of the periodic abstinence method of contraception in 725 couples in 5 countries: New Zealand, India, Ireland, the Phillipines, and El Salvador.[10–14] The objectives were to determine whether the method could be taught to women of widely different educational and socioeconomical status and to document the effectiveness. 97% of the subjects learned the method well.

The WHO defined failures with periodic abstinence as follows:

- Method-related (pregnancies that occur despite correct application of the rules).
- Inadequate teaching.
- Inaccurate application of instructions.
- Conscious departure from the rules.
- Uncertain.

Among those who learned the method, the pregnancy rate was 22.5 per 100 woman-years; however, almost all failures could be attributed to a conscious departure from the rules. Abstinence was necessary for about 17 days in each cycle.

Using the WHO data and a strict application of the definitions for method and use failure, method failure during the first year was associated with only a 3.1% pregnancy rate, but imperfect use with a 86.4% rate.[14] *Thus, if used perfectly, the method is very effective, but all methods of periodic abstinence are extremely unforgiving of imperfect use.*

The probability of pregnancy is greatest when any of the following 3 rules are broken:[15]

- No intercourse during mucus days.
- No intercourse within 3 days after peak fecundity.
- No intercourse during times of stress.

267

Analysis of the periodic abstinence experience provides these conclusions:[15]

1. Periodic abstinence is associated with good efficacy when used correctly and consistently, but the method is very unforgiving of imperfect use.
2. There is an increased risk of pregnancy during periods of stress.
3. Couples with a poor attitude towards the rules are more likely to take risks.
4. Those couples who get away with taking risks are more likely to take risks again.

A multicenter trial in the 1970s of the cervical mucus method in the U.S. documented over a 2-year period of time, a method failure rate of 1.2 pregnancies per 100 woman-years, and a user failure rate of 19.3 pregnancies per 100 woman-years.[16] In the 1990s, the pregnancy rates reported throughout the world have ranged from 2 to 11 pregnancies per 100 woman-years.[17]

The cervical mucus method has been compared to the symptothermal method.[18,19] Again, most pregnancies came from conscious departure from the rules. The two methods were comparable, with pregnancy rates of 20–24%.

Couples who do practice periodic abstinence successfully report no significant increase in marital-domestic friction, and some argue that the cooperation and communication required for the use of this method improve a relationship.

Concerns

A lingering concern is that because of periodic abstinence, inadvertent fertilization could occur with aged gametes. Is pregnancy from aged gametes more likely to result in birth defects, spontaneous abortions, and chromosome abnormalities?

No differences have been noted in the frequency of monosomic or trisomic abnormalities in relation to the timing of conception; however, conceptions with post-ovulatory aged ova appear to be at increased risk of polyploidy.[20] Furthermore, there is evidence, although not conclusive, to suggest that aged gametes have an increased risk of spontaneous abortions, as well as chromosomal defects.[21] In one cohort of women, an effect of aging sperm or oocytes on the risk of spontaneous abortion was present only in women who had a history of recurrent pregnancy losses.[22] In what is regarded as a well-designed, case-control study, increased relative risks for cleft lip and palate, and congenital hydrocele were associated with periodic abstinence.[23] However, because of small numbers and the very difficult problem of recall bias, it is uncertain if this later observation is real or due to chance.

It is worth emphasizing that the well-done and large WHO prospective trial observed no increase in congenital malformations, stillbirths, or spontaneous abortions.[13]

Evidence does support the idea that the further away from the time of highest fertility fertilization occurs, the more likely a male child will be conceived.[24] If this is true, the effect is not great, a ratio of approximately 58 males to 42 females. Here too, the WHO prospective clinical trial failed to detect any difference in the male to female ratio.[13] Others have also reported that the day of conception does not influence the sex ratio.[1]

Conclusion

In our view, periodic abstinence is best suited for married couples who are united in their motivation to practice this method. Use of periodic abstinence is possible during lactation, but scrupulous attention is required to detect impending ovulation. With typical practice of the method, the pregnancy rate is about the same as with diaphragm and spermicides.

The problem of a long period of abstinence can be overcome by using a barrier method or spermicides during the fertile period. This combination is associated with an efficacy rate that is surpassed only by oral contraception, the IUD, and the sustained release methods.[25]

References

1. **Wilcox AJ, Weionberg CR, Baird DD,** Timing of sexual intercourse in relation to ovulation. Effects on the probability of conception, survival of the pregnancy, and sex of the baby, New Engl J Med 333:1517, 1995.

2. **Simpson JL, Gray RH, Queenan JJ, Mena P, Perez A, Kambic RT, Paredo F, Barbato M, Spieler J,** Timing of intercourse, Hum Reprod 10:2176, 1995.

3. **WHO,** Temporal relationships between ovulation and defined changes in the concentration of plasma estradiol-17beta, luteinizing hormone, follicle-stimulating hormone and progesterone. I. Probit analysis, Am J Obstet Gynecol 138:383, 1980.

4. **Mosher WD, Pratt WF,** Contraceptive use in the United States, 1973–88. Advance data from vital and health statistics; No. 182, National Center for Health Statistics, Hyattsville, Maryland, 1990.

5. **Forrest J, Fordyce R,** U.S. women's contraceptive attitudes and practice: How have they changed in the 80s? Fam Plann Perspect 20:112, 1988.

6. **Labbok MH, Queenan JT,** The use of periodic abstinence for family planning, Clin Obstet Gynecol 32:387, 1989.

7. **Drouin J, Guilbert EE, Désaulniers G,** Contraceptive application of the Bioself fertility indicator, Contraception 50:229, 1994.

8. **Billings EL, Billings JJ, Catarinich M,** *Atlas of the Ovulation Method,* 2nd edition, Advocate Press, Melbourne, 1974.

9. **Frank-Hermann P, Freundl G, Baur S, Bremme M, Döring GK, Godehart EAJ, Sottong V,** Effectiveness and acceptability of the symptothermal method of natural family planning in Germany, Am J Obstet Gynecol 165:2052, 1991.

10. **WHO,** A prospective multicenter trial of the ovulation method of natural family planning. I. The teaching phase, Fertil Steril 36:152, 1981.

11. **WHO,** A prospective multicenter trial of the ovulation method of natural family planning. II. The effectiveness phase, Fertil Steril 36:591, 1981.

12. **WHO,** A prospective multicenter trial of the ovulation method of natural family planning. III. Characteristics of the menstrual cycle and of the fertile phase, Fertil Steril 40:773, 1983.

13. **WHO,** A prospective multicenter trial of the ovulation method of natural family planning. IV. The outcome of pregnancy, Fertil Steril 41:593, 1984.

14. **WHO,** A prospective multicenter trial of the ovulation method of natural family planning. V. Psychosexual aspects, Fertil Steril 47:765l, 1987.

15. **Trussell J, Grummer-Strawn L,** Contraceptive failure of the ovulation method of periodic abstinence, Fam Plann Perspect 22:65, 1990.

16. **Klaus H. Goebel JM, Muraski B, Egizio MT, Wetzel D, Taylor RS, Fagan MU, Ek K, Hobday K,** Use-effectiveness and client satisfaction in six centers teaching the Billings ovulation method, Contraception 19:613, 1979.

17. **Ryder B, Campbell H,** Natural family planning in the 1990s, Lancet 346:233, 1995.

18. **Medina JE, Cifuentes A, Abernathy JR, Spieler SM, Wade ME,** Comparative evaluation of two methods of natural family planning in Columbia, Am J Obstet Gynecol 138:1142, 1980.

19. **Wade ME, McCarthy P, Braunstein GD, Abernathy JR, Suchindram CM, Harris GS, Danzer HC, Vricchio WA,** A randomized prospective study of the use-effectiveness of two methods of natural family planning, Am J Obstet Gynecol 141:368, 1981.

20. **Boue J, Boue A, Lazar P,** Retrospective and prospective epidemiological studies of 1500 karyotyped spontaneous abortions, Teratology 12:11, 1975.

21. **Gray RH, Kambic RT,** Epidemiologial studies of natural family planning, Hum Reprod 3:693, 1988.

22. **Gray RH, Simpson JL, Kambic RT, Queenan JT, Mena P, Perez A, Barbato M,** Timing of conception and the risk of spontaneous abortion among pregnancies occurring during the use of natural family planning, Am J Obstet Gynecol 172:1567, 1995.

23. **Bracken MB, Vita K,** Frequency of nonhormonal contraception around conception and association with congenital malformations in offspring, Am J Epidemiol 117:281, 1983.

24. **Kambic R, Gray RH, Simpson JL,** Outcome of pregnancy in users of natural family planning, Int J Gynecol Obstet Suppl 1:99, 1989.

25. **Rogow D, Rintoul EJ, Greenwood S,** A year's experience with a fertility awareness program: a report, Adv Plann Parenthood 15:27, 1980.

9

The Postpartum Period, Breastfeeding and Contraception

BREASTFEEDING PROTECTS infants against infection, offers an inexpensive supply of nutrition, contributes to maternal-infant bonding, and provides contraception. The relationship between lactation and fertility is an important public health issue. A birth interval of two or more years improves infant survival and reduces maternal morbidity.[1] In developing countries, breastfeeding provides protection from pregnancy and is important for achieving the two-year birth interval.

Giving up breastfeeding was a misguided notion of civilized times. Urbanization, education, and modernization all contributed to a decline in breastfeeding, which, fortunately, has been somewhat reversed. Even in ancient Greek and Roman societies, breastfeeding was disdained by the elite. The tradition of wet nursing (the practice of breastfeeding by someone other than the mother) was popular from the days of the ancient Greeks to the time of medieval Europe.[2] A further decline in breastfeeding came with the introduction of bottle feeding.

The domestication of cattle dates back thousands of years, but the use of animal milk for infant feeding is recent. In the U.S., modification of cow's milk for infant feeding was not established until 1900. In the early 1900s, milk banks were popular, using freezing techniques to keep the milk sterile. But it wasn't until the 1930s that the preparation of infant "formulas" moved from the home kitchen to commercial production and promotion. Breast milk substitutes were initially developed to meet specific needs (allergies and intolerance with cow's milk), but eventually came to be viewed as a means to free women from the responsibility of breastfeeding.

A decline in breastfeeding began in the 1930s (in 1922, about 90% of infants were still being breastfed at one year of age). By the 1950s, the prevalence of breastfeeding on discharge from the hospital fell to 30%, and the downward trend reached its nadir (22%) in 1972.[3] This trend was followed in Europe a decade or two later.

A higher mortality rate in artificially fed infants was observed in the 1900s. By the 1940s, the mortality difference between early and late weaned infants was recognized to be due to conditions of hygiene and general care. In the developed parts of the world, where infants receive good health supervision, the mortality difference is no longer a significant problem. However, in the developing world, excess mortality due to early weaning continues to be high.

The revival of breastfeeding can be attributed to the growth of knowledge regarding the health of infants. The following reasons emerged as motivations to encourage breastfeeding:

1. Breastfeeding has a child-spacing effect, which is very important in the developing world as a means of limiting family size.
2. Human milk prevents infections in infants, both by the transmission of immunoglobulins and by modifying the bacterial flora of the infant's gastrointestinal tract.
3. Breastfeeding enhances the bonding process between mother and child.
4. Breastfeeding provides some (not a great amount) of protection against breast cancer, perhaps limited to premenopausal breast cancer.

Breastfeeding is a personal choice, but one influenced by custom and social and economic circumstances. Beginning in the 1960s, breastfeeding became more popular in the U.S., Sweden, Canada, and the U.K.[3,4] Even in the developing world there was evidence of increased breastfeeding. In general, the knowledge that breastfeeding is superior was being spread. But this upward trend in the U.S. peaked in 1982 (at 61% for initiation and 40% for 3 or more months).[3]

Unfortunate, and somewhat perplexing (does it represent more women in the workforce?), is the fact that during the 1980s, there was a steady decline in breastfeeding, reaching 52% for initiation by 1989.[3] By age 6 months, only 19.6% of infants were still breastfeeding. The average duration remains short, usually under 6 months, and most often only 2–3 months. This still provides a significant benefit for the infant, but as we shall see, it is not so good from a contraceptive point of view.

Breast Physiology

The basic component of the breast is the hollow alveolus or milk gland lined by a single layer of milk-secreting epithelial cells. Each alveolus is encased in a crisscrossing mantle of contractile myoepithelial strands. Also surrounding the milk gland is a rich capillary network. Growth of this milk-producing system is dependent on numerous hormonal factors which occur first at puberty and then in pregnancy.

The major influence on breast growth at puberty is estrogen. In most girls, the first response to the increasing levels of estrogen is an increase in size and pigmentation of the areola and the formation of a mass of breast tissue just underneath the areola. Breast tissue binds estrogen in a manner similar to the uterus and vagina; however, the development of estrogen receptors in the breast does not occur in the absence of prolactin. The primary effect of estrogen according to animal studies is to stimulate growth of the ductal portion of the gland system. Progesterone in these animals influences growth of the alveolar components of the lobule. However, neither hormone alone, or in combination, is capable of yielding optimal breast growth and development.

The pubertal response is a manifestation of closely synchronized central (hypothalamus-pituitary) and peripheral (ovary-breast) events. This suggests a paracrine interaction between gonadotrophs and lactotrophs, linked by estrogen, ultimately with an impact on the breast. Changes occur routinely in response to the estrogen-progesterone sequence of a normal menstrual cycle. Maximal size of the breast occurs late in the luteal phase. Fluid secretion, mitotic activity, and DNA production of nonglandular tissue and glandular epithelium peak during the luteal phase.[5-7] This accounts for cystic and tender premenstrual changes.

Final differentiation of the alveolar epithelial cell into a mature milk cell during pregnancy is accomplished in the presence of prolactin, but only after prior exposure to cortisol and insulin. The complete reaction depends on the availability of minimal quantities of thyroid hormone. Thus, the endocrinologically intact individual in whom estrogen, progesterone, thyroxine, cortisol, insulin, prolactin, and growth hormone are available can have appropriate breast growth and function.[8,9] Mild deficiencies in any of the hormones, short of severe restrictions or total absence, can be compensated for by excess prolactin.

Lactation

During pregnancy, prolactin levels rise from the normal level of 10–25 ng/mL to high concentrations, beginning about 8 weeks and reaching a peak of 200–400 ng/mL at term.[10,11] Made by the placenta and actively secreted into the maternal circulation from the 6th week of pregnancy, human placental lactogen (HPL) rises progressively reaching a level of approximately 6,000 ng/mL at term. HPL, though displaying less activity than prolactin, is produced in such large amounts that it may exert a lactogenic effect.

Although prolactin stimulates significant breast growth, and is available for lactation, only colostrum (composed of desquamated epithelial cells and transudate) is produced during gestation. Full lactation is inhibited by progesterone which interferes with prolactin action at the alveolar cell prolactin receptor level. Both estrogen and progesterone are necessary for the expression of the lactogenic receptor, but progesterone antagonizes the positive action of prolactin on its own receptor while progesterone and pharmacologic amounts of androgens reduce prolactin binding.[12–14] The effective use of high doses of estrogen to suppress postpartum lactation suggests that pharmacologic amounts of estrogen also block prolactin action.

The principal hormone involved in milk biosynthesis is prolactin. Without prolactin, synthesis of the primary protein, casein, and the major carbohydrate, lactose, will not occur, and true milk secretion will be impossible. The hormonal trigger for initiation of milk production within the alveolar cell and its secretion into the lumen of the gland is the rapid disappearance of estrogen and progesterone from the circulation after delivery. The clearance of prolactin is much slower, requiring 7 days to reach nonpregnant levels in a nonbreastfeeding woman. These discordant hormonal events result in removal of the estrogen and progesterone inhibition of prolactin action on the breast. Breast engorgement and milk secretion begin 3–4 days postpartum when steroids have been sufficiently cleared. Maintenance of steroidal inhibition or rapid reduction of prolactin secretion (e.g., with the administration of bromocriptine) is effective in preventing postpartum milk synthesis and secretion.

In the first postpartum week, prolactin levels in breastfeeding women decline approximately 50% (to about 100 ng/mL). Suckling elicits increases in prolactin, which are important in initiating milk production. Until 2–3 months postpartum, basal levels are approximately 40–50 ng/mL, and there are large (about 10–20-fold) increases after suckling. Subsequently, throughout breastfeeding, baseline prolactin levels remain slightly elevated, and suckling produces a two-fold increase that is essential for continuing milk production.[15]

Secretion of calcium into the milk of lactating women approximately doubles the daily loss of calcium.[16] In women who breastfeed for 6 months or more, this is accompanied by significant bone loss even in the presence of a high calcium intake.[17] However, bone density rapidly returns to baseline levels in the 6 months after weaning.[17,18] The bone loss is due to increased bone resorption, probably secondary to the relatively low estrogen levels associated with lactation. It is possible that recovery is impaired in women with inadequate calcium intake; total calcium intake during lactation should be at least 1500 mg per day.

Antibodies are present in breast milk and contribute to the health of an infant. Human milk prevents infections in infants both by transmission of immunoglobulins and by modifying the bacterial flora of the infant's gastrointestinal tract. Viruses are transmitted in breast milk, and although the actual risks are unknown, women infected with cytomegalovirus, hepatitis B, or human immunodeficiency virus are advised not to breastfeed. Vitamin A, vitamin B_{12}, and folic acid are significantly reduced in the breast milk of women with poor dietary intake. As a general rule approximately 1% of any drug ingested by the mother appears in breast milk.

Maintenance of milk production at high levels is dependent on the joint action of anterior and posterior pituitary factors. Suckling causes the release of both prolactin and oxytocin.[19,20] Prolactin sustains the secretion of casein, fatty acids, lactose and the volume of secretion, while oxytocin contracts myoepithelial cells and empties the alveolar lumen, thus enhancing further milk secretion and alveolar refilling. Frequent emptying of the lumen is important for maintaining an adequate level of secretion. Indeed, after the 4th postpartum month, suckling appears to be the only stimulant required; however, environmental and emotional states also are important for continued alveolar activity.

The ejection of milk from the breast does not occur as the result of a mechanically induced negative pressure produced by suckling. Tactile sensors concentrated in the areola activate, via thoracic sensory nerve roots, an afferent sensory neural arc which stimulates the paraventricular and supraoptic nuclei of the hypothalamus to synthesize and transport oxytocin to the posterior pituitary. The efferent arc (oxytocin) is blood-borne to the breast alveolus-ductal systems to contract myoepithelial cells and empty the alveolar lumen. Milk contained in major ductal repositories is ejected from openings in the nipple. This rapid release of milk is called "letdown." In many instances, the activation of oxytocin release leading to letdown does not require initiation by tactile stimuli. The central nervous system can be conditioned to respond to the presence of the infant, or to the sound of the infant's cry, by inducing activation of the efferent arc. The release of oxytrocin is also important for uterine contractions that contribute to involution of the uterus.

The oxytocin effect is a release phenomenon acting on secreted and stored milk. Prolactin must be available in sufficient quantities for continued secretory replacement of ejected milk. This requires the transient increase in prolactin associated with suckling. The amount of milk produced correlates with the amount removed by suckling. The breast can store milk for a maximum of 48 hours before production diminishes.

Suckling suppresses the formation of a hypothalamic substance, prolactin inhibiting factor (PIF). This intrahypothalamic effect is either mediated by dopamine, or, in contrast to the peptide nature of other hypothalamic hormones, PIF is dopamine itself.[21] Dopamine is secreted by the basal hypothalamus into the portal system and conducted to the anterior pituitary. Dopamine binds specifically to lactotroph cells and suppresses the secretion of prolactin into the general circulation; in its absence, prolactin is secreted. Suckling, therefore, acts to refill the breast by activating both portions of the pituitary (anterior and posterior) causing the breast to produce new milk and to eject milk.

Lactation can be terminated by discontinuing suckling. The primary effect of this cessation is loss of milk letdown via the neural evocation of oxytocin. With passage of a few days, the swollen alveoli depress milk formation probably via a local pressure effect. With resorption of fluid and solute, the swollen engorged breast diminishes in size in a few days. In addition to the loss of milk letdown the absence of suckling reactivates dopamine (PIF) production so that there is less prolactin stimulation of milk secretion.

The Contraceptive Efficacy of Lactation

In primitive human societies, the duration of the birth interval has been very important for the survival of the young. Throughout human history, no preliterate society has achieved a fertility rate at the maximal level possible. The hunter-gatherer, nomadic !Kung women had a high suckling frequency and gave birth about every 4 years.[22] Lactation amenorrhea, lasting up to 2 years, has been nature's most effective form of contraception.[23] Indeed, lactation is the mechanism that maintains a reasonable interval between pregnancies in all non-seasonally breeding animals. In Africa and Asia breastfeeding reduces the fertility rate by an average of about 30%.[1] Birth intervals of less than 2 years are associated with a greater incidence of low birth weight, preterm birth, and neonatal death.[24] The contraceptive effectiveness of lactation, i.e., the length of the interval between births, depends on the level of nutrition of the mother (if low, the longer the contraceptive interval), the intensity of suckling, and the extent to which supplemental food is added to the infant diet.

Mechanism of Action

Prolactin concentrations are increased in response to the repeated suckling stimulus of breastfeeding. Given sufficient intensity and frequency, prolactin levels will remain elevated. Under these conditions, follicle-stimulating hormone (FSH) concentrations are in the normal range (having risen from extremely low concentrations at delivery to follicular range in the 3 weeks postpartum) and luteinizing hormone (LH) values are in the low normal range. Despite the presence of gonadotropins, the ovary during lactational hyperprolactinemia does not display follicular development and does not secrete estrogen. Therefore, vaginal dryness and dyspareunia are commonly reported by breastfeeding women. *The use of vaginal estrogen preparations is discouraged because absorption of the estrogen can lead to inhibition of milk production. Vaginal lubricants should be used until ovarian function and estrogen production return.*

Earlier experimental evidence suggested that the ovaries might be refractory to gonadotropin stimulation during lactation, and in addition, the anterior pituitary might be less responsive to GnRH stimulation. Other studies, done later in the course of lactation, indicated, however, that the ovaries as well as the pituitary were responsive to adequate tropic hormone stimulation.[25]

These observations suggest that high concentrations of prolactin work at both central and ovarian sites to produce lactational amenorrhea and anovulation. Prolactin appears to affect granulosa cell function in vitro by inhibiting synthesis of progesterone. It also may change the testosterone:dihydrotestosterone ratio, thereby reducing aromatizable substrate and increasing local antiestrogen concentrations. Nevertheless, a direct effect of prolactin on ovarian follicular development does not appear to be a major factor. The central action predominates.

Elevated levels of prolactin inhibit the pulsatile secretion of GnRH.[26,27] Prolactin excess has stimulatory feedback effects on dopamine. Increased dopamine reduces GnRH by suppressing arcuate nucleus function, apparently in a mechanism mediated by endogenous opioid activity.[28] However, blockade of dopamine receptors with a dopamine antagonist or the administration of an opioid antagonist in breastfeeding women does not always affect gonadotropin secretion.[29] The exact mechansim for the suppression of gonadotropin secretion remains to be unraveled.

At weaning, as prolactin concentrations fall to normal, gonadotropin concentrations increase and estradiol secretion rises. This prompt resumption of ovarian function is also indicated by the occurrence of ovulation within 14–30 days of weaning.

Resumption of Ovulation

The resumption of ovulation in the postpartum period has been well studied in recent times.

Nonbreastfeeding Women. In nonbreastfeeding women, gonadotropin levels remain low during the early puerperium and return to normal concentrations during the 3rd to 5th week when prolactin levels have returned to baseline. In an assessment of this important physiologic event (in terms of the need for contraception), the mean delay before first ovulation was found to be approximately 45 days, while no woman ovulated before 25 days after delivery.[30,31] Of the 22 women, 11 ovulated before the 6th postpartum week, underscoring the need to move the traditional postpartum medical visit to the 3rd week after delivery. In addition, two-thirds of the women ovulated before their first menses. The suppression of prolactin secretion with a dopamine agonist (e.g., bromocriptine), not surprisingly, is associated with the return of gonadotropin secretion in the 2nd postpartum week, and an earlier return to ovulation and menses.[32] In women who receive dopamine agonist treatment at or immediately after delivery, contraception is required a week earlier, in the 2nd week postpartum.[33]

Breastfeeding Women. In Scotland, no ovulation could be detected in women during exclusive breast-feeding.[34] However, in Chile, 14% of women ovulated during full breastfeeding, although full nursing provided effective contraception up to 3 months postpartum.[35,36] It has been argued that the threshold for suppression of ovulation is at least 5 feedings for a total of at least 65 minutes per day suckling duration.[37] However in the studies from Chile, the frequency of nursing was the same in breastfeeders who ovulated and those who did not.

In Mexico, a study of 29 breastfeeding mothers and 10 nonbreastfeeders observed that in the absence of bleeding and supplementary feedings, 100% of the breastfeeders remained anovulatory for 3 months postpartum, and 96% up to 6 months.[38] The median time from delivery to first ovulation was 259 days for breastfeeders compared to 119 days for nonbreastfeeders. However, by the third postpartum month, 18% of the breastfeeders had ovulated.

In a well-nourished population in Australia, less than 20% of breastfeeding women ovulated by the 6th postpartum month, and less than 25% menstruated.[39] Neither time of first supplement nor the amount of supplement predicted the return of ovulation or menstruation. In other words, even in women giving their infants supplemental feedings, there is effective inhibition of ovulation during the first 6 months of breastfeeding.

Risk of Pregnancy

Over the years, Roger Short, more than anyone, has increased our appreciation for the importance of breastfeeding. He has documented from Australia that among women who have unprotected intercourse during lactation amenorrhea and use contraception when menses resume, 1.7% become pregnant in the first 6 months of breastfeeding, 7% after 12 months, and 13% after 24 months.[40]

In a study of 422 middle-class women in Santiago, Chile, there was only one pregnancy (in month 6) when lactational amenorrhea was consciously relied upon for contraception.[41] This was equal to a cumulative 6-month life-table pregnancy rate of 0.45%. However, this accomplishment required an extensive program of education and support. In this study, 9% of exclusively breastfeeding women had resumption of menses by the end of 3 months and 19% by the end of 6 months. This increased suppression of fertility undoubtedly reflected the intensity of the breastfeeding program and the motivation of the participants.

In Chile, the probability of pregnancy in breastfeeding women has been measured as follows:[42]

Amenorrheic women:	**0.9% at 6 months;**
	17% at 12 months.
Menstruating women:	**36% at 6 months;**
	55% at 12 months.

In Pakistan, women who deliberately chose lactational amenorrhea as a method of contraception experienced a pregnancy rate of only 1.1% at 12 months if they remained amenorrheic.[43] It is apparent that while lactation provides a contraceptive effect, it is variable and not reliable for every woman, especially in view of the variablity in intensity of breastfeeding and the use of supplemental feeding.

An international group of researchers in the area of lactational infertility reached the following consensus in 1989, called the Bellagio Consensus (after the site of the conference at Bellagio, Italy):[44]

"The maximum birth spacing effect of breastfeeding is achieved when a mother 'fully' or nearly fully breastfeeds and remains amenorrheic. When these two conditions are fulfilled, breastfeeding provides more than 98% protection from pregnancy in the first six months."

Full breastfeeding means that the infant's total suckling stimulus is directed to the mother. There is no diminution of suckling by supplementation or the use of a pacifier.

Only amenorrheic women who exclusively breastfeed at regular intervals, including nighttime, during the first 6 months have the contraceptive protection equivalent to that provided by oral contraception; with menstruation or after 6 months, the risk of ovulation increases.[45] Supplemental feeding increases the risk of ovulation (and pregnancy) even in amenorrheic women.[42] Total protection against pregnancy is achieved by the exclusively breastfeeding woman for a duration of only 10 weeks.

Choice of Contraception

When to Start

Additional contraception is necessary during lactation for most women. That is not to say that full breastfeeding shouldn't be encouraged and that the protection obtained in the first 6 months of breastfeeding shouldn't be emphasized. But after 3 months, the first ovulation can precede the first menstrual bleed.

The Rule of 3's.

In the presence of FULL breastfeeding, a contraceptive method should be used beginning in the *3rd postpartum month.*

With PARTIAL breastfeeding or NO breastfeeding, a contraceptive method should begin during the *3rd postpartum week.*

After the termination of a pregnancy of less than 12 weeks, oral contraception can be started immediately. After a pregnancy of 12 or more weeks, the 3rd postpartum week rule should be followed if the pregnancy is term or near term. The latter delay has been based on a theoretical concern over an increased risk of thrombosis early in the postpartum period. This is probably no longer an issue with low-dose oral contraception. *We believe that oral contraception can be initiated immediately after a second trimester abortion or premature delivery.*

The Postpartum Visit. Contraception is usually on the mind of both patient and clinician at the first postpartum visit. A recent pregnancy and a new infant provide strong motivation to consider contraception. Traditionally, the first medical visit after delivery has been scheduled at 6 weeks, a time when good involution of the uterus and healing have occurred. Unfortunately in nonbreastfeeding women, ovulation can occur during the 4th postpartum week. We urge clinicians and patients to start a new tradition: schedule the first postpartum visit during the *3rd week after delivery.* Even breastfeeding women should be evaluated at this time, to consider whether breastfeeding is full and exclusive, or whether an additional contraceptive method is necessary.

Oral Contraception

Oral contraception even in low-dose formulations has been demonstrated to diminish the quantity and quality of lactation in postpartum women. Also of concern is the potential hazard of transfer of contraceptive steroids to the infant (a significant amount of the progestational component is secreted into breast milk);[46,47] however, no adverse effects have thus far been identified. Women who use oral contraception have a lower incidence of breastfeeding after the 6th postpartum month, regardless of whether oral contraception is started at the first, second, or third postpartum month.[48-50]

In adequately nourished women, no impairment of infant growth and development can be detected; presumably compensation is achieved either through supplementary feedings or increased suckling.[51-53] In an 8-year follow-up study of children breastfed by mothers using oral contraceptives, no effect could be detected on diseases, intelligence, or psychological behavior.[54] This study also found that mothers on birth control pills lactated a significantly shorter period of time than controls, a mean of 3.7 months vs 4.6 months in controls.

Because of the concerns regarding the impact of oral contraceptives on breastfeeding, a useful alternative is to combine the contraceptive effect of lactation with the progestin-only minipill (See Chapter 3). In contrast to the combined oral contraceptive, the progestin-only minipill provides a modest boost to milk production, and women using the minipill breastfeed longer and add supplementary feeding at a later time.[51,55,56] The combination of lactation and the progestin-only minipill is associated with near total contraceptive efficacy. Because of the positive impact on breastfeeding, the minipill can be started immediately after delivery at or near term. In addition, the minipill can protect against the bone loss associated with lactation, a potential advantage in undernourished women.[18]

In patients who prefer the standard low-dose combined oral contraceptive, the full breastfeeder should begin during the 3rd postpartum month; all others during the 3rd postpartum week. Starting oral contraception during the 3rd postpartum week safely avoids the hypercoaguable state immediately after delivery.

Long-Acting Methods

Depo-Provera. Depo-Provera does not affect breast feeding.[57] Medroxyprogesterone acetate is transferred into the infant circulation; however, no adverse effects have been reported. A large WHO study failed to find any effects on infant growth or development with any progestin-only contraceptive method, including Depo-Provera.[52,53] This is an excellent choice for postpartum contraception. Although studies have not been reported with use within 30 days after delivery, there are no effects associated with this method that require caution. Depo-Provera can be administered immediately postpartum, and certainly should be utilized no later than the 3rd postpartum week.

Contraceptive Implants. Although not well-studied, it is possible to draw some conclusions about the effects of implant contraceptives like Norplant on breastfeeding. Suppression of estradiol is more profound with Depo-Provera compared with Norplant, and the relative dose of the progestin with Depo-Provera is greater. The effect on lactation that these differences in estrogen and progestin levels would predict should place Norplant users somewhere between Depo-Provera and nonusers of contraception.

Discontinuation of Breastfeeding Due to No Milk Secretion[58]

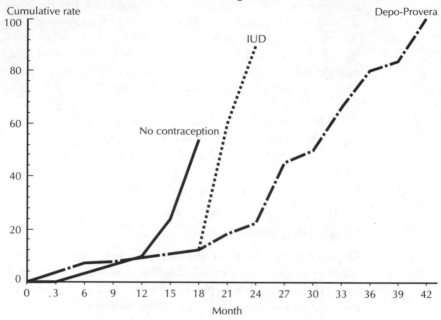

Cumulative rate

Depo-Provera

IUD

No contraception

Month

Studies in Egypt indicate that when Norplant is inserted at least 30–42 days postpartum, the only difference in lactation or infant growth and development comparing Norplant users and controls is that infant weight gain in the first few months with exclusively breastfeeding Norplant users is slightly less.[59,60] In Indonesian women whose infants were followed for 6 months after their mothers received Norplant 4–6 weeks postpartum, there was no adverse effect on infant growth.[61] A study of 100 Chilean women who received Norplant from 52–58 days postpartum was associated, as in Egypt, with a slightly lower infant weight gain in the first 4–6 months of breastfeeding, but after 6 months, weights were similar comparing Norplant users to controls.[62]

These findings with Norplant can be compared to those from studies of the effects of progestin-only minipills on lactation because the serum concentrations of levonorgestrel are comparable in the two methods. As noted above, women using levonorgestrel-only minipills have been documented to begin supplementary feeding about one month later and are one-third as likely to discontinue breastfeeding compared to women using nonhormonal contraceptives.[54,55]

The transfer of progestin from the mother's circulation to her milk and thence to the infant's blood has been studied with 3 delivery systems for levonorgestrel (minipill, implant, and intrauterine contraception).[46,47] Transfer from maternal serum to breast milk was highest for the levonorgestrel IUD (12%), and lower for Norplant and the oral minipill, 7% and 8%, respectively. Transfer from breast milk to the infants' sera averaged 75% for the levonorgestrel IUD, 75% for Norplant, and only 32% for the Minipill.[46] These infant sera concentrations are about 25% of those reported for levonorgestrel-containing combination oral contraceptives.[47] This transfer is relatively low, and no adverse effects have been reported.

No studies have been reported examining the effects of Norplant administered prior to 30 days after delivery, and, therefore, the package advisory insert cautions against immediate postpartum use. In some situations, however, the delivery may provide the only opportunity to receive Norplant. Since another pregnancy within a year of delivery poses a far greater health hazard to both mother and infant, in our view such caution is not warranted. If the new mother will not have access to implant contraception 30 days after delivery, we believe it is appropriate to provide it immediately postpartum.

Periodic Abstinence

Women skilled in the cervical mucus method can detect evidence of fertile type mucus prior to the first menses in the postpartum period. However, there are many false positive and false negative interpretations.[63] This method cannot be used with a great deal of confidence until regular menses are resumed.

Barrier Methods

Barrier methods, of course, have no impact on breastfeeding, and they are an excellent choice for motivated couples. Lubricated condoms are especially helpful for the vaginal dryness experienced by some breastfeeding women. Spermicides and foam products can also help with the dryness and dyspareunia. It is difficult to fit a diaphragm or cervical cap before healing and involution are complete (about 6 weeks), and it is not advisable to use a sponge, cap, or diaphragm while still bleeding. Therefore spermicides, foam, and condoms should be used in the immediate postpartum period, and use of the sponge, cap, or diaphragm can be started about the 6th postpartum week.

The Postpartum IUD

Expulsion rates were higher when the older, large plastic IUDs were inserted sooner than 8 weeks postpartum; however, studies indicate that the copper IUDs can be inserted between 4 and 8 weeks postpartum without an increase in pregnancy rates, expulsion, uterine perforation, or removals for bleeding and/or pain.[64,65] Insertion can even occur immediately after a vaginal delivery; it is not associated with an increased risk of infection, uterine perforation, postpartum bleeding, or uterine subinvolution.[66] This is not recommended if intrauterine infection is present, and a slightly higher expulsion rate is to be expected compared to insertion 4–8 weeks postpartum. The IUD can also be inserted at cesarean section; the expulsion rate is slightly lower than that with insertion immediately after vaginal delivery.[67]

Insertion of an IUD in breastfeeding women is relatively easier, and is associated with a lower removal rate for bleeding or pain.[66] An early suggestion that uterine perforation is more common in lactating women has not been substantiated.[66,68]

An IUD can be inserted immediately after a first trimester abortion, but after a second trimester abortion, it is recommended to wait until uterine involution occurs.[69,70]

References

1. Thapa S, Short RV, Potts M, Breastfeeding, birthspacing and their effects on child survival, Nature 335:679, 1988.

2. Davidson WD, Durham NC, A brief history of infant feeding, J Pediatrics 43:74, 1953.

3. National Academy of Sciences, *Nutrition During Lactation,* National Academy Press, Washington, D.C., 1991.

4. Ryan AS, Pratt WF, Wysong JL, Lewandowski G, McNally JW, Krieger FW, A comparison of breast-feeding data from the National Surveys of Family Growth and the Ross Laboratories Mothers Surveys, Am J Public Health 81:1049, 1991.

5. Ferguson DP, Anderson TJ, Morphological evaluation of cell turnover in relation to menstrual cycle in the "resting" human breast, Br J Cancer 44:177, 1988.

6. Longacre TA, Bartow SA, A correlative morphologic study of human breast and endometrium in the menstrual cycle, Am J Surg Path 10:382, 1986.

7. Going JJ, Anderson TJ, Battersby S, MacIntyre CC, Proliferative and secretory activity in human breast during natural and artificial menstrual cycles, Am J Path 130:193, 1988.

8. Topper YL, Freeman C, Multiple hormone interactions in the developmental biology of the mammary gland, Physiol Rev 60:1049, 1980.

9. Klineberg DL, Niemann W, Flamm E, Cooper P, Babitsky G, Primate mammary development, J Clin Invest 75:1943, 1985.

10. Tyson JE, Hwang P, Guyda H, Friesen HG, Studies of prolactin secretion in human pregnancy, Am J Obstet Gynecol 113:14, 1972.

11. Kletzky OA, Marrs RP, Howard WF, McCormick W, Mishell DR Jr, Prolactin synthesis release during pregnancy and puerperium, Am J Obstet Gynecol 136:545, 1980.

12. Murphy LJ, Murphy LC, Stead B, Sutherland RL, Lazarus L, Modulation of lactogenic receptors by progestins in cultured human breast cancer cells, J Clin Endocrinol Metab 62:280, 1986.

13. Simon WE, Pahnke VG, Holzel F, In vitro modulation of prolactin binding to human mammary carcinoma cells by steroid hormones and prolactin, J Clin Endocrinol Metab 60:1243, 1985.

14. Kelly PA, Kjiane J, Postel-Vinay M-C, Edery M, The prolactin/growth hormone receptor family, Endocrin Rev 12:235, 1991.

15. Battin DA, Marrs RP, Fleiss PM, Mishell DR Jr, Effect of suckling on serum prolactin, luteinizing hormone, follicle-stimulating hormone, and estradiol during prolonged lactation, Obstet Gynecol 65:785, 1985.

16. **Kumar R, Cohen WR, Epstein FH,** Vitamin D and calcium hormones in pregnancy, New Engl J Med 302:1143, 1980.

17. **Sowers M, Corton G, Shapiro B, Jannausch ML, Crutchfield M, Smith ML, Randolph JF, Hollis B,** Changes in bone density with lactation, JAMA 269:3130, 1993.

18. **Caird LE, Reid-Thomas V, Hannan WJ, Gow S, Glasier AF,** Oral progestogen-only contraception may protect against loss of bone mass in breast-feeding women, Clin Endocrinol 41:739, 1994.

19. **Dawood MY, Khan-Dawood FS, Wahl RS, Fuchs F,** Oxytocin release and plasma anterior pituitary and gonadal hormones in women during lactation, J Clin Endocrinol Metab 52:678, 1981.

20. **McNeilly AS, Robinson KA, Houston MJ, Howe PW,** Release of oxytocin and prolactin in response to suckling, Br Med J 286:257, 1983.

21. **Ben-Jonathan N,** Dopamine: a prolactin-inhibiting hormone, Endocrin Rev 6:564, 1985.

22. **Kolata G,** !Kung hunter-gatherers: feminism, diet and birth control, Science 185:932, 1974.

23. **Short RV,** Lactation — The central control of reproduction, Ciba Found Symp 45:73, 1976.

24. **Miller JE,** Birth intervals and perinatal health: an investigation of three hypotheses, Fam Plann Perspect 23:62, 1991.

25. **Tyson JE, Carter JN, Andreassen B, Huth J, Smith B,** Nursing mediated prolactin and luteinizing hormone secretion during puerperal lactation, Fertil Steril 30:154, 1978.

26. **Sauder SE, Frager M, Case GD, Kelch RP, Marshall JC,** Abnormal patterns of pulsatile luteinizing hormone secretion in women with hyperprolactinemia and amenorrhea: responses to bromocriptine, J Clin Endocrinol Metab 59:941, 1984.

27. **Tay CCK, Glasier A, McNeilly AS,** Twenty-four hour secretory profiles of gonadotropins and prolactin in breastfeeding women, Hum Reprod 7:951, 1992.

28. **Petraglia F, De Leo V, Nappi C, Facchinetti F, Montemagno U, Brambilla F, Genazzani AR,** Differences in the opioid control of luteinizing hormone secretion between pathological and iatrogenic hyperprolactinemic states, J Clin Endocrinol Metab 64:508, 1987.

29. **Tay CCK, Glasier AF, McNeilly AS,** Effect of antagonists of dopamine and opiates on the basal and GnRH-induced secretion of luteinizing hormone, follicle stimulating hormone and prolactin during lactational amenorrhea in breastfeeding women, Hum Reprod 8:532, 1993.

30. **Gray RH, Campbell OM, Zacur HA, Labbok MH, MacRae SL,** Postpartum return of ovarian activity in nonbreastfeeding women monitored by urinary assays, J Clin Endocrinol Metab 64:645, 1987.

31. **Campbell OM, Gray RH,** Characteristics and determinants of postpartum ovarian function in women in the United States, Am J Obstet Gynecol 169:55, 1993.

32. **Kremer JAM, Thomas CMG, Rolland R, Lancranjan I, van der Heijden PFM,** Return of gonadotropin function in postpartum women during bromocriptine treatment, Fertil Steril 51:622, 1989.

33. **Haartsen JE, Heineman MJ, Elings M, Evers JLH, Lancranjan I,** Resumption of pituitary and ovarian activity post-partum: endocrine and ultrasonic observations in bromocriptine-treated women, Hum Reprod 7:746, 1992.

34. **Howie PW, McNeilly AS, Houston MJ, Cook A, Boyle H,** Effect of supplementary food on suckling patterns and ovarian activity during lactation, Br Med J 283:757, 1981.

35. **Perez A, Vela P, Masnick GS, Potter RG,** First ovulation after childbirth: the effect of breastfeeding, Am J Obstet Gynecol 114:1041, 1972.

36. **Diaz S, Peralta O, Juez G, Salvatierra AM, Casado ME, Duran E, Croxatto HB,** Fertility regulation in nursing women. I. The probablity of conception in full nursing women living in an urban setting, J Biosoc Sci 14:329, 1982.

37. **McNeilly AS, Glasier A, Howie PW,** Endocrine control of lactational infertility, in Dobbing J (ed): *Maternal Nutrition and Lactational Infertility,* Nevey/Raven Press, New York, 1985, p. 177.

38. **Rivera R, Kennedy KI, Ortiz E, Barrera M, Bhiwandiwala PP,** Breastfeeding and the return to ovulation in Durango, Mexico, Fertil Steril 49:780, 1988.

39. **Lewis PR, Brown JB, Renfree MB, Short RV,** The resumption of ovulation and menstruation in a well-nourished population of women breastfeeding for an extended period of time, Fertil Steril 55:529, 1991.

40. **Short RV, Lewis PR, Renfree MB, Shaw G,** Contraceptive effects of extended lactational amenorrhoea: beyond the Bellagio Consensus, Lancet 337:715, 1991.

41. **Pérez A, Labbok MH, Queenan JT,** Clinical study of the lactational amenorrhoea method for family planning, Lancet 339:968, 1992.

42. **Diaz S, Aravena R, Cardenas H, Casado ME, Miranda P, Schiappacasse V, Croxatto HB,** Contraceptive efficacy of lactational amenorrhea in urban Chilean women, Contraception 43:335, 1991.

43. **Kazi A, Kennedy KI, Visness CM, Khan T,** Effectiveness of the lactational amenorrhea method in Pakistan, Fertil Steril 64:717, 1995.

44. **Kennedy KI, Rivera R, McNeilly AS,** Consensus statement on the use of breastfeeding as a family planning method, Bellagio, Italy, Contraception 39:477, 1989.

45. **Gray RH, Campbell OM, Apelo R, Eslami SS, Zacur H, Ramos RM, Gehret JC, Labbok MH,** Risk of ovulation during lactation, Lancet 335:25, 1990.

46. **Shikary ZK, Bertrabet S, Patel ZM, Paytel S, Joshi JV, Toddywala VS, Toddywala SP, Patel DM, Jhaveri K, Saxena BN,** ICMR task force study on hormonal contraception. Transfer of levonorgestrel administered through different drug delivery systems from the maternal circulation into the newborn's circulation via breast milk, Contraception 35:477, 1987.

47. **Betrabet SS, Shikary ZK, Toddywalla VS, Toddywalla SP, Patel D, Saxena BN,** Transfer of norethisterone (NET) and levonorgestrel (LNG) from a single tablet into the infant's circualtion through the mother's milk, Contraception 35:517, 1987.

48. **Diaz S, Peralta O, Juez G, Herreros C, Casado ME, Salvatierra AM, Miranda P, Durn E, Croxatto HB,** Fertility regulation in nursing women: III. Short-term influence of a low-dose combined oral contraceptive upon lactation and infant growth, Contraception 27:1, 1982.

49. **Croxatto HB, Diaz S, Peralta O, Juez G, Herreros C, Casado ME, Salvatierra AM, Miranda P, Durn E,** Fertility regulation in nursing women: IV. Long-term influence of a low-dose combined oral contraceptive initiated at day 30 postpartum upon lactation and child growth, Contraception 27:13, 1983.

50. **Peralta O, Diaz S, Juez G, Herreros C, Casado ME, Salvatierra AM, Miranda P, Durn E, Croxatto HB,** Fertility regulation in nursing women: V. Long-term influence of a low-dose combined oral contraceptive initiated at day 90 postpartum upon lactation and infant growth, Contraception 27:27, 1983.

51. **WHO Special Programme of Research, Development, and Research Training in Human Reproduction, Task Force on Oral Contraceptives,** Effects of hormonal contraceptives on milk volume and infant growth, Contraception 30:505, 1984.

52. **WHO Task Force for Epidemiological Research on Reproductive Health; Special Programme of Research, Development and Research Training in Human Reproduction,** Progestogen-only contraceptives during lactation. I. Infant growth, Contraception 50:35, 1994.

53. **WHO Task Force for Epidemiological Research on Reproductive Health; Special Programme of Research, Development and Research Training in Human Reproduction,** Progestogen-only contraceptives during lactation. II. Infant development, Contraception 50:55, 1994.

54. **Nilsson S, Mellbin T, Hofvander Y, Sundelin C, Valentin J, Nygren KG,** Long-term follow-up of children breast-fed by mothers using oral contraceptives, Contraception 34:443, 1986.

55. **McCann MF, Moggia AV, Hibbins JE, Potts M, Becker C,** The effects of a progestin-only oral contraceptive (levonorgestrel 0.03 mg) on breast-feeding, Contraception 40:635, 1989.

56. **Moggia AV, Harris GS, Dunson TR, Diaz R, Moggia MS, Ferrer MA, McMullen SL,** A comparative study of a progestin-only oral contraceptive versus non-hormonal methods in lactating women in Buenos Aires, Argentina, Contraception 44:31, 1991.

57. **Jimenez J, Ochoa M, Soler MP, Portales P,** Long-term follow-up of children breast-fed by mothers receiving depot-medroxyprogesterone acetate, Contraception 30:5232, 1984.

58. **Zacharias S, Aguilera E, Assenzo JR, Zanartu J,** Effects of hormonal and nonhormonal contraceptives on lactation and incidence of pregnancy, Contraception 33:203, 1986.

59. **Shabaan MM, Salem HT, Abdullah KA,** Influence of levonorgestrel contraceptive implants, Norplant, initiated early postpartum upon lactation and infant growth, Contraception 32:623, 1985.

60. **Shaaban MM,** Contraception with progestogens and progesterone during lactation, J Steroid Biochem Mol Biol 40:705, 1991.

61. **Affandi B, Karmadibrata S, Prihartono J, Lubis F, Samil RS,** Effect of Norplant on mother and infants in the postpartum period, Adv Contracept 2:371, 1986.

62. **Diaz S, Herreros C, Juez G, Casado ME, Salvatierra AM, Miranda P, Peralto O, Croxatto HB,** Fertility regulation in nursing women: influence of Norplant levonorgestrel implants upon lactation and infant growth, Contraception 32:53, 1985.

63. **Gross BA,** Natural family planning indicators of ovulation, Clin Reprod Fertil 5:91, 1987.

64. **Mishell DR Jr, Roy S,** Copper intrauterine contraceptive device event rates following insertion 4 to 8 weeks post partum, Am J Obstet Gynecol 143:29, 1982.

65. **Zhuang L, Wang H, Yang P,** Observations of the clinical efficacies and side effects of six different timings of IUD insertions, Clin J Obstet Gynecol 22:350, 1987.

66. **Chi I-c, Farr G,** Postpartum IUD contraception — A review of an international experience, Adv Contracept 5:127, 1989.

67. **Zhou S, Chi I-c,** Immediate postpartum IUD insertions in a Chinese hospital — A two-year follow-up, Int J Gynaecol Obstet 35:157, 1991.

68. **Chi I-c, Potts M, Wilkens L, Champion C,** Performance of the TCu-380A device in breastfeeding and non-breastfeeding women, Contraception 39:603, 1989.

69. **Nielsen NC, Nygren K-G, Allonen H,** Three years of experience after post-abortal insertion of Nova-T and Copper-T-200, Acta Obstet Gynecol Scand 63:261, 1984.

70. **QueridoL, Ketting E, Haspels AA,** IUD insertion following induced abortion, Contraception 31:603, 1985.

Clinical Guidelines for Contraception at Different Ages

MODERN SOCIETY is coping with two contraceptive problems, each at the opposite end of the reproductive lifespan. In the early years, we are struggling with the high rate of unwanted teenage pregnancies. In the later years, we face a growing demand for reversible contraception as the post World War II baby boom generation ages. It is entirely appropriate, therefore, that we give special attention to these age groups: adolescence and the transition years (ages 35 to menopause).

Contraception for Adolescents

Providing contraception or information about contraception for young people under age 20 is an important obligation for clinicians. More young women (over 1 million teenagers) become pregnant in the United States than do their contemporaries in other developed parts of the world, and young American women have a slightly higher abortion rate than young European women.[1] More than 50% of the 1.5 million abortions per year in the United States are obtained by women younger than age 25, with the rate peaking at ages 18–19.[2,3]

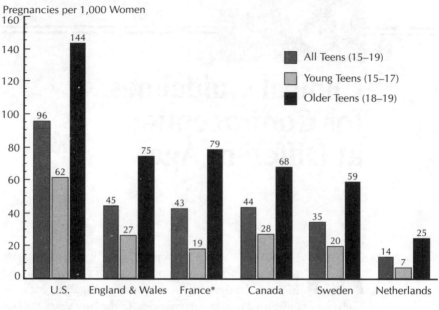

**1981 Teenage Pregnancy Rates in
the U.S. vs. Other Developed Countries** [19]

Pregnancies per 1,000 Women

Legend:
- All Teens (15–19)
- Young Teens (15–17)
- Older Teens (18–19)

U.S.: 96, 62, 144
England & Wales: 45, 27, 75
France*: 43, 19, 79
Canada: 44, 28, 68
Sweden: 35, 20, 59
Netherlands: 14, 7, 25

*1980 data

There was a marked increase in teenage sexual activity in the United States during the 1980s, and contrary to common opinion, much of that increase occurred among white and nonpoor adolescents.[4] Approximately 56% of young women and 73% of young men have had sexual intercourse by age 18.[5] Within a relatively short period of time after becoming sexually active, 58% of adolescent females have had sex with 2 or more partners (and thus, increase their risk of sexually transmitted diseases [STDs]). After the increase that occurred over the last 3 decades, sexual behavior among U.S. high school students has remained relatively unchanged in the 1990s.[6,7] The good news is that the use of oral contraceptives and condoms has increased in the 1990s; however, at least half of sexually active teenagers do not use condoms, placing them at increased risk for STDs.

The adolescent pregnancy rate in the U.S. has been stable in recent years.[5] A decline in the pregnancy rate in sexually experienced teenagers is balanced by an increase in the proportion of adolescents sexually active. Approximately 85% of teenage pregnancies are unintended.[5]

Characteristics of Teen Pregnancy in the United States[8–12]
1. 3,000 teen pregnancies occur every day.
2. One of every 10 teens aged 15–19 gets pregnant.
3. Half of teen pregnancies occur in the first 6 months after first intercourse.
4. 20% of teen pregnancies occur in the first month after first intercourse.
5. Half who give birth do not graduate from high school.
6. Teen pregnancies are associated with increased risks of obstetrical and neonatal complications and mortality.
7. The children of teen mothers are more likely to have behavioral and social problems when they are adolescents.

Adolescence is a time for "trying your wings," a time for experimenting and testing. Most of the 25 million teenagers in the United States will make it, but unfortunately for many, the consequences of this time of trying things will be a lasting problem for health and life. Unwanted pregnancy (premature parenthood) and the STDs are the risks of sexual experimentation. Teenaged girls carry the burdens of unprotected sexual activity: unwanted pregnancy, undetected STDs, and pelvic inflammatory disease. Their male partners, who are often not themselves teenagers, must be made aware of these consequences through public education that reaches all young people, not just those in school, and through social programs that enforce male responsibility for child support and disease prevention.

Teenagers are noted for their sense of invincibility and their risk-taking behavior, both of which denote the inability of immature people to connect present action with future consequences. It is not surprising that adolescents often have sex and do not use contraception. Contraception takes planning and premeditation about having sex, but television and movies present teenagers with unrealistic examples of romantic liaisons that disconnect sex, pregnancy, and STDs from contraception. More than half of female teenagers have risked pregnancy and infertility by having unprotected intercourse at least once. The onset of fertility following menarche cannot be predicted for individuals; any sexually active teenager is at risk for pregnancy, as well as STDs. It is worth emphasizing that there is no evidence that provision of contraception leads to adolescents having sex earlier or more frequently. Studies have repeatedly documented a constant finding: most adolescents seeking contraception usually do so many months to a year or more *after* initiating sexual activity.[5]

Among the obstacles to earlier use of contraception are exaggerated perceptions about the risks of contraceptive methods, as well as a deep dread of the misunderstood "pelvic exam."[13] We clinicians can do much to remove these obstacles by talking with teenagers and adjusting our practices to suit their special needs.

Our objective is to get adolescents to realistically assess their sexual futures, not to just let sex "happen." The fact that European adolescents use contraception at a rate higher than in the United States argues that we can do better. Unfortunately, secrecy usually surrounds a young person's decision to use contraception. Adolescent involvement in sex often occurs without an opportunity for discussion with family, other adults, peers, or even the partner. Access to contraception (physical and psychological) and motivation to use are the keys. Success in achieving our goals requires specific approaches and skills in communicating with adolescents. Greater openness about sexual discussion in the family, church, or school can all lead to a better consideration of the health and social risks of early sexual activity by a teenager.

School-Based Programs. Many school-based (or school-linked) educational programs and clinics have been developed to prevent adolescent pregnancies. These vary in focus and content, including abstinence and contraception. Unfortunately, the overall impact of these programs is questionable. A review of school-based programs concluded that it was uncertain if a focus on abstinence is effective.[14] School clinics by themselves do not seem to lower pregnancy rates, but an associated educational effort does seem effective.[14–16] However, at least one comprehensive community-wide program (in South Carolina) that included school interventions, public education, and emphasis of both abstinence and contraception did result in a reduction of the teenage pregnancy rate.[17] To counter a common criticism, it is worth noting that school-based programs and clinics do not affect the initiation or frequency of sexual activity.[14,16]

Topics Teenagers Would Like to Discuss with Physicians [18]

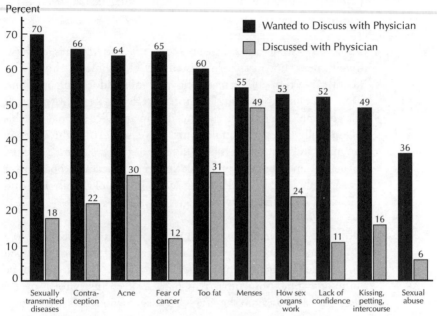

Percent

Legend:
- ■ Wanted to Discuss with Physician
- ▨ Discussed with Physician

Topic	Wanted to Discuss	Discussed
Sexually transmitted diseases	70	18
Contraception	66	22
Acne	64	30
Fear of cancer	65	12
Too fat	60	31
Menses	55	49
How sex organs work	53	24
Lack of confidence	52	11
Kissing, petting, intercourse	49	16
Sexual abuse	36	6

Communication with Adolescents

Teenagers want to talk about STDs and contraception, but clinicians usually don't bring these subjects up for discussion.[18] Clinicians can be sure that 75% of adolescents will be interested in discussing STDs and contraception by age 15. No matter what brings an adolescent into the office, contraception and continuation (compliance) are issues that should be addressed.

Our goals are to promote abstinence among teenagers who are not yet ready to cope with responsibility, and to promote behavior to prevent pregnancy and STDs in sexually active adolescents. Building trust is a requirement for a successful interaction between clinician and adolescent. A teenager must be assured that a discussion about sexuality and contraception will be strictly confidential. This must be stated in plain words. One reason European countries are able to provide better contraceptive services to adolescents is the guarantee by law of complete confidentiality (other reasons are dissemination of information via public media and distribution of contraceptives through free or low-cost services).[19] Research confirms that requiring parental notification or consent deters young people from using contraception.[5]

Successful use of contraception (continuation) requires teenager involvement, not just passive listening. The clinician should frequently interrupt talking by asking questions and seeking opinions. Don't wait until the physical examination to initiate conversation. It is a good practice to see all patients first in an office setting, but this is especially true with adolescents. Give some thought to body language and position. It is helpful to sit next to a patient; avoid the formality (and obstacle) of a desk between clinician and patient. A teenager should be asked about success in school, family life, and behaviors indicative of risk taking.

Don't miss the chance to point out the wisdom of abstinence to a young person who is not yet sexually active, but leave the door open for protection against pregnancy and STDs. Be careful to be nonjudgmental. Sometimes it is hard to keep disapproval over a teenager's activity from showing. A teenager who senses disapproval won't listen to instructions or advice.

A good way to introduce the subject of contraception is to ask an adolescent *when* he or she would like to have children. Then follow with: what plans do you have to avoid getting pregnant until then? Elicit objections, concerns, fears, and address each of them. The clinician must anticipate those concerns and fears that will lead to poor continuation. They must be identified and addressed in advance.

Contraceptive use is a private matter, and therefore, instruction comes from the clinician, not from peers. Be very concrete; demonstrate the use of pill packages, foam aerosols, and condom application. This seems like oversimplification, but clinicians working with adolescents have found that this approach is both necessary and appreciated by their young patients. Nevertheless, family involvement that results in improved emotional support of a teenager is associated with better contraceptive behavior.[20]

Adolescents must be convinced that having sex means you are at risk of becoming pregnant. Adolescents are immersed in conflicting messages about sexuality in our society. A clinician may be the only resource for information and guidance, but clinicians must give the right signals to adolescents and must initiate communication. No matter what the chief complaint, any interaction with an adolescent is an opportunity to discuss sexuality and contraception.

Choice of Method

Oral Contraception. The combined oral contraceptive is by far the most popular and most requested method of contraception by teenagers.[4,5] This is appropriate because oral contraceptives are almost never medically contraindicated in healthy adolescents. The risk of death from oral contraceptive use by adolescents is virtually nil. This is a good match; adolescents are at highest risk for unwanted pregnancies and are at lowest risk for complications. Thus, the high efficacy of combined oral contraception is the best choice for teenagers.

Adolescents certainly don't know the history of oral contraception. It is important to point out the change in dosage and the new safety. But teenagers do have concerns regarding oral contraception, citing most often a fear of cancer, concern with impact on future fertility, and problems with weight gain and acne.[21]

The cancer issue is a difficult one. We believe it is appropriate to state that there is no definitive evidence demonstrating a link between breast cancer and oral contraception. On the other hand, patients deserve to know of our concern, and the findings regarding long duration of use and the possible increased risk of early, premenopausal breast cancer (Chapter 2). As long as inconsistencies exist in the epidemiologic evidence, the clinician is justified in being optimistic, stating that risk is possible, but it has not been proven. Cervical cancer also continues to be a concern, although confounding factors have been difficult to control, and Pap smear surveillance must be emphasized. It is worth pointing out that these data on breast and cervical cancer are derived from older, higher dose pills.

By the time of menarche, growth and reproductive development are essentially complete. There is no evidence that early use of oral contraception has any inhibiting impact on growth or any adverse effects on the reproductive tract. With great confidence, a clinician can tell adolescents that there is no impact on future fertility with the use of oral contraception.[22] Indeed, one can emphasize that oral contraception preserves future fertility by its protection against PID and ectopic pregnancies. While oral contraception protects against PID, it does not protect against contracting STDs, hence the recommendation to combine oral contraception use with barrier methods. *Because it is now relatively common for young women to have changing relationships, a dual approach is recommended, combining the contraceptive efficacy and protection against PID offered by oral contraception with the use of a barrier method (and spermicide) for prevention of viral STDs.*

Repeatedly, it is worth emphasizing to adolescents that studies with low-dose oral contraception, even studies in adolescents,[23] do not indicate a problem of weight gain, and that acne is usually improved. Weight gain as it is perceived by the teenager deserves attention at every visit.[24]

Adolescents are especially receptive to hearing about the beneficial impact of oral contraception on menstrual problems: cramps, bleeding, and iron-deficiency anemia. Relief of dysmenorrhea in teenagers has been documented to be associated with better and more consistent use of oral contraceptives.[25] Although irregular bleeding on oral contraceptives can distress teenagers, it will not by itself cause improper use if teenagers are well prepared and instructed.

Teenage smoking continues to be a big problem. The number of American adults who smoke dropped from 40% in 1965 to 26% in 1991.[26] Smoking initiation has decreased markedly in men, but unfortunately has remained essentially unchanged in women.[27] In addition, female smokers begin smoking at a younger age. More young women (including teenagers) smoke than young men. It is important to note that smoking appears to have a greater adverse effect on women compared to men.[28,29] Women who smoke only 1 to 4 cigarettes per day have a 2.5-fold increased risk of fatal coronary heart disease.[30]

The relative risk of cardiovascular events is increased for women of all ages who smoke and use oral contraceptives. However, because the actual incidence of cardiovascular events is so low at a young age, the real risk is very, very low for young women. Given the lack of impact on clotting parameters of 20 µg estrogen in smokers,[31,32] it is worth considering a 20 µg formulation for all smoking women, regardless of age. This recommendation also applies to all women using nicotine-containing products as an aid to stop smoking. Exsmokers (for at least one year) should be regarded as nonsmokers. However, keep in mind that the theoretical greater safety of 20 µg estrogen has not been confirmed by epidemiologic data.

Estimated Annual Mortality Rates Associated with Oral Contraceptive Use and Smoking Compared to Pregnancy

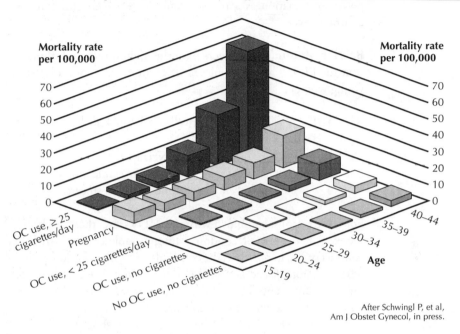

After Schwingl P, et al,
Am J Obstet Gynecol, in press.

Adolescents with diabetes mellitus uncomplicated with vascular changes can use oral contraception. Other conditions with which oral contraception is acceptable include cystic fibrosis and sickle cell disease.

Serial monogamy is common among teens, and this often is associated with episodic use of contraception. With oral contraception, it is helpful to instruct the adolescent that the minor side effects diminish in frequency with use, and therefore, there is an advantage to staying on the oral contraceptive. It is also good advice to tell teenagers to continue taking oral contraceptives for at least two months after "breaking up" with a boyfriend, by then a new relationship is likely to have begun.

One reason the average teenager waits months to a year after initiating sexual activity before seeking contraception is fear about the pelvic exam.[13] Furthermore, anxiety over the pelvic exam is a barrier to comprehending contraceptive instructions. Thus, letting teenagers know that the pelvic exam can be delayed until the 3rd or 6th month will encourage them to seek contraceptive advice. This approach requires a completely normal history (an absence of risk factors for STDs) and a limited prescription. We advocate the elimination of the pelvic examination as a requirement for teenagers to obtain oral contraceptives.

Barrier Methods. Teenagers have the highest rates of hospitalization for PID. The following statistics are cited about adolescent, young women:[33]

1. 8–25% of sexually active adolescent females are infected with Chlamydia.
2. 0.4–12% are infected with Neisseria.
3. 15–38% have human papillomavirus infection.
4. 16% of adolescents have abnormal Pap smears.

For these reasons, combined with the AIDS scare, there has been an increase in the use of condoms among adolescents.[4,5] After oral contraception, in our view, the condom used with a spermicide is the next best choice for adolescents. And this obviously is the only choice for male adolescents. *Indeed, we strongly advocate combining condoms with oral contraception to provide maximum protection against pregnancy and STDs.* Sexually active young women should be examined every 6 months, with Pap smear and STD screening.

The advantage of condoms with spermicide is that neither a prescription nor a consultation with a clinician is required. The problem, then, is achieving sufficient education and motivation without the intervention of clinicians. We believe this is a social problem, not a medical problem, and we are strongly supportive of public education efforts in schools and the media to accomplish this important public and individual health objective.

Many teenagers rely on condoms, and of course their contribution to preventing STDs is important. Condom failures, unfortunately, are about 10 times as high among teenagers as among older, married couples. Don't assume that teenagers know how to use a condom; use a model and demonstrate. Furthermore, young women need to know that they are in charge; they can insist on condom use.

The female condom provides a young woman with a female-controlled method, but its expense and complexity are obstacles for teenagers. Its use by teenagers has not been studied, and its effects on STDs are not documented.

Diaphragms or cervical caps are not good choices for adolescents. Adolescents are not comfortable with body interventions, and the insertion is too willful an act linked with coitus. Furthermore, this method requires privacy for insertion. Adolescents are discouraged by complicated methods. The diaphragm and cervical cap should be reserved for very motivated and mature young people.

The Intrauterine Device. Traditionally, IUDs have not been recommended for nulliparous women and those who have a high risk of STDs. This eliminated it from consideration for most teenagers. However, we wish to emphasize that age and parity are not the critical factors; the risk for STDs is the most important consideration. The IUD can and should be considered for the older teenager who is in a stable monogamous relationship and has had a child, and even in the appropriate nulliparous young woman. It is also a good choice in a patient with a chronic illness, such as diabetes mellitus or systemic lupus erythematosus, or in mentally retarded individuals.

Vaginal Contraceptives. The creams, foams, suppositories, and jellies are not ideal for adolescents. They require proper timing and placement (consistent use) for good efficacy.

Norplant and Depo-Provera. Although a long-acting method is an excellent answer to continuation problems, the many minor side effects represent a difficult problem for teenagers. Acne, weight change, and irregular bleeding are more common among Norplant and Depo-Provera users compared to oral contraception (however, the difference is not great). In addition the cost and the surgical procedure with Norplant are major difficulties for adolescents.[34] Nevertheless, both Depo-Provera and Norplant have proven to be relatively popular and successful with teenagers, especially among those who have experienced previous pregnancies or have used oral contraception in the past.[35-37] The long-acting feature and the ease of continuation are attractive to teenagers.[38] Effective counseling and education are critical for the successful use of these long-acting methods. The problems experienced with Norplant are identical in adolescent and adult women.[39] In properly prepared adolescent mothers, the use of Norplant has been reported to have a higher continuation rate and a lower failure rate compared to oral contraceptives, and the rate of condom use continued unchanged (in other words, condom use for protection against STDs was not diminished in Norplant users).[40]

There are special candidates to consider for long-acting contraception: teens who have failed oral contraception and teens who are mentally retarded or who have chronic illnesses.

There is some concern that the blood levels of estrogen with the use of Depo-Provera are relatively lower over a period of time compared to a normal menstrual cycle, and therefore patients can lose bone to some degree.[41] Another possible mechanism is displacement of cortisol by the progestin from its binding globulin in the circulation, resulting in elevated levels of free cortisol.

The subsequent risk of fracture from osteoporosis will depend upon bone mass at the time of menopause and the rate of bone loss following menopause. Although the peak bone mass is influenced by heredity and endocrine factors, it is now recognized that there exists only a relatively narrow window of opportunity for acquiring bone mass. Almost all of the bone mass in the hip and the vertebral bodies will be accumulated by late adolescence (age 18).[42] After adolescence, there is only a slight gain in total skeletal mass that ceases around age 30, and in many individuals a decline in bone mass in the hip and spine begins after age 18.[42] After age 30 in most people, there is a slow decline in bone mass density, about 0.7% per year. The importance of a normal diet and a normal hormonal environment during adolescence cannot be overrated.

In a study of bone density in adolescents using different methods of contraception, the use of Depo-Provera was associated with a decrease in bone density compared to an increase observed with Norplant or oral contraceptives.[43] However, bone density measurements in women who stopped using Depo-Provera indicated that the loss is regained even after long-term use.[44] This concern will require on-going surveillance, especially of past users, but at the present time, this should not be a reason to avoid this method of contraception. It is not known whether any significant amount of bone is permanently lost, and thus whether the risk of osteoporosis later in life is affected.

Postcoital Contraception. Because adolescents often have unplanned sexual intercourse, access to emergency postcoital contraception is important. The failure rate is approximately 2%. Treatment should be initiated as soon after exposure as possible, but no later than 72 hours. Side effects reflect the high-doses used: nausea, vomiting, headache, dizziness. We recommend a regimen (Chapter 3) that uses oral contraceptives as follows:

Ovral: 2 tablets followed by 2 tablets 12 hours later.

Lo Ovral, Nordette, Levlen, Triphasil, Trilevlen:
4 tablets followed by 4 tablets 12 hours later.

Clinicians should consider providing emergency contraceptive kits to patients (a kit can be a simple envelope containing instructions and the appropriate number of oral contraceptives) to be taken when needed. It would be a major contribution to our efforts to avoid unwanted pregnancies for all patients without contraindications to oral contraceptives to have emergency contraception available for use when needed. In our view, this would be much more effective in reducing the need for abortion than waiting for patients to call.

Adolescent Continuation

Knowing that contraception is available is not enough to prevent adolescent pregnancy. Adolescents have higher failure rates with all methods. Adolescent continuation with oral contraception has been particularly well-studied.[21,45] Factors associated with good continuation include: older age, suburban residence, health care in a private practice, payment status, prior use of contraception, mother's *unawareness* of oral contraception, married parents, older boyfriend, and satisfaction with pill use. Good continuation is also associated with educational goals and an absence of side effects. Inner city teens express more concern with side effects and safety, while suburban patients are more worried about weight gain and the effect of smoking. Surprisingly, in a study of 214 patients, only 11 reported reading the written instruction sheets which were provided.[45]

These studies indicate the importance of verbal instructions and the need to allow for questions. Long-term continuation is associated with an adolescent's career goals; it is worth bringing this up in conversation. Because adolescents tend to switch methods, all methods should be discussed with adolescents at each visit. Studies demonstrate that the extra time and effort required to meet the needs of adolescents result in improved contraceptive use and lower pregnancy rates.[24,46]

307

1. Establish and maintain confidentiality.
2. Do not lecture; make the patient visit a conversation; build trust.
3. Identify and address fears and concerns in advance.
4. Emphasize benefits.
5. Emphasize that minor side effects with oral contraception diminish with use.
6. Give instructions for managing side effects, missing pills.
7. Demonstrate package and pill taking (use the 28-day package), condom application.
8. Incorporate pill taking into patient's daily routine.
9. Don't let patient run out of pills.
10. Request that you be called before oral contraception is discontinued.
11. Identify and educate office personnel to interact with adolescents.
12. Frequent visits (every 3 months the first year), short waiting time, convenient hours.

Contraception for Older Women

Women of the post World War II generation have faced an unique evolutionary change. They were the first to be able to exercise control over their fertility, and then as they aged and deferred pregnancy, they had to deal with the problem of unintended infertility. After World War II, the U.S. total fertility rate reached a modern high of 3.8 births per woman. The last women born in this period won't be reaching their 45th birthday until around 2010. For approximately a 20-year period, therefore, there will be an unprecedented number of women in the later child-bearing years. The aging of the World War II population boom is giving current times a greater number of women who are delaying marriage and childbirth. This demographic change has 3 specific impacts on couples.

1. A need for effective contraception.
2. The problem of achieving pregnancy later in life.
3. The problem of being pregnant later in life.

This combination of increasing numbers, deferment of marriage, and postponement of pregnancy in marriage is responsible for the fact that we will be seeing more and more older women who will need reversible contraception. This is underscored by the fact that from ages 20–44, American women have the highest proportion of pregnancies aborted compared to other countries, indicating an unappreciated, but real, problem of unintended pregnancy existing beyond the teenage years, especially after age 35. More than half of all pregnancies in the U.S. are estimated to be unplanned, and more than half of these are aborted.[1] The best way to minimize the number of induced abortions is effective contraception.

The Ortho Pharmaceutical Corporation performs an annual birth control study involving thousands of women.[47] According to this study, the current use of oral contraception by U.S. women aged 15–44 increased from 21% in 1984 to 25% in 1993, followed by a slight decline to 24% in 1994. Women are using oral contraception for longer durations (the average length of time in the 1994 Ortho Study was 5.8 years), and more older women are using oral contraception. Oral contraceptive use quadrupled from 1990 to 1993 in women aged 40–45. These changes undoubtedly reflect clinician and patient awareness of the greater safety in low-dose formulations. IUD use decreased from 4% in 1984 to 1% in 1989, and this percentage has remained stable since then. Most IUD users (73%) are in the age group 35–50.

Oral Contraception for the Transitional Years

The years from age 35 to menopause can be referred to as the transition years. During this period of time, there are several medical needs which must be addressed: the need for contraception, the management of persistent anovulation, and finally, menopausal and postmenopausal hormone therapy.

At approximately 40 years of age, the frequency of ovulation decreases. This initiates a period of waning ovarian function called the climacteric that will last several years, carrying a woman through decreased fertility and menopause to the postmenopausal years. Prior to menopause, the remaining follicles perform less well. As cycles become irregular, vaginal bleeding occurs at the end of an inadequate luteal phase or after a peak of estradiol without subsequent ovulation and corpus luteum formation. Eventually, many women will live through a period of anovulation. Occasionally corpus luteum formation and function occur, and therefore the older woman is not totally safe from the threat of an unplanned and unexpected pregnancy.

Fortunately clinicians and patients have recognized that low-dose oral contraception is very safe for healthy, nonsmoking older women. However, their use is still not sufficient to meet the need. Besides fulfilling a need, we would argue that this population of women has a series of benefits to be derived from oral contraception that tilts the risk/benefit ratio to the positive side. The following benefits are especially pertinent for older women:

Effective Contraception.
- **less need for induced abortion.**
- **less need for surgical sterilization.**

Less Endometrial Cancer.
Less Ovarian Cancer.
Fewer Ectopic Pregnancies.
More Regular Menses.
- **less flow.**
- **less dysmenorrhea.**
- **less anemia.**

Less Salpingitis.
Less Rheumatoid Arthritis.
Increased Bone Density.
Probably Less Endometriosis.
Possibly Less Benign Breast Disease.
Possibly Protection against Atherosclerosis.
Possibly Fewer Fibroids.
Possibly Fewer Ovarian Cysts.

Thromboembolic disease is a consequence of pharmacologic administration of estrogen, and the level of risk is related to the estrogen dose (reviewed in Chapter 2). *It is likely that a slight increase of nonfatal venous thromboembolism is still present at estrogen doses less than 50 μg, but the actual incidence is low (about 15 per 100,000 woman-years), lower than that associated with pregnancy.*[48–50]

Smoking continues to be a difficult problem, not only for patient management, but for analysis of data as well. In large national surveys in 1982 and 1988, the decline in the prevalence of smoking was similar in users and nonusers of oral contraception; however, 24.3% of 35 to 45-year old women who used oral contraceptives were smokers![51] In this group of smoking, oral contraceptive-using women, 85.3% smoked 15 or more cigarettes per day (heavy smoking). Despite the widespread teaching and publicity that smoking is a contraindication to oral contraceptive use over the age of 35, more older women who use oral contraceptives smoke and smoke heavily, compared to young women. This strongly implies that older smokers are less than honest with clinicians when requesting oral contraception, and this further raises serious concern over how well this confounding variable can be controlled in case-control and cohort studies. *A former smoker must have stopped smoking for at least 12 consecutive months to be regarded as a nonsmoker. Women who have nicotine in their bloodstream obtained from patches or gum should be regarded as smokers.*

Smokers over age 35 should continue to be advised that combined oral contraceptives are not a good choice, regardless of the number of cigarettes smoked. In view of the unreported high rate of smoking in older women who use oral contraceptives, clinicians should consider using 20 μg estrogen products for women over age 35.

The minimal risk of thrombosis associated with oral contraceptive use does not justify the cost of routine screening for deficiencies in the coagulation system. **If a patient has a family history of idiopathic thrombosis or develops a thrombotic complication while taking oral contraceptives, an evaluation to search for an underlying abnormality in the coagulation system is warranted (measurement of antithrombin III, protein C, activated protein C resistance, protein S, activated partial thromboplastin time, fibrinogen, and plasminogen).**[52]

Combination oral contraception is contraindicated in women who have a history of idiopathic venous thrombosis, and also in women who have a family history of idiopathic venous thrombosis. These women will have a higher incidence of congenital deficiencies in important clotting measurements, especially antithrombin II, protein C, protein S, and resistance to activated protein C.[53]

Presently there is no reason why low-dose oral contraception cannot be utilized by appropriate patients until menopause. Menopause occurs in American women between the ages of 48 and 55, with the average age being approximately 51. Because the age of menopause occurs over such a relatively large age range, it is difficult to know when it is safe to transfer from oral contraception to a hormonal replacement program. And it should be emphasized that such transfer is important because the estrogen dose in even the lowest contraceptive formulations available is at least four times greater than what is needed for postmenopausal treatment. However, even this

311

dose of estrogen has an insignificant impact on the coagulation system.[54,55]

The therapeutic principle remains to utilize the formulation which gives effective contraception and the greatest margin of safety. Because we now appreciate the dose-response relationship between the steroid components and side effects, it makes sense to use the lowest doses that are still effective. For this reason products with less than 30 μg of estrogen might be especially useful for older women.

Over the years, the debate over the cause of circulatory complications attributed to oral contraception turned from thrombosis to atherosclerosis. Today, belief is firmly back in the camp of thrombosis. A significant reason is the failure to detect any lingering risk of cardiovascular disease in former pill users. Most noteworthy is the Nurses' Health Study.[56] Now that the nurses initially enrolled in this follow-up study have aged sufficiently, we have statistically and clinically significant data from women who have reached the age of major risk for cardiovascular disease. Even the use of higher-dose oral contraceptives is not associated with a subsequent increased risk of coronary heart disease and stroke. The fact that an increased risk of cardiovascular disease is limited to current use is a very strong indicator that the mechanism is a short-term acute mechanism, specifically thrombosis, an estrogen-related effect. Therefore, coming back to the belief that cardiovascular disease is linked to thrombosis makes the role, and the dose, of estrogen very important.

A product containing 20 μg ethinyl estradiol and 150 μg desogestrel has been demonstrated in multicenter studies of women over age 30 to have the same efficacy and side effects as pills containing 30 and 35 μg of estrogen.[57–60] In a randomized study of women over age 30, this formulation was associated with the virtual elimination of any effects on coagulation factors.[55] Indeed, the 20 μg formulation has no significant impact on the measurements of clotting factors, even in smokers.[31,32,54,55]

While it is true that the implied safety of the lowest estrogen dose remains to be documented by epidemiologic studies, it seems clinically prudent to maximize the safety margin in this older age group of women. Although there may be some increase in breakthrough bleeding, we believe that older women who understand the increased safety implicit in the lowest estrogen dose are more willing to endure breakthrough bleeding and maintain continuation. With avoidance of risk factors and use of lowest dose pills, health risks are probably negligible for healthy, nonsmoking women. For healthy nonsmoking women, no specific laboratory screening is necessary, beyond that which is usually incorporated in a program of preventive health care.

We should also mention the progestin-only minipill (Chapter 3). Because of reduced fecundity, the minipill achieves near total efficacy in women over age 40. Therefore, the progestin-only minipill is a good choice for older woman, and especially for those women in whom estrogen is contraindicated. Older women are more accepting of irregular menstrual bleeding when they understand its mechanism, and thus, are more accepting of the progestin-only minipill.

When to Change from Oral Contraception to Postmenopausal Hormone Therapy. One approach to establish the onset of the postmenopausal years is to measure the FSH level, beginning at age 50, on an annual basis, being careful to obtain the blood sample on day 6 or 7 of the pill-free week. Friday afternoon works well in women on Sunday start packages. By then, the steroid levels will have declined sufficiently to allow FSH to rise. When FSH is greater than 30 IU/L it is time to transfer to a postmenopausal hormone program. Because of the variability in FSH levels experienced by women around the menopause, this method is not always accurate. But there is no harm in another year or two on low-dose oral contraceptives. Some clinicians are comfortable allowing patients to enter their mid-fifties on low-dose oral contraception, and then empirically switching to a postmenopausal hormone regimen.

Anovulation and Bleeding. Throughout the transitional period of life there is a significant incidence of dysfunctional uterine bleeding due to anovulation. While the clinician is usually alerted to this problem because of irregular bleeding, clinician and patient often fail to diagnose anovulation when bleeding is not abnormal in schedule, flow, or duration. As a woman approaches menopause, a more aggressive attempt to document ovulation is warranted. A serum progesterone level measured approximately one week before menses is simple enough to obtain and worth the cost. The prompt diagnosis of anovulation (serum progesterone less than 300 ng/dL) will lead to appropriate therapeutic management which will have a significant impact on the risk of endometrial cancer.

In an anovulatory woman with proliferative or hyperplastic endometrium (unaccompanied by atypia), periodic oral progestin

313

therapy is mandatory, such as 10 mg medroxyprogesterone acetate given daily the first 10 days of each month. If hyperplasia is already present, follow-up aspiration office curettage after 3–4 months is required. If progestin treatment is ineffective and histological regression is not observed, more aggressive treatment is warranted.

Monthly progestin treatment should be continued until withdrawal bleeding ceases or menopausal symptoms are experienced. These are reliable signs (in effect, a bioassay) indicating the onset of estrogen deprivation and the need for the addition of estrogen in a postmenopausal hormone program.

If contraception is desired, the clinician and patient should seriously consider the use of oral contraception. The anovulatory woman cannot be guaranteed that spontaneous ovulation and pregnancy will not occur. The use of a low-dose oral contraceptive will at the same time provide contraception and prophylaxis against irregular, heavy anovulatory bleeding and the risk of endometrial hyperplasia and neoplasia. In some patients, oral contraceptive treatment achieves better regulation of menses than monthly progestin administration.

Clinicians have been made so wary of providing oral contraceptives to older women that a traditional postmenopausal hormone regimen is often utilized to treat a woman with the kind of irregular cycles usually experienced in the transitional years. This addition of exogenous estrogen when a woman is not amenorrheic or experiencing menopausal symptoms is inappropriate, and even risky (exposing the endometrium to excessively high levels of estrogen). *And something that is often unappreciated, the standard doses of estrogen and progestin in a postmenopausal regimen will not suppress gonadotropins and prevent ovulation.* The appropriate response is to regulate anovulatory cycles with monthly progestational treatment or to utilize low-dose oral contraception.

Long-Acting Methods for Older Women

The long-acting methods of hormonal contraception (Norplant and Depo-Provera) deserve consideration in those situations where combination estrogen-progestin is unacceptable because of health problems (where estrogen is contraindicated), or where oral contraception has already proved to be unsuccessful. These methods are especially advantageous for smokers and for women with a history of thromboembolic disease. Progestin-only contraception is a good choice for women with hypertriglyceridemia, for diabetic women (even if they are older and smoke), and for women with severe migraine headaches.

Older women, as they approach the menopause, may be more comfortable with the irregular bleeding or amenorrhea associated with these methods. However, the irregular bleeding patterns associated with these methods can cause more concern in some women regarding possible pathology. Hormone treatment can be initiated if menopausal symptoms develop or when annual measurement of the FSH level (beginning at age 50) indicates a rise above 30 IU/L.

The IUD for Older Women

The growing need for reversible contraception would also be served by increased utilization of the IUD. After several years of use, efficacy with the IUD is similar to that of oral contraceptives. The decline in IUD use in the U.S. is in direct contrast to the experience in the rest of the world, a complicated response to publicity and litigation. An increased risk of pelvic infection with contemporary IUDs in use is limited to the act of insertion and the transportation of pathogens to the upper genital tract. This risk is effectively minimized by careful screening with preinsertion cultures and the use of good technique. A return to IUD use by American couples is both warranted and desirable.

The IUD is a good reversible contraceptive choice for older women. An older woman is more likely to be mutually monogamous and less likely to develop PID, and for those women who have already had their children, concern with fertility and problems with cramping and bleeding are both lesser issues. If protection from STDs is not a concern, insertion of a copper IUD can provide very effective contraception until the menopause without the need to do anything other than check the string occasionally. On the other hand, because alterations of bleeding patterns become more common in this age group, it may be necessary to remove an IUD. Because many older women have diabetes mellitus, it is worth emphasizing that no increase in adverse events has been observed with copper IUD use in women with either insulin-dependent or non-insulin-dependent diabetes.[61,62] The IUD is not a good choice when the uterine cavity is distorted by leiomyomata.

Barrier Methods for Older Couples

Some women use barrier methods throughout their reproductive years, but most change to easier, more effective methods as their sexual lives become more stable, their risk of STDs decreases accordingly, and they need contraception for avoiding rather than spacing pregnancies. Some women begin new relationships as they age and may require reminding about the risks of STDs and the need to use condoms with new partners whose sexual and drug use histories are unknown. Perimenopausal women whose earlier use of contraception was not directed at avoiding HIV infection may need to learn how and with whom to use condoms.

Preventive Health Care for Older Women

Preventive health care for women is especially important during the transition years. The issues of preventive health care are familiar ones. They include contraception, cessation of smoking, prevention of heart disease and osteoporosis, maintenance of mental well-being (including sexuality), and cancer screening. Management of the transition years should be significantly oriented to preventive health care, and the use of low-dose oral contraception can now legitimately be viewed as a component of preventive health care. A discussion of the noncontraceptive health benefits of low-dose oral contraception is especially important with patients in their transition years. This group of women appreciates and understands decisions made with the risk-benefit ratio in mind. For example, a useful observation to bring to our patient's attention is the following: continuous use of oral contraception for 10 years by women with a positive family history for ovarian cancer can reduce the risk of epithelial ovarian cancer to a level equal to or less than that experienced by women with a negative family history.[63]

Contraceptive advice is a component of good preventive health care, and the clinician's approach is a key. This is an era of informed choice by the patient. Patients deserve to know the facts and need help in dealing with the state of the art and the uncertainty. But there is no doubt that patients are influenced in their choice by their clinician's advice and attitude. While the role of a clinician is to provide the education necessary for the patient to make proper choices, one should not lose sight of the powerful influence exerted by the clinician in the choices ultimately made.

References

1. Westoff CF, Unintended pregnancy in America and abroad, Fam Plann Perspect 20:254, 1988.

2. Koonin L, Smith J, Ramick M Abortion surveillance — United States, 1991, MMWR 44:23, 1995.

3. Henshaw SK, Van Vort J, Abortion services in the United States, 1991 and 1992, Fam Plann Perspect 26:100, 1994.

4. Forrest JD, Singh S, The sexual and reproductive behavior of American women, 1982–1988, Fam Plann Perspect 22:206, 1990.

5. The Alan Guttmacher Institute, *Sex and America's Teenagers,* The Alan Guttmacher Institute, New York, New York, 1994.

6. Centers for Disease Control and Prevention, *Adolescent Health: State of the Nation — Pregnancy, Sexually Transmitted Diseases and Related Risk Behaviors Among U.S. Adolescents,* U.S. Department of Health and Human Services, Public Health Service, DHHS Publication No. (CDC) 099-4630, 1995.

7. Centers for Disease Control and Prevention, Trends in sexual behavior among high school students — United States, 1990, 1991, 1993, MMWR 44:124, 1995.

8. Zabin LS, Kanatner JF, Zelnick M, The risk of adolescent pregnancy in the first months of intercourse, Fam Plann Perspect 11:215, 1979,

9. Trussell J, Teenage pregnancy in the United States, Fam Plann Perspect 20:262, 1989.

10. Ahn N, Teenage childbearing and high school completion: accounting for individual heterogeneity, Fam Plann Perspect 26:17, 1994.

11. McAnarney ER, Hendee WR, Adolescent pregnancy and its consequences, JAMA 262:74, 1989.

12. Furstenberg FF, Brooks-Gunn J, Morgan SP, Adolescent mothers and their children in later life, Fam Plann Perspect 19:142, 1987.

13. Zabin LS, Stark HA, Emerson MR, Reasons for delay in contraceptive clinic utilization, J Adolesc Health 12:225, 1991.

14. Kirby D, Short L, Collins J, Rugg D, Kolbe L, Howard M, Miller B, Sonenstein F, Zabin LS, School-based programs to reduce sexual risk behaviors: a review of effectiveness, Public Health Reports 109:339, 1994.

15. Kirby D, Waszak C, Ziegler, Six school-based clinics: their reproductive health services and impact on sexual behavior, Fam Plann Perspect 23:6, 1991.

16. Kirby D, Resnick MD, Downes B, Kocher T, Gunderson P, Potthoff S, Zelterman D, Blum RW, The effects of school-based health clinics in St. Paul on school wide birthrates, Fam Plann Perspect 25:12, 1993.

17. **Vincent ML, Clearie AF, Schluchter MD,** Reducing adolescent pregnancy through school and community-based education, JAMA 257:3382, 1987.

18. **Malus M, LaChance PA, Lamy L, Macaulay A, Vanasse M,** Priorities in adolescent health care: the teenager's viewpoint, J Fam Pract 25:159, 1987.

19. **Jones EF, Forrest JD, Goldman N, Henshaw SK, Lincoln R, Rosoff J, Westoff CF, Wulf D,** Teenage pregnancy in developed countries: determinants and policy implications, Fam Plann Perspect 17:53, 1985.

20. **Hanson SL,** Involving families in programs for pregnant teens: consequences for teens and their families, J Appl Fam Child Stud 41:303, 1992.

21. **Jay MS, DuRant RH, Litt IF,** Female adolescents' compliance with contraceptive regimens, Ped Clinics N Am 36:731, 1989.

22. **Bagwell MA, Coker AL, Thompson SJ, Baker ER, Addy CL,** Primary infertility and oral contraceptive steroid use, Fertil Steril 63:1161, 1995.

23. **Carpenter S, Neinstein LS,** Weight gain in adolescent and young adult oral contraceptive users, J Adoles Health Care 7:342, 1986.

24. **Grace E, Emans SJ, Havens KK, Merola JL, Woods ER,** Contraceptive compliance with a triphasic and a monophasic norethindrone-containing oral contraceptive pill in a private adolescent practice, Adolesc Pediatr Gynecol 7:29, 1994.

25. **Robinson JC, Plichter S, Weisman CS, Nathanson CA, Ensminger M,** Dysmenorrhea and use of oral contraceptives in adolescent women attending a family planning clinic, Am J Obstet Gynecol 166:578, 1992.

26. **Centers for Disease Control and Prevention,** Prevalence of adults with no known major risk factors for coronary heart disease—behavioral risk factor surveillance system, 1992, JAMA 271:741, 1994.

27. **Fiore MC, Novotny TE, Pierce JP, Hatziandreu EJ, Patel KM, Davis RM,** Trends in cigarette smoking in the United States, JAMA 261:49, 1989.

28. **Risch HA, Howe GR, Jain M, Burch JD, Holowaty EJ, Miller AB,** Are female smokers at higher risk for lung cancer than male smokers? A case-control analysis by histologic type, Am J Epidemiol 138:281, 1993.

29. **Davis DL, Dinse GE, Hoel DG,** Decreasing cardiovascular disease and increasing cancer among whites in the United States from 1973 through 1987, JAMA 271:431, 1994.

30. **Willett WC, Green A, Stampfer MJ, Speizer FE, Colditz GA, Rosner B, Monson RR, Stason W, Hennekens CH,** Relative and absolute excess risks of coronary heart disease among women who smoke cigarettes, New Engl J Med 317:1303, 1987.

31. **Fruzzetti F, Ricci C, Fioretti P,** Haemostasis profile in smoking and nonsmoking women taking low-dose oral contraceptives, Contraception 49:579, 1994.

32. **Basdevant A, Conard J, Pelissier C, Guyene T-T, Lapousterle C, Mayer M, Guy-Grand B, Degrelle H,** Hemostatic and metabolic effects of lowering the ethinyl-estradiol dose from 30 mcg to 20 mcg in oral contraceptives containing desogestrel, Contraception 48:193, 1993.

33. **Werner MJ, Biro FM,** Contraception and sexually transmitted diseases in adolescent females, Adoles Pediatr Gynecol 3:127, 1990.

34. **Darney PD, Klaisle CM, Tanner S, Alvarado AM,** Sustained-release contraceptives, Curr Probl Obstet Gynecol Fertil 13:95, 1990.

35. **Smith RD, Cromer BA, Hayes JR, et al,** Medroxyprogesterone acetate (Depo-Provera) use in adolescents: uterine bleeding and blood pressure patterns, patient satisfaction, and continuation rates, Adolesc Pediatr Gynecol 8:24, 1995.

36. **Berenson AB, Wiemann CM,** Use of levonorgestrel implants versus oral contraceptives in adolescence: a case-control study, Am J Obstet Gynecol 172:1128, 1995.

37. **Weisman CS, Plichta SB, Tirado DE, et al,** Comprison of contraceptive implant adopters and pill users in a family planning clinic in Baltimore, Fam Plann Perspect 25:224, 1993.

38. **Cromer BA, Smith RD, Blair JM, Dwyer J, Brown RT,** A prospective study of adolescents who choose among levonorgestrel implant (Norplant), medroxyprogesterone acetate (Depo-Provera), or the combined oral contraceptive pill as contraception, Pediatrics 94:687, 1994.

39. **Cullins VE, Remsburg RE, Blumenthal PD, Huggins GR,** Comparison of adolescent and adult experience with Norplant levonorgestrel contraceptive implants, Obstet Gynecol 83:1026, 1994.

40. **Polaneczky M, Slap G, Forke C, Rappaport A, Sondheimer S,** The use of levonorgestrel implants (Norplant) for contraception in adolescent mothers, New Engl J Med 331:1201, 1994.

41. **Cundy T, Evans M, Roberts H, Wattie D, Ames R, Reid IR,** Bone density in women receiving depot medroxyprogesterone acetate for contraception, Br Med J 303:13, 1991.

42. **Matkovic V, Jelic T, Wardlaw GM, Ilich J, Goel PK, Wright JK, Andon MB, Smith KT, Heaney RP,** Timing of peak bone mass in caucasian females and its implication for the prevention of osteoporosis: inference from a cross-sectional model, J Clin Invest 93:799, 1994.

43. **Blair JM, Cromer B, Mahan J, et al,** Bone density in adolescent girls on Depo-Provera and Norplant, J Adolesc Health 16:164, 1995.

44. **Cundy T, Cornish J, Evans MC, Roberts H, Reid IR,** Recovery of bone density in women who stop using medroxyprogesterone acetate, Br Med J 308:247, 1994.

45. **Emans SJ, Grace E, Woods ER, Smith DE, Klein K, Merola J,** Adolescents' compliance with the use of oral contraceptives, JAMA 257:3377, 1987.

46. **Winter L, Breckenmaker LC,** Tailoring family planning services to the special needs of adolescents, Fam Plann Perspect 23:24, 1991.

47. **Ortho Pharmaceutical Corporation,** Annual birth control study, 1994.

48. **Lidegaard Ø,** Oral contraception and risk of a cerebral thromboembolic attack: results of a case-control study, Br Med J 306:956, 1993.

49. **Farmer RDT, Preston TD,** The risk of venous thromboembolism associated with low estrogen oral contraceptives, J Obstet Gynaecol 15:195, 1995.

50. **WHO Collaborative Study of Cardiovascular Disease and Steroid Hormone Cosntraception,** Venous thromboembolic disease and combined oal contraceptives: results of international multicentre case-control study, Lancet 348:1575, 1995.

51. **Barrett DH, Anda RF, Escobedo LG, Croft JB, Williamson DF, Marks JS,** Trends in oral contraceptive use and cigarette smoking, Arch Fam Med 3:438, 1994.

52. **Vandenbroucke JP, Koster T, Briët E, Reitsma PH, Bertina RM, Rosendaal FR,** Increased risk of venous thrombosis in oral-contraceptive users who are carriers of factor V Leiden mutation, Lancet 344:1453, 1994

53. **Pabinger I, Schneider B, and the GTH Study Group,** Thrombotic risk of women with hereditary antithrombin III, protein C, and protein S deficiency taking oral contraceptive medication, Thromb Haemost 5:548, 1994.

54. **Gordon EM, Williams SR, Frenchek B, Mazur CH, Speroff L,** Dose-dependent effects of postmenopausal estrogen/progestin on antithrombin III and factor XII, J Lab Clin Med 111:52, 1988.

55. **Melis GB, Fruzzetti F, Nicoletti I, Ricci C, Lammers P, Atsma WJ, Fioretti P,** A comparative study on the effects of a monophasic pill containing desogestrel plus 20 mcg ethinylestradiol, a triphasic combination containing levonorgestel and a monophasic combination containing gestodene on coagulatory factors, Contraception 43:23, 1991.

56. **Colditz, GA and the Nurses' Health Study Research Group,** Oral contraceptive use and mortality during 12 years of follow-up: the Nurses' Health Study, Ann Intern Med 120:821, 1994.

57. **Volpe A, Silferi M, Genazzani AD, Genazzani AR,** Contraception in older women, Contraception 47:229, 1993.

58. **Kirkman RJE, Pedersen JH, Fioretti P, Roberts HE,** Clinical comparison of two low-dose oral contraceptives, Minulet and Mercilon, in women over 30 years of age, Contraception 49:33, 1994.

59. **Fioretti P, Fruzzetti F, Navalesi R, Ricci C, Moccoli R, Cerri FM, Orlandi MC, Melis GB,** Clinical and metabolic study of a new pill containing 20 mcg ethinylestradiol plus 0.150 mg desogestrel, Contraception 35:229, 1987.

60. **Steffensen K,** Evaluation of an oral contraceptive containing 0.150 desogestrel and 0.020 mg ethinylestradiol in women aged 30 years or older, Acta Obstet Gynecol Scand Suppl 144:23, 1987.

61. **Kimmerle R, Weiss R, Berger M, Kurz K,** Effectiveness, safety, and acceptability of a copper intrauterine deivce (Cu Safe 300) in type I diabetic women, Diabetes Care 16:1227, 1993.

62. **Kjos SL, Ballagh SA, La Cour M, Xiang A, Mishell DR Jr,** The copper T380A intrauterine device in women with Type II diabetes mellitus, Obstet Gynecol 84:1006, 1994.

63. **Gross TP, Schlesselman JJ,** The estimated effect of oral contraceptive use on the cumulative risk of epithelial ovarian cancer, Obstet Gynecol 83:419, 1994.

11

Sterilization

C ONTRACEPTIVE METHODS today are very safe and effective, however, we remain decades away from a perfect method of contraception for either women or men. Because reversible contraceptive methods are not perfect, more than a third of American couples use sterilization instead, and sterilization is now the predominate method of contraception in the world.[1]

Over the past 20 years, nearly a million Americans each year have undergone a sterilization operation, and recently, more women than men. By 1988, 24% of reproductive aged women relied on contraceptive sterilization, 17% by tubal occlusion and 7% depended upon their partner's vasectomy.[2,3] This same trend has occurred in Great Britain, where by age 40, just over 20% of men and women have had a sterilization procedure.[4] In Spain and Italy, sterilization rates are very low, but the use of oral contraceptives and the IUD is very high.[5]

Americans use sterilization for contraceptive purposes more than the people of most countries, in our view, because the intrauterine device (the IUD) and oral contraception have a worse reputation here than in the rest of the world. Publicity about side effects and litigation have frightened prospective users, and it is little wonder that Americans turn to sterilization more often and at an earlier age, and, we believe, before they really want to. A significant increase in both female and male sterilization occurred between 1973 and 1988, a period during which the use of IUDs declined, and the use of oral contraception decreased substantially, although since the late 1980s, oral contraception has regained some of its popularity.[6]

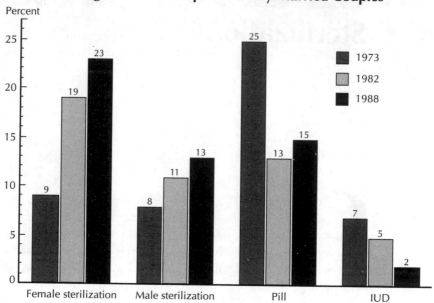

Changes in Contraceptive Use by Married Couples[1,2]

History

James Blundell proposed in 1823, in lectures at Guy's Hospital in London, that tubectomy ought to be performed at cesarean section to avoid the need for repeat sections.[7] He also proposed a technique for sterilization which he later described so precisely that he must actually have performed the operation, although he never wrote about it. The first report was published in 1881 by Samuel Lungren of Toledo, Ohio, who ligated the tubes at the time of cesarean section, as Blundell had suggested 58 years earlier.[8] The Madlener procedure was devised in Germany in 1910 and reported in 1919. Because of many failures, the Madlener technique was supplanted in the U.S. by the method of Ralph Pomeroy, a prominent physician in Brooklyn, New York. This method, still popular today, was not described to the medical profession by Pomeroy's associates until 1929, 4 years after Pomeroy's death. Frederick Irving of the Harvard Medical School described his technique in 1924, and the Uchida method was not reported until 1946.

Few sterilizations were performed until the 1930s when "family planning" was first suggested as an indication by Baird in Aberdeen. He required women to be over 40 and to have had 8 or more children. Mathematical formulas of this kind persisted through the 1960s. In 1965, Sir Dugald Baird delivered a remarkable lecture, entitled "The Fifth Freedom," calling attention to the need to alleviate the fear of unwanted pregnancies, and the important role of sterilization.[9] By the end of the 1960s, sterilization was a popular procedure.

The Pomeroy

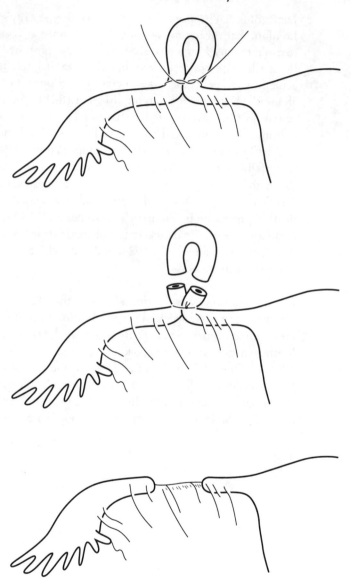

The Irving

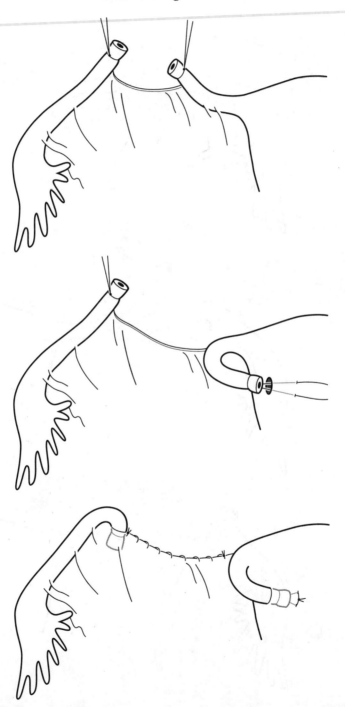

The Uchida

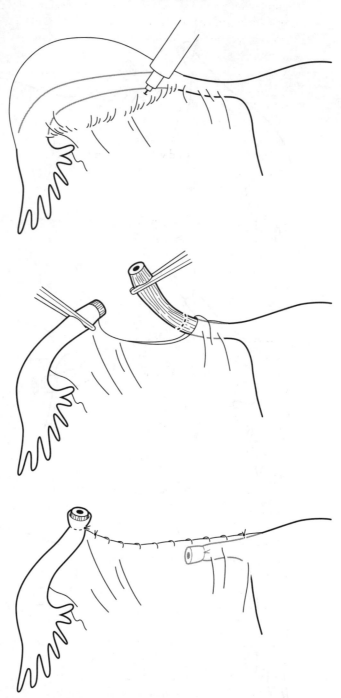

Laparoscopic methods were introduced in the early 1970s. The annual number of vasectomies began to decline, and the number of tubal occlusion operations increased rapidly. By 1973, more sterilization operations were performed for women than for men. This is accurately attributed to dramatic decreases in costs, hospital time, and pain due to the introduction of laparoscopy and minilaparotomy methods. The use of laparoscopy for tubal occlusion increased from only 0.6% of sterilizations in 1970 to more than 35% by 1975.[10] Since 1975, minilaparotomy, a technique popular in the less developed world, has been increasingly performed in the U.S. These methods have allowed women to undergo sterilization operations at times other than immediately after childbirth or during major surgery.

Laparoscopy and minilaparotomy have led to a profound change in the convenience and cost of sterilization operations for women. In 1970, the average woman stayed in the hospital 6.5 days for a tubal sterilization. By 1975, this had declined to 3 days, and today, women rarely remain in the hospital overnight. The shorter length of stay achieved from 1970 to 1975 represented a savings of more than 200 million dollars yearly in health care costs and a tremendous increase in convenience for women eager to return to work and their families.[11] Unlike some advances in technology, laparoscopy and minilaparotomy sterilization are technical innovations which have resulted in large savings in medical care costs. New methods are currently being investigated employing hysteroscopy and transcervical application of substances to obstruct the fallopian tubes.

The great majority of sterilization procedures are accomplished in hospitals by physicians in private practice, but a rapidly increasing proportion are performed outside of hospitals in ambulatory surgical settings, including physician's offices. In either hospital or outpatient settings, female sterilization is a very safe operation. Deaths specifically attributed to sterilization now account for a fatality rate of only 1.5 per 100,000 procedures, a mortality rate that is lower than that for childbearing (about 10 per 100,000 births in the U.S.).[12] When the risk of pregnancy from contraceptive method failure is taken into account, sterilization is the safest of all contraceptive methods.

Vasectomy has long been more popular in the U.S. than anywhere else in the world, but why don't more men use it? One explanation is that women have chosen laparoscopic sterilization in increasing numbers. Another is that men have been frightened by reports, often from animal data, of associations with autoimmune diseases, athero-sclerosis, and most recently, prostatic cancer. Large epidemiologic studies have failed to confirm any of these associations. When patients consider sterilization, we can assure them that vasectomy has not been demonstrated to have any harmful effects on men's health.[13] In addition, vasectomy is less expensive, morbidity is less, and mortality is essentially zero.

Efficacy of Sterilization

Laparoscopic and minilaparotomy sterilization are not only conve-nient, they are almost as effective at preventing pregnancy as were the older, more complex operations. Vasectomy is also highly effective once the supply of remaining sperm in the vas deferens is exhausted. After 6 weeks or 15 ejaculations, essentially all men are sterile.

Failure Rates During the First Year, United States [14]

Method	Percent of Women with Pregnancy Lowest Expected	Typical
Female sterilization	0.2%	0.4%
Male sterilization	0.1%	0.15%

Besides the specific operation employed, the skill of the operator and characteristics of the patient make important contributions to the efficacy of female sterilization. Up to 50% of failures are due to technical errors. The methods employing complicated equipment, such as spring-loaded clips and Silastic rings, fail for technical reasons more commonly than did simpler procedures such as the Pomeroy tubal sterilization.[15] Minilaparotomy failures, therefore, occur much less frequently due to technical errors.

It is hardly surprising that more complicated techniques of tubal occlusion have higher technical failure rates. What is surprising is the finding that characteristics of the patient influence the likelihood of failure even when technical problems are considered. In a careful study of this issue, two patient characteristics, age and lactation, demonstrated a significant impact.[16] Patients younger than 35 years were 1.7 times more likely to become pregnant, and women who were not breastfeeding following sterilization were 5 times more likely to become pregnant. These findings probably reflect the greater fecundity of younger women and the contraceptive contribution of lactation.

Significant numbers of pregnancies following tubal occlusion are present before the procedure. For this reason, some clinicians routinely perform a uterine evacuation or curettage prior to tubal occlusion. It seems more reasonable (and cost effective) to exclude pregnancy by careful history taking, physical examination, and an appropriate pregnancy test prior to the sterilization procedure.[17]

Because method, operator, and patient characteristics all influence sterilization failures, it is difficult to predict which individual will experience a pregnancy after undergoing a tubal occlusion. Therefore, during the course of counseling, all patients should be made aware of the possibility of failure as well as the intent to cause permanent, irreversible sterility. It is important to avoid giving patients the impression that the tubal occlusion procedure is foolproof or guaranteed. Individual clinicians must be cautious judging their own success in accomplishing sterilization because failure is infrequent and many patients who become pregnant following sterilization never reveal the failure to the original surgeon.

Ectopic pregnancies can occur following tubal occlusion, and the incidence is much higher with some types of tubal occlusion.[18,19,20] Bipolar tubal coagulation is more likely to result in ectopic pregnancy than is mechanical occlusion.[15,21] The probable explanation is that microscopic fistulae in the coagulated segment connecting to the peritoneal cavity permit sperm to reach the ovum. Ectopic pregnancies following tubal sterilization are more likely to occur 2 or more years after sterilization, rather than immediately after. In the first year after sterilization, about 6% of pregnancies will be ectopic, but the majority of pregnancies which occur 2–3 years after occlusion will be ectopic.[22] The rate of intrauterine pregnancies decreases with time, but ectopic rates remain constant. Overall, however, the risk of an ectopic pregnancy in sterilized women is lower than if they had not been sterilized. Nevertheless, about 30% of the pregnancies in previously sterilized women are ectopics.[23]

Vaginal procedures have higher failure rates than laparoscopy or minilaparotomy, but the principal disadvantage is higher infection rates, and this approach is not favored. Intraperitoneal infection is a rare complication of minilap or laparoscopic techniques. In vaginal procedures, abscess formation approaches 1%.[24] This risk can be reduced by the use of prophylactic antibiotics administered intraoperatively, but open laparoscopy is usually easier and safer even in obese women.

Sterilization and Ovarian Cancer — A Benefit of Sterilization

Evidence from the Nurses' Health Study suggests that tubal sterilization strongly protects against ovarian cancer.[25] In addition, case-control data have consistently supported this finding.[26-28] The mechanism for such an effect is not clear, but this information is worth sharing with patients.

Female Sterilization Techniques

Because laparoscopy permits direct visualization and manipulation of the abdominal and pelvic organs with minimal abdominal disruption, it offers many advantages. Hospitalization is not required; most patients return home within a few hours, and the majority return to full activity within 24 hours. Discomfort is minimal, the incision scars are barely visible, and sexual activity need not be restricted. In addition, the surgeon has an opportunity to inspect the pelvic and abdominal organs for abnormalities. The disadvantages of laparoscopic sterilization include the cost, the expensive, fragile equipment, the special training required, and the risks of inadvertent bowel or vessel injury.

Laparoscopic sterilization can be achieved with any of these methods:

1. Occlusion and partial resection by unipolar electrosurgery.
2. Occlusion and transection by unipolar electrosurgery.
3. Occlusion by bipolar electrocoagulation.
4. Occlusion by mechanical means (clips or Silastic rings).

All of these methods can use an operating laparoscope alone, or the diagnostic laparoscope with operating instruments passed through a second trocar, or both the operating laparoscope and secondary puncture equipment. All can be employed using the "open" laparoscopic technique in which the laparoscopic instrument is placed into the abdominal cavity under direct vision to avoid the risk of bowel or blood vessel puncture on blind entry. Patient acceptance and recovery are approximately the same with all methods.

Female Tubal Sterilization Methods
Ten-Year Cumulative Failure Rates [23]

Unipolar coagulation	0.75%
Postpartum tubal excision	0.75%
Silastic (Falope or Yoon) ring	1.78%
Interval tubal excision	2.01%
Bipolar coagulation	2.48%
Hulka-Clemens clip	3.65%

Early reports of laparoscopic sterilization revealed that electrocoagulation was not without hazard. Complications were attributed to defective coagulation equipment or inadvertent coagulation of the bowel.[29] These complications can be reduced by establishing a consistent operating protocol and an education program for all operating room personnel, particularly with respect to electrosurgical principles and techniques.

Tubal Occlusion by Electrosurgical Methods

If electrons from an electrosurgical generator are concentrated in one location, heat within the tissue increases sharply and desiccates the tissue until resistance is so high that no more current can pass. Unipolar methods of sterilization create a dense area of current under the grasping forceps of the unipolar electrode. In order to complete the circuit, however, these electrons must spread through the body and be returned to the generator via a return electrode (the ground plate) which has a broad surface to minimize the density of the current to avoid burns as the electrons leave the body. "Unipolar" refers to the method which requires the patient ground plate.

With the unipolar method, if tissue resistance is high and the electrical pressure (voltage) relatively low, current may cease to flow or may search out alternate pathways with lower resistance. When the

333

voltage is increased, the electrons have more "push" to find another pathway, therefore the surgeon must use the lowest possible voltage necessary to completely coagulate. The return electrode (the ground plate) must be in good contact with the patient.

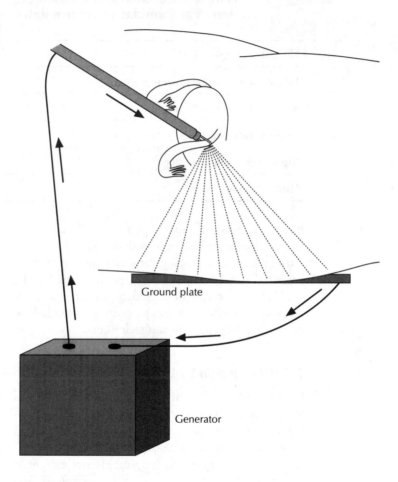

Ground plate

Generator

Unipolar electrosurgery can create a unique electrical "capacitance" problem when an operating laparoscope is used with unipolar forceps. A capacitor is any device that can hold an electric charge, and can exist wherever an insulated material separates two conductors that have different potentials. This property of capacitance explains some of the inadvertent bowel burns that have occurred with laparoscopic sterilization. The operating laparoscope is a hollow metal tube surrounding an active electrode, the forceps used to grasp and coagulate the tubes. When current passes through the active electrode, the laparoscope itself becomes a capacitor. Up to 70% of the current passed through the active electrode can be induced into the laparoscope. Should bowel or other structures touch a laparoscope which is insulated from the abdominal incision (for example, by a fiberglass cannula), the stored electrons will be discharged at high density directly into the vital organ. This potential hazard is eliminated by using a metal trocar sleeve rather than a nonconductive sleeve like fiberglass. Because there is little pressure behind the electrons from a low-voltage generator, not enough heat is generated to burn the skin as the capacitance current leaks out into the patient's body through the sleeve. Even if the active electrode comes in direct contact with the laparoscope, as when a two-incision technique is employed, the current will leak harmlessly through the metal trocar sleeve. The risk of inadvertent coagulation of bowel or other organs cannot be completely eliminated because all body surfaces offer a path back to the ground plate.

The unipolar electrosurgical technique is straightforward. The isthmic portion of the fallopian tube is grasped, elevated away from the surrounding structures and the electrical energy applied until the tissue blanches, swells, and then collapses. The tube is then grasped, moving toward the uterus, recoagulated, and the steps repeated until 2–3 cm of tube have been coagulated. Some surgeons advise against cornual coagulation for fear it may increase the risk of ectopic pregnancy due to fistula formation.

The coagulation and transection technique is performed in a similar fashion with the same instruments. In order to transect the tube, however, an instrument designed to cut tissue must be utilized. The transection of tissue increases the risk of possible bleeding and does not, by itself, reduce the failure rate over coagulation alone. The specimens obtained by this method are usually coagulated beyond microscopic recognition, and therefore, will not provide pathological evidence of successful sterilization. Unipolar coagulation has a very low failure rate, but a high risk of inadvertant bowel damage compared to other techniques.

The bipolar method of sterilization eliminates the ground plate required for unipolar electrosurgery and employs a specially designed forceps. One jaw of the forceps is the active electrode and the other jaw is the ground electrode. Current density is great at the point of forceps contact with tissue, and the use of a low voltage, high-frequency current prevents the spread of electrons. By eliminating the return electrode, the chance of an aberrant pathway through bowel or other structures is greatly reduced. There is, however, a disadvantage with this technique. Since electron spread is decreased, more applications of the grasping forceps are necessary to coagulate the same length of tube than with unipolar coagulation. As desiccation occurs at the point of high current density, tissue resistance increases, and the coagulated area eventually provides resistance to flow of the low-voltage current. Should the resistance increase beyond the voltage's capability to push electrons through the tissue, incomplete coagulation of the endosalpinx can result.[30] In addition, the desiccated tissue can adhere to the bipolar forceps, making it difficult to remove from the surface of the tube.

The bipolar method can be used with either a single incision operating laparoscope or with dual incision instruments. The forceps are, however, more delicate than unipolar equipment and must be kept meticulously clean. Damage to the instruments can alter the ability to coagulate, and inadequate or incomplete electrocoagulation is the main cause of failure.

Bipolar cautery is safer than unipolar cautery with regard to burns of abdominal organs, but most studies indicate higher failure rates. Although the bipolar forceps will not burn tissues that are not actually grasped, care must be taken to avoid coagulating structures adherent to the tubes. For example, the ureter can be damaged when the tube is adherent to the pelvic side wall.

Tubal Occlusion with Clips and Rings

Female sterilization by mechanical occlusion eliminates the safety concerns with electrosurgery. However, mechanical devices are subject to flaws in material, defects in manufacturing, and errors in design; all of which can alter efficacy. Three mechanical devices have been widely used and have low failure rates with long-term follow-up: the Hulka-Clemen's (spring) clip, the Filshie Clip, and the Silastic (Falope or Yoon) ring. Each of the three requires an understanding of its mechanical function, a working knowledge of the intricate applicator necessary to apply the device, meticulous attention to maintenance of the applicators, and skillful tubal placement.

Hulka-Clemens Spring Clip. The spring clip consists of two plastic jaws made of Lexan, hinged by a small metal pin 2 mm from one end. Each jaw has teeth on the opposed surface, and a stainless steel spring is pushed over the jaws to hold them closed over the tube. A special laparoscope for one incision application is most commonly employed, although the spring clip can also be used in a two incision procedure. The spring clip destroys 3 mm of tube and has one year pregnancy rates of 2 per 1,000 women, but the highest 10-year cumulative failure rate.[15,23]

Complications unique to spring clip sterilization result from mechanical difficulties. Should the clip be dislodged or dropped into the abdomen during the procedure, it should be retrieved. Usually it can be removed laparoscopically, but sometimes laparotomy is necessary. Should incomplete occlusion or incorrect alignment of the clip occur, a second clip can be applied without hazard. This clip offers a good chance for reanastomosis, better than electrosurgical methods which destroy more tube, hence the higher failure rate over time.

The Hulka-Clemens Spring Clip

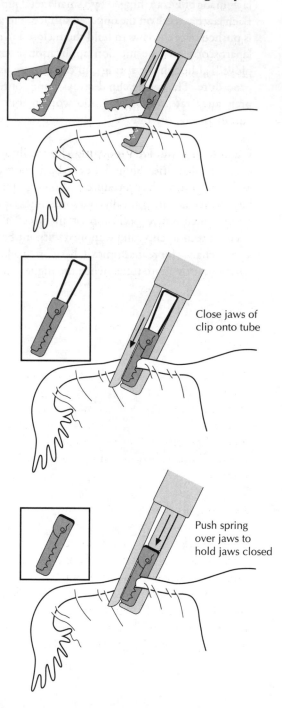

Close jaws of
clip onto tube

Push spring
over jaws to
hold jaws closed

338

Filshie Clip. The Filshie clip is made of titanium lined with silicone rubber. The hinged clip is locked over the tube using a special applicator through a second incision or operating laparoscope. The rubber lining of the clip expands on compression to keep the tube blocked. Only 4 mm of the tube is destroyed. Failure rates with the newest model approximate 2 per 1,000 women.[20] Because the Filshie clip is longer, it is reported to occlude dilated tubes more readily than does the spring clip. Both the spring clip and the Filshie clip provide good chances for tubal reanastomosis.

Silastic (Falope or Yoon) Ring. The nonreactive Silastic rubber band has an elastic memory of 100% if stretched to no more than 6 mm for a brief time (a few minutes at most). A special applicator, 6 mm in diameter, can be placed through a second cannula, or through an offset operating laparoscope. The applicator is designed to grasp a knuckle of tube and release the Silastic band onto a 2.5 cm loop of tube. The avascular loop of tube can be resected with biopsy forceps to provide a pathology specimen, but this is rarely done (it does not increase efficacy). Ten to 15% of patients experience severe postoperative pelvic cramping from the tight bands (which can be alleviated by the application of a local anesthetic to the tube before or after banding).

The ring applicator consists of two concentric cylinders. Within the inner cylinder is a forceps for grasping, elevating, and retracting a segment of the tube. The Silastic ring is stretched around the exposed end of the inner cylinder by means of a special ring loader and ring guide. The outer cylinder moves the ring from the inner cylinder on to the tube, a loop of which is held within the inner cylinder by the forceps.

As with application of clips, the ring should be placed at the junction of the proximal and middle third of each fallopian tube. Once the tube is grasped, it is gently withdrawn into the inner cylinder by slowly squeezing the handles of the applicator together. A final strong pull is needed to slide the ring from the inner applicator cylinder onto the loop of tube. Necrosis occurs promptly and a 2–3 cm segment of the tube is destroyed. Failure rates are about 1% after two years, and the 10-year cumulative rate is only better with unipolar coagulation and postpartum tubal excision.[23]

The Silastic (Falope-Yoon) Ring

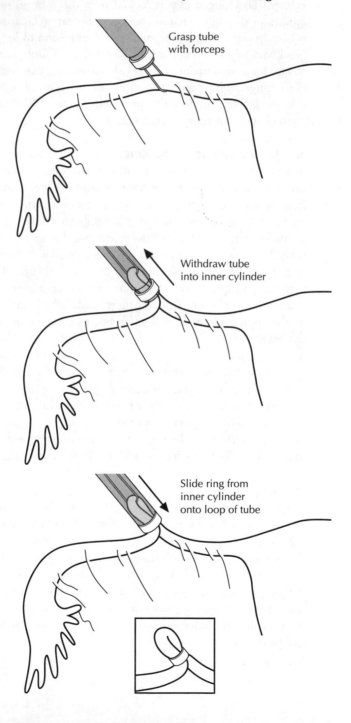

Grasp tube
with forceps

Withdraw tube
into inner cylinder

Slide ring from
inner cylinder
onto loop of tube

Mesosalpingeal bleeding is the most common complication of Silastic ring application. It usually occurs when the forceps grabs not only the tube but also a vascular fold of mesosalpinx. The mesosalpinx can also be torn on the edge of the stainless steel cylinder as the tube is drawn into the applicator. If bleeding is noted, application of the Silastic band often controls it. If the placement of additional bands or electrocoagulation fails to stop bleeding, laparotomy may be required.

Silastic rings are occasionally placed on structures other than the tube. If this mistake is recognized, the band can usually be removed from the round ligament or mesosalpingeal folds by grasping the band with the tongs of the applicator and applying gradual, increasing traction. If a gentle attempt fails, removal is not necessary. If rings are inadvertently discharged into the peritoneal cavity, they can safely be left behind.

Surgeons should be prepared to use electrosurgical instruments in case bands or clips cannot be applied (because of adhesions or bleeding).

Minilaparotomy

Tubal sterilization accomplished through a small suprapubic incision, "minilaparotomy," is the most frequent method of interval female sterilization around the world. In the U.S. and most of the developed world, laparoscopy is more popular, but minilaparotomy is gaining in favor because of its safety, simplicity, and adaptability to ambulatory surgical settings (particularly when local anesthesia is used).[31]

The fallopian tubes can be occluded through the minilaparotomy incision with bands or clips, but a simple Pomeroy-type tubal sterilization is the method most commonly used. Patient characteristics such as obesity, previous pelvic infection, or previous surgery are the principal determinants of complications.[32]

Minilaparotomy is accomplished through an incision which usually measures 3–5 cm in length. Tubal sterilization through a suprapubic incision can be accomplished for obese patients, but the incision will necessarily exceed the usual length. Forceful retraction increases the pain associated with the procedure and the time of recovery. For these reasons, we believe that minilaparotomy for ambulatory tubal occlusion should be limited to patients who are not obese (usually less than 150–160 pounds, 70 kg).

Patients who are likely to have adhesions from previous surgery or pelvic infection will probably have a shorter operating and recovery time (and less pain) with open laparoscopic tubal occlusion. In addition, the wide view provided by the laparoscope will make possible a precise description of the pelvic abnormalities which may be useful should the patient develop chronic pelvic pain or recurrent infection.

Tubal occlusion is difficult to accomplish through a minilaparotomy if the uterus is immobile. Laparoscopic tubal occlusion, on the other hand, does not require extreme uterine elevation or rotation, and is a better choice for a patient with a uterus fixed in position.

The Vaginal Approach

Although vaginal techniques are still used for tubal sterilization, high rates of infection and occasional pelvic abscesses following these operations have caused most clinicians to abandon them.[24] An apparent advantage in obese patients is sometimes deceptive because omental fat can block access to the fallopian tubes. Open laparoscopy is usually easier and safer in obese women.

Counseling for Sterilization

All patients undergoing a surgical procedure for permanent contraception should be aware of the nature of the operation, its alternatives, efficacy, safety, and complications. The operation can be described using drawings or pelvic models, as well as films, slides, or video tapes. The description of the operation should emphasize its similarities to and differences from laparoscopy and pelvic surgery, especially hysterectomy or ovariectomy which may be confused with simple tubal sterilization. Alternatives, including vasectomy, oral contraception, long-acting hormone methods, barrier methods, and IUDs should be specified. It should be emphasized to the patient that tubal sterilization is not intended to be reversible, and that it cannot be guaranteed to prevent intrauterine or ectopic pregnancy. Informed consent is best obtained at a time when a patient is not distracted or distraught, for example, not immediately before or after an induced abortion.

Sexuality. There is no detrimental effect on sexuality specifically due to sterilization procedures.[33] Indeed, sexual life is usually positively affected. Many couples are less inhibited and more spontaneous in love making when they don't have to worry about an unwanted pregnancy.

Menstrual Function. The effects on menstrual function are less clear, and therefore more difficult to explain. The first well-controlled studies of this issue demonstrated no change in menstrual patterns, volume, or pain.[34,35] Subsequently these same authors reported an increase in dysmenorrhea and changes in menstrual bleeding.[36,37] However, these authors failed to agree in their findings (a change found by one group was not confirmed by the other). Adding to the confusion, the incidence of hysterectomy for bleeding disorders in women after tubal sterilization was reported to be increased by some,[38] but not by others.[39] In a large cohort of women in a group health plan, hospitalization for menstrual disorders was significantly increased; however, the authors believed this reflected bias by patient and physician preference for surgical treatment.[40] These discordant reports do not make patient counseling about the long-term effects of tubal sterilization an easy task.

It is possible that extensive electrocoagulation of the fallopian tubes can change ovarian steroid production. Perhaps this is why menstrual changes were detected with longer (4 years) follow-up, while no changes have been noted with the use of rings or clips.[40–42] However, attempts to relate poststerilization menstrual changes with extent of tissue destruction fail to find a correlation, and an increase in hospitalization for menstrual disorders after unipolar cautery cannot be documented.[40,42] Still another long-term follow-up study (3–4.5 years) failed to document any significant changes in menstrual cycles.[43] This inconsistency can reflect differences in sterilization techniques, as well as the fact that a surgical solution is more likely to be chosen if continuing fertility is no longer an issue.

More studies with careful attention to the type of tubal occlusion procedure will be necessary. The best answer for now is that some women experience menstrual changes, but most do not.

Reversibility. An important objective of counseling is to help couples make the right decision about an irreversible decision to become sterile. The active participation of both spouses is a critical factor.[44] Not all couples are pleased following sterilization; in one series, 2% of U.S. women expressed regret one year later, and 2.7% after two years.[45] At the two year mark, the main factors associated with regret were age less than 30 and sterilization at the convenient time of a cesarean section. In Europe where tubal sterilization is less common, the most important risk factor for regret was an unstable marriage.[46] A change in marital status is undoubtedly an important reason for a desire to reverse sterilization.[47]

Young women in unstable relationships need special attention in counseling, and both partners should participate in the counseling. Furthermore, for many couples tubal occlusion at the time of cesarean section or immediately after a difficult labor and delivery is not the best time for the procedure.

It is important to know that sterilized women have not been observed to develop psychological problems at a greater than expected rate.[48,49]

Microsurgery for tubal anastomosis is associated with excellent results if only a small segment of the tube has been damaged. Pregnancy rates correlate with the length of remaining tube, a length of 4 cm or more is optimal. Thus, the pregnancy rates are lowest with electrocoagulation, and reach 70–80% with clips, rings, and surgical methods such as the Pomeroy.[50] About 2 per 1,000 women will eventually undergo tubal anastomosis.[47]

Male Sterilization: Vasectomy

Vasectomy is safer, easier, and less expensive than female steriliza-tion.[51] Some 50 million men around the world have relied on vasectomy for contraception. The operation is almost always per-formed under local anesthesia, usually by a urologist in a private office. Surgeons who do more than 10 operations yearly have lower complication rates.[52]

Hematomas and infection occur rarely, and are easily treated with heat, scrotal support, and antibiotics. Most men will develop sperm antibodies following vasectomy, but no long-term sequelae have been observed, including no increased risk of cardiovascular dis-ease.[53,54] Adverse psychological and sexual effects have not been reported. Since the other constituents of semen are made down-stream from the testes, men do not notice a decreased volume or velocity of ejaculate.

Prostate cancer is the most frequent cancer among men, with a lifetime risk of 1 in 11 in the United States. An increased risk of prostate cancer after vasectomy has been reported in several cohort and case-control studies.[55–58] However, there is disagreement as other studies could not support an association between prostate or testicular cancer risk and vasectomy.[59–61] In a very large mixed racial/ethnic (black and white; Chinese-Americans and Japanese-Americans) case-control study of prostate cancer, no statistically significant increase in risk could be identified after vasectomy, including no effect of age at vasectomy or years since vasectomy.[62] Reviews of 6 cohort studies and 5 case-control studies concluded that there is no increased risk of cancer of the testis following vasectomy, and consideration of the studies examining the possible association between prostate cancer and vasectomy (6 cohort and 7 case-control studies), found the evidence to be equivocal and weak.[63,64] Observational studies cannot totally avoid potential biases, and the disagreement in regards to prostate cancer is consistent with either no effect or an effect too small to escape confounding biases. It is worth noting that the countries with the highest vasectomy rates (China and India) do not have the highest rates of prostate cancer. Screening for prostate cancer should be no different in men who have had a vasectomy.

Vasectomy Methods

Providers of vasectomy worldwide have adopted the "no scalpel" technique perfected over the past 30 years by Li in Sichuan Province of China.[65] This approach is faster, less invasive, and requires only a few simple instruments. In a one-day comparison in Bangkok, 680 vasectomies were performed using the no scalpel method with 3 complications, and 523 vasectomies were performed with a standard technique with 16 complications.[66] The method is no easier to reverse than other vasectomies. A video tape and instruments for this method can be obtained from AVSC International, 79 Madison Avenue, New York, NY 10016 (FAX 212-779-9439).

Reversibility

Vasectomy reversal is associated with pregnancy rates greater than 50%.[67,68] The prospect for pregnancy diminishes with time elapsed from vasectomy, decreasing significantly to 30% after 10 years; the best results are achieved when reversal is performed within 3 years after vasectomy.

Medical Methods for the Male

A reversible method of contraception for men has been sought for years. Hormonal contraception for men is inherently a difficult physiologic problem because, unlike cyclic ovulation in women, spermatogenesis is continuous.[69] Investigational approaches to inhibit production of sperm include the administration of sex steroids, the use of GnRH analogs, and the administration of gossypol, a derivative of cotton seed oil.

The sex steroids reduce testosterone synthesis which leads to loss of libido and development of female secondary sexual characteristics. Furthermore, despite the use of large doses, sperm counts are not adequately reduced in all subjects. GnRH analogs also decrease the endogenous synthesis of testosterone, and supplemental testosterone must be provided.

Gossypol effectively decreases sperm counts to contraceptive levels, apparently by incapacitating the sperm producing cells. Gossypol pills are taken daily for 2 months until sperm are no longer observed in the ejaculate, and then the pills are taken weekly. Fertility returns to normal 3 months after discontinuation. Although the experience in China has been largely positive, animal studies in the U.S. indicate that gossypol, or contaminants of the preparation, are toxic. Analogs of gossypol may offer potential but are years away from development.

Future Developments with Sterilization

Although current methods of sterilization are safe and effective, they require skillful surgeons and, in the case of laparoscopic operations, elaborate and expensive equipment. Simpler approaches could make sterilization available and acceptable to more people. Female transcervical methods have used electrocoagulation, cryosurgery, or laser to destroy the interstitial portion of the tube, to inject sclerosing agents or tissue adhesives through the tubal ostia, and to mechanically obstruct the tubal lumen. Most of these methods, and the formed-in-place silicone plugs applied either hysteroscopically or with the "Femcept" intrauterine device, are either too complicated or have high failure rates. The most practical approach is the application of sclerosing agents to the tubal openings using cannulae or an intrauterine device. Transcervical insertion of quinicrine pellets during the proliferative phase of the menstrual cycle occludes the tubes and is the most promising of the "non-surgical" approaches, but the long-term effects of quinicrine have not been assessed.[70–72]

References

1. **Parker-Mauldin W, Segal S,** Prevalence of contraceptive use: trends and issues, Stud Fam Plann 6:335, 1988.

2. **Mosher WD, Pratt WF,** Contraceptive use in the United States, 1973–88, Advance data from vital and health statistics; No. 182, National Center for Health Statistics, Hyattsville, Maryland, 1990.

3. **Mosher WD,** Use of family planning services in the United States: 1982 and 1988, Advance data from vital and health statistics, No. 184, National Center for Health Statistics, Hyattsville, Maryland, 1990.

4. **Murphy M,** Sterilisation as a method of contraception: recent trends in Great Britain and their implications, J Biosoc Sci 27:31, 1995.

5. **Riphagen FE, Fortney JA, Koelb S,** Contraception in women over forty, J Biosoc Sci 20:127, 1988.

6. **Ortho Pharmaceutical Corporation,** Annual birth control study, 1994.

7. **Speert H,** *Obstetric and Gynecologic Milestones,* The Macmillan Company, New York, 1958, pp 619–629.

8. **Lungren SS,** A case of cesarean section twice successfully performed on the same patient, with remarks on the time, indications, and details of the operation, Am J Obstet 14:78, 1881.

9. **Baird D,** The Fifth Freedom, Br Med J 1:234, 1966.

10. **Centers for Disease Control and Prevention** Surgical sterilization surveillance: tubal sterilization 1976–1978, 1981.

11. **Layde PM, Ory HW, Peterson HB, Scally MJ, Greenspan JR, Smith JC, Fleming D,** The declining lengths of hospitalization for tubal sterilizations, JAMA 245:714, 1981.

12. **Escobedo LG, Peterson HB, Grubb GS, Franks AL,** Case fatality rates for tubal sterilization in U.S. hospitals, Am J Obstet Gynecol 160:147, 1989.

13. **Peterson HB, Huber DH, Belker AM,** Vasectomy: an appraisal for the obstetrician-gynecologist, Obstet Gynecol 76:568, 1990.

14. **Trussell J, Hatcher RA, Cates W Jr, Stewart FH, Kost K,** Contraceptive failure in the United States: an update, Stud Fam Plann 21:51, 1990.

15. **Chi I-c, Laufe L, Gardner SD, Tolbert M,** An epidemiologic study of risk factors associated with pregnancy following female sterilizations, Am J Obstet Gynecol 136:768, 1980.

16. **Cheng M, Wong YM, Rochat R, Ratnam SS,** Sterilization failures in Singapore: an examination of ligation techniques and failure rates, Stud Fam Plann 8:109, 1977.

17. **Lichterg E, Laff S, Friedman E,** Value of routine dilatation and curettage at the time of interval sterilization, Obstet Gynecol 67:763, 1986.

18. **World Health Organization,** A multicenter case-control study of ectopic pregnancy, Clin Reprod Fertil 3:131, 1985.

19. **Holt V, Chu J, Daling JR, Stergacis AS, Weiss NS,** Tubal sterilization and subsequent ectopic pregnancy, JAMA 266:242, 1991.

20. **Chick PH, Frances M, Paterson PJ,** A comprehensive review of female sterilisation tubal occlusion methods, Clin Reprod Fertil 3:81, 1985.

21. **McCausland A,** High rate of ectopic pregnancy following laparoscopic tubal coagulation failure, Am J Obstet Gynecol 136:977, 1980.

22. **Chi I-c, Laufe LE, Atwed R,** Ectopic pregnancy following female sterilization procedures, Adv Plann Parenthood 16:52, 1981.

23. **Peterson HB and the U.S. Collaborative Review of Sterilization Working Group,** The risk of pregnancy after tubal sterilization, Am J Obstet Gynecol, 1996, in press.

24. **Miesfeld R, Gaarontans R, Moyers T,** Vaginal tubal sterilization. Is infection a significant risk? Am J Obstet Gynecol 137:183, 1980.

25. **Hankinson SE, Hunter DJ, Colditz GA, Willett WC, Stampfer MJ, Rosner B, Hennekens CH, Speizer FE,** Tubal sterilization, hysterectomy, and risk of ovarian cancer. A prospective study, JAMA 270:2813, 1993.

26. **Mori M, Harabuchi I, Miyake H, Casagrande JT, Henderson BE, Ross RK,** Reproductive, genetic, and dietary risk factors for ovarian cancer, Am J Epidemiol 128:771, 1988.

27. **Irwin KL, Weiss NS, Lee NC, Peterson HB,** Tubal sterilization, hysterectomy, and the subsequent occurrence of epithelial ovarian cancer, Am J Epidemiol 134:362, 1991.

28. **Whittemore AS, Harris R, Itnyre J, and the Collaborative Ovarian Cancer Group,** Characteristics relating to ovarian cancer risk: collaborative analysis of 12 US case-control studies. II: invasive epithelial ovarian cancers in white women, Am J Epidemiol 136:1184, 1992.

29. **Centers for Disease Control and Prevention,** Deaths following female sterilization with unipolar electrocoagulating devices, MMWR 30:150, 1981.

30. **Soderstrom RM, Levy BS, Engel T,** Reducing bipolar sterilization failures, Obstet Gynecol 74:60, 1989.

31. **McCann M, Cole L,** Laparoscopy and minilaparotomy: two major advances in female sterilization, Stud Fam Plann 11:119, 1980.

32. **Layde PM, Peterson HB, Dicker RC, DeStefano F, Ruben GL, Ory HW,** Risk factors for complications of interval tubal sterilization by laparotomy, Obstet Gynecol 62:180, 1983.

33. **Kjer J,** Sexual adjustment to tubal sterilization, Eur J Obstet Gynecol 35:211, 1990.

34. **Rulin MC, Turner JH, Dunworth R, Thompson D,** Post tubal sterilization syndrome: a misnomer, Am J Obstet Gynecol 151:13, 1985.

35. **DeStefano F, Huezo CM, Peterson HB, Rubin GL, Layde PM, Ory HW,** Menstrual changes after tubal sterilization, Obstet Gynecol 62:673, 1983.

36. **Rulin MC, Davidson AR, Philliber SG, Graves WL, Cushman LF,** Changes in menstrual symptoms among sterilized and comparison women: a prospective study, Obstet Gynecol 79:749, 1989.

37. **DeStefano F, Perlman J, Peterson HB, Diamond E,** Long-term risk of menstrual disturbances after tubal sterilization, Am J Obstet Gynecol 152:835, 1985.

38. **Kjer J, Knudsen L,** Hysterectomy subsequent to laparoscopic sterilization, Eur J Obstet Gynecol 35:63, 1990.

39. **Stergachis A, Shy KK, Gouthaus LC, Wagner EH, Hecht JA, Anderson G, Normand EH, Raboud J,** Tubal sterilization and the long-term risk of hysterectomy, JAMA 264:2893, 1990.

40. **Shy KK, Stergachis A, Grothaus LG, Wagner EH, Hecth J, Anderson G,** Tubal sterilization and risk of subsequent hospital admission for menstrual disorders, Am J Obstet Gynecol 166:1698, 1992.

41. **Thranov I, Hertz JB, Kjer JJ, Andresen A, Micic S, Nielsen J, Hancke S,** Hormonal and menstrual changes after laparoscopic sterilization by Falope-rings or Filshie-clips, Fertil Steril 57:751, 1992.

42. **Wilcox LS, Martinez-Schnell B, Peterson HB, Ware JH, Hughes JM,** Menstrual function after tubal sterilization, Am J Epidemiol 135:1368, 1992.

43. **Rulin MC, Davidson AR, Philliber SG, Graves WL, Cushman LF,** Long-term effect of tubal sterilization on menstrual indices and pelvic pain, Obstet Gynecol 82:118, 1993.

44. **Miller WB, Shain RN, Pasta DJ,** Tubal sterilization or vasectomy: how do married couples make the decision? Fertil Steril 56:278, 1991.

45. **Grubb G, Refoser H, Layde PM, Rubin GL,** Regret after decision to have a tubal sterilization, Fertil Steril 44:248, 1985.

46. **Vemer HM, Colla P, Schoot DC, Willensen WN, Bierkens PB, Rolland R,** Women regretting their sterilization, Fertil Steril 46:724, 1986.

47. **Wilcox LS, Chu SY, Peterson HB,** Characteristics of women who considered or obtained tubal reanastomosis: results from a prospective study of tubal sterilization, Obstet Gynecol 75:661, 1990.

48. **Vessey M, Huggins G, Lawless M, McPherson K, Yeates D,** Tubal sterilization: findings in a large prospective study, Br J Obstet Gynaecol 90:203, 1983.

49. **World Health Organization,** Mental health and female sterilization: report of a WHO collaborative study, J Biosc Sci 16:1, 1984.

50. Siegler AM, Hulka J, Peretz A, Reversibility of female sterilization, Fertil Steril 43:499, 1985.

51. Smith GL, Taylor GP, Smith KF, Comparative risks and costs of male and female sterilization, Am J Public Health 75:370, 1985.

52. Kendrick JS, Gonzales B, Huber DH, Grubb GS, Rubin G, Complications of vasectomies in the United States, J Fam Pract 25:245, 1987.

53. Schuman LM, Coulson AH, Mandel JS, Massey FJ Jr, O'Fallon WM, Health status of American men — a study of post-vasectomy sequelae, J Clin Endocrinol 46:697, 1993.

54. Giovannucci E, Tosteson TD, Speizer FE, Vessey MP, Colditz GA, A long-term study of mortality in men who have undergone vasectomy, New Engl J Med 326:1392, 1992.

55. Giovanucci E, Ascherio A, Rimm EB, Colditz GA, Stampfer MJ, Willett WC, A prospective cohort study of vasectomy and prostate cancer in US men, JAMA 269:873, 1993.

56. Giovanucci E, Tosteson TD, Speizer FE, Ascherio A, Vessey MP, Colditz GA, A retrospective cohort study of vasectomy and prostate cancer in US men, JAMA 269:878, 1993.

57. Hayes RB, Pottern LM, Greenberg R, Schoenberg J, Swanson GM, Liff J, Schwartz AG, Brown LM, Hoover RN, Vasectomy and prostate cancer in US blacks and whites, Am J Epidemiol 137:263, 1993.

58. Hsing AW, Wang RT, Gu FL, Lee M, Wang T, Leng TJ, Spitz M, Blot WJ, Vasectomy and prostate cancer risk in China, Cancer Epidemiol Biomarkers Prev 3:285, 1994.

59. Sidney S, Quesenberry CP Jr, Sadler MC, Guess HA, Lydick EG, Cattolica EV, Vasectomy and the risk of prostate cancer in a cohort of multiphasic health-checkup examinees: second report, Cancer Causes Control 2:113, 1991.

60. Moller H, Knudsen LB, Lynge E, Risk of testicular cancer after vasectomy: cohort study of over 73,000 men, Br Med J 309:295, 1994.

61. Rosenberg L, Palmer JR, Zauber AG, Warshauer E, Strom BL, Harlap S, Shapiro S, The relation of vasectomy to risk of cancer, Am J Epidemiol 140:431, 1994.

62. John EM, Whittemore AS, Wu AH, Kolonel LN, Hislop TG, Howe GR, West DW, Hankin J, Dreon DM, The C-Z, Burch JD, Paffenbarger RS Jr, Vasectomy and prostate cancer: results from a multiethnic case-control study, J Natl Cancer Inst 87:662, 1995.

63. Lynge E, Knudsen LB, Møller H, Vasectomy and testis and prostate cancer, Fertil Control Rev 3:8, 1994.

64. Healey B, Does vasectomy cause prostate cancer? JAMA 269:2620, 1993.

65. Li S-q, Goltein M, Zhu J, Huber DH, The no scalpel vasectomy, J Urol 145:341, 1991.

66. **Nirapathpongporn A, Huber DH, Krieger JN,** No scalpel vasectomy at the King's birthday vasectomy festival, Lancet 335:894, 1990.

67. **Belker AM, Thomas AJ, Fuchs EF, Konnak JM, Sharlip ID,** Results of 1,469 microsurgical vasectomy reversals by the vasovasostomy group, J Urol 145:505, 1991.

68. **Hendry WF,** Vasectomy and vasectomy reversal, Br J Urol 73:337, 1994.

69. **Winters SJ, Marshall GR,** Hormonally-based male contraceptives: will they ever be a reality? J Clin Endocrinol Metab 73:464A, 1991.

70. **Mumford S, Kessel E,** Sterilization needs in the 1990s: the case for the quinicrine nonsurgical female sterilization, Am J Obstet Gynecol 167:1203, 1992.

71. **Hiei DT, Tan TT, Tan DN, Nguyet PT, Than P, Vinh DQ,** 31,781 cases of nonsurgical female sterilization with quinicrine pellets in Vietnam, Lancet 342:213, 1993.

72. **El Kady AA, Nagib HS, Kessel E,** Efficacy and safety of repeated transcervical quinicrine pellet insertions for female sterilization, Fertil Steril 59:301, 1993.

12

Induced Abortion

CONTRACEPTION IS MORE EFFECTIVE and convenient than ever, but our modern methods are far from perfect. Even the most conscientious couples can experience contraceptive failure. In the past, failure of contraception meant another, sometimes unwanted, birth or recourse to dangerous, clandestine abortion. The most ancient medical texts indicate that abortion has been practiced for thousands of years. Induced abortion did not become illegal until the 19th century, as a result of changes in the teachings of the Catholic Church (life begins at fertilization), and in the U.S., the efforts of the American Medical Association to have greater regulation of the practice of medicine.

In the 1950s, vacuum aspiration led to much safer abortion, and beginning in Asia, induced abortion was gradually legalized in the developed countries of the world. This trend reached the U.S. from Western Europe in the late 1960s when California, New York, and other states rewrote their abortion laws. The U.S. Supreme Court followed the lead of these states in 1973 in the "Roe versus Wade" decision that limited the circumstances under which "the right of privacy" could be restricted by local abortion laws.

In the years since the 1973 U.S. Supreme Court decision, induced abortion has become the most commonly reported surgical procedure, with rates leveling off by 1980. In 1992, 1, 529,000 abortions gave a rate of 26 abortions for every 1,000 women 15–44 years of age, and a ratio of approximately 340 abortions for every 1,000 births.[1,2] The number estimated by the Alan Guttmacher Institute[1] (1.5 million) is higher than that reported by the Centers for Disease Control and Prevention (1.39 million)[2] because the CDC depends on legal abortions reported while the Guttmacher Institute actually surveys abortion providers, probably yielding a more accurate measurement.

These rates and ratios place the U.S. between the countries of Eastern Europe that rely heavily on abortion as a means of family planning, and those of Western Europe that provide contraception so effectively that abortion, although easily available, is not frequently used.[3]

Complications of Induced Abortion

Public health authorities have demonstrated that the legalization of induced abortion has reduced maternal morbidity and mortality more than any single development since the advent of antibiotics to treat puerperal infection and blood banking to treat hemorrhage. The number of American women reported as dying from abortion declined from nearly 300 deaths in 1961, to only 6 in 1987, or 0.4 deaths for every 100,000 legal abortions.[4] For comparison, in 1987, maternal death rates for childbirth in the U.S. were about 9 per 100,000 births, and for ectopic pregnancy about 50 per 100,000 cases.[4,5]

The most important determinants of abortion mortality rates are duration of gestation and type of anesthesia; later abortions and general anesthesia are more hazardous.[6,7,8] The most important determinants of complications of abortion (fever, hemorrhage, infection, retained products of conception, uterine perforation, and need for major surgery) are the training and experience of abortion providers and the general health of the patients. More experienced surgeons and younger, healthier women are less likely to have complications.

Major and minor complications in a series of 170,000 first trimester abortion patients were as follows:[9]

Major Complications (Hospitalization Required)

Retained tissue	27.7 per 100,000 induced abortions
Sepsis	21.2
Uterine perforation	9.4
Hemorrhage	7.1
Inability to complete	3.5
Intrauterine plus tubal pregnancy	2.4

Minor Complications (Managed in Clinic or Office)

Mild infection	462.0 per 100,000 induced abortions
Reaspiration same day	180.8
Reaspiration later	167.8
Cervical stenosis	16.5
Cervical tear	10.6
Underestimated gestation	6.5
Convulsive seizure	4.0

The possibility that induced abortion may result in longer-term complications such as spontaneous abortion, cervical incompetence, infertility, or ectopic pregnancy has been examined in over 150 studies.[10] There is no evidence for any adverse consequences of vacuum aspiration abortion for subsequent fertility,[11,12] pregnancies,[13,14] or increased risk for ectopic pregnancy,[15] It is not yet clear if second trimester abortions or several first trimester abortions can affect the outcome of later pregnancies. The long-term effects of second trimester abortion may depend on the method used (see later).[16]

The psychological sequelae of elective abortion have been studied and debated. The unequivocal evidence indicates that depression is less frequent among women postabortion compared with postpartum, that women denied abortion experience resentment for years, and that the children born after abortion is denied have social, occupational, and interpersonal difficulties lasting into early adulthood.[17]

Case-control studies have suggested an increased risk of breast cancer associated with the number of induced and spontaneous abortions experienced by individual patients, implying an initial proliferative stimulation that is not followed by the protective effect achieved with full term pregnancies early in life. However, the results are not consistent, and the results may be influenced by recall bias.[18,19]

First Trimester Abortion Procedures

More than 90% of the 1.5 million induced abortions performed in the U.S. yearly are carried out during the first trimester of pregnancy.[1,2] During the first trimester, abortion morbidity and mortality rates are less than one tenth those of abortions performed in the later midtrimester.[4] The vast majority of these operations occur in freestanding abortion clinics, although in recent years physicians have performed larger numbers in their offices where women are less subject to the harassment that has plagued clinics.[1] The safety of outpatient abortion under local anesthesia for abortion is well-established.[20]

Patient Selection

Nearly all patients who want to terminate a pregnancy in the first trimester are good candidates for an office or clinic procedure under local anesthesia. Possible exceptions include women with severe cardiorespiratory disease, severe anemias or coagulopathies, a mental disorder severe enough to preclude patient cooperation, and those who are so afraid of pain under local anesthesia that they cannot be reassured. These patients require consultation with the clinician managing their primary disease and sometimes hospital admission so that complications can be promptly treated or general anesthesia administered.

Women who have known uterine anomalies (duplicated cervix, double uterus) or cervical myomata or who have previously had difficult first trimester abortion procedures should have their operations where ultrasonography is immediately available and the surgeon is experienced in its intraoperative use. Previous cesarean section or other pelvic surgery is not a contraindication to outpatient first trimester abortion.

Counseling and Informed Consent

Whether first trimester abortion is accomplished in a clinic, office, or a hospital, the functions of the counselor must be fulfilled to ensure quality patient care. These include discussion of alternatives, help with decision-making, giving information about the abortion procedure, obtaining informed consent, provision of emotional support to the patient and her family before, during, and after the operation, and education about contraception.[21]

The counselor must be able to make judgments about duration of gestation using the last menstrual period and reports from other clinicians, must be aware of referral opportunities for prenatal care or adoption for women who choose to carry an unplanned pregnancy to term, must know about the abortion operation itself, must be skilled and sensitive at obtaining informed consent after presenting understandable estimates of risk, must be able to give pre- and postoperative instructions and serve as a contact person for problems that arise during these periods, and must provide realistic information about contraception. Informed consent is important both for the patient's understanding of the risks of first trimester abortion and for the legal protection of the physician when outcomes are unsatisfactory.

Each clinic or office should have a first trimester abortion informed consent document that defines risks such as incomplete abortion, infection, uterine perforation, transfusion, laparotomy, ectopic pregnancy, and failed abortion.

First Trimester Abortion Technique

A standard set of simple instruments is satisfactory for termination of most first trimester pregnancies:

Graves medium open-sided vaginal speculum.
Bierer atraumatic tenaculum.
Foerster sponge forceps, curved.
Pratt or Denniston cervical dilators, sizes 13 through 43 French.
Medicine bowl (50 mL) for local anesthetic.
Stainless steel bowl (500 mL) for antiseptic solution.
Uterine curette, size 2 Sims.

Disposable equipment and supplies recommended for each procedure:

Chloroprocaine (Nesacaine) 1%, 15 mL.
Atropine, 0.4 mg (1 mL).
Syringe, 10 cc plastic with control grip for paracervical block.
Syringe, 5 cc for intravenous administration of analgesics.
Needle, 25-gauge (1.5 inch) for paracervical block.
Needle, 25-gauge (0.5 inch) for intravenous medications.
Gauze sponges, 4 x 4.
Cotton balls.
Clear plastic collection tubing with clear plastic handle, 11 mm inside diameter (or a hand-held 50 cc uterine evacuation syringe with double valves).
Cannulas for uterine evacuation; rigid, clear plastic, 8 mm through 12 mm outside diameter, straight and curved.
Cannulas; whistle-tip, flexible plastic, 5 mm through 8 mm outside diameter.

The instrument tray should be kept as simple as possible because unnecessary instruments disturb patients, increase costs, and waste time. For example, if hydrophilic dilators (Laminaria or Dilapan) are inserted preoperatively, it is not necessary to have cervical dilators in the tray.[22,23]

The treatment room should be equipped with an electric vacuum pump that reaches adequate negative pressures (60 mm Hg) quietly and rapidly. The operating table should provide comfortable knee support for the patient in lithotomy position. Foot slings or stirrups are not desirable; knee crutches are much better because the patient can relax her legs, allowing the crutches to hold them apart. Ideally, the table should provide Trendelenburg position so that the surgeon can alter the angle of vision and vasovagal reactions can be treated by lowering the patient's head. A wheeled bucket should stand at the end of the table in front of the surgeon's stool which must be height adjustable and have wheels. Two stools or tall chairs should be set at the head of the operating table for the counselor and the patient's support person, if one is with her.

The Uterine Aspiration Procedure

Patient Preparation. Correct position on the operating table will help the patient to relax and the surgeon to complete the procedure quickly; both factors are critical for pain relief. The patient should be invited to empty her bladder before she enters the treatment room (unless a full bladder is needed for intraoperative sonography). She should recline on the table and rest her legs in the padded knee crutches, achieving a comfortable dorsal lithotomy position with her buttock margins beyond the end of the table. Obese women should be positioned even further down so that the handle of the speculum can lie between the buttocks. Intravenous premedications are administered immediately before or after assuming the lithotomy position but not prior to reclining on the table because their relaxing effect will be disturbed by ambulation. Oral medications are used cautiously because gastrointestinal absorption is unpredictable, and some of them (e.g., diazepam) can have long-lasting effects. Analgesic medications can be most comfortably administered by direct intravenous push with a 25-gauge, 0.5 inch needle. A continuous infusion is necessary only in special circumstances, when patients with sickle cell disease or severe hyperemesis need hydration, for example, or when venous access might be difficult in an emergency.

Analgesia can be obtained with intravenous fentanyl (Sublimaze) 0.1 mg, or butorphanol (Stadol) 2 mg. Atropine, 0.4 mg (1 mL), mixed with the analgesic agent or with the local anesthetic for the paracervical block provides protection against vasovagal responses to cervical manipulation. Under special circumstances, such as seizure disorders or extreme anxiety, midazolam (Versed), 1–3 mg, is preferable to diazepam because it does not irritate veins, has a faster onset of action, and is eliminated sooner than diazepam. It can be mixed with the other agents, but when given with a narcotic like fentanyl, the mixture must be injected more slowly, over a period of 1–2 minutes, depending on the dose.

Cervical Assessment, Exposure, and Local Anesthesia. Promptly after intravenous premedication, a bimanual examination is performed, during which any previously placed hydrophilic dilators and sponges can be removed and the size and position of the uterus assessed. The degree of cervical dilation present can be estimated with an examining finger. After the exam, gloves are exchanged for new sterile ones, and a "no touch" technique is followed with intrauterine instruments throughout the remainder of the abortion procedure. It is best to avoid scrubbing the vulva or labia because it does not reduce the incidence of infection and makes relaxation difficult for the patient. A Weissman-Graves open-sided speculum is slowly and gently placed in the vagina and opened as widely as possible without causing the patient discomfort in order to fully expose the cervix. After receiving intravenous analgesia, most patients will not find a widely-opened speculum painful. The cervix can then be gently cleaned with a non-staining antiseptic such as chlorhexidine (Hibiclens).

Paracervical Block Technique. A well-placed paracervical block relieves the pain of cervical dilation and is important even for the patient whose cervix is already dilated because it also relieves the pain of cervical manipulation. The block should be placed at least 2 minutes before uterine evacuation begins; a longer wait is preferable. A 10 cc control grip syringe is filled with 1% chloroprocaine (Nesacaine) and a 25-gauge, 0.5 inch needle is attached. A deeply-placed block provides better pain relief than a shallow one.[24] Inject about 2 mL, 1 cm deep into the cervical lip, the anterior lip for an anteverted uterus or posterior lip for a retroverted uterus. The injected lip is grasped with a Bierer atraumatic tenaculum so that the curve of the tenaculum does not obscure the view of the cervix (curve up for an anterior uterus, down for a posterior uterus). Apply traction to the tenaculum and observe the angle at which the cervix passes back into the lateral fornices. Bend the needle at its hub to about the same angle by pressing it on a sterile surface. Hold the syringe lightly at the end of the plunger and select a point at 3 o'clock, 1–2 cm lateral to the external os. Insert the needle tip at this point immediately beneath the cervical mucosa and slide it under the mucosa to the needle's hub so that the needle is completely buried. This will place the needle tip at or near the paracervical plexus. Inject 3–4 mL in the plexus and another 1 mL as the needle is withdrawn from under the mucosa, so that the nerves that pass between the stroma and mucosal layers after leaving the plexus will be anesthetized. The procedure is repeated on the other side at 9 o'clock.

If extensive cervical dilation is anticipated, injection of the uterosacral ligaments at 5 and 7 o'clock in the posterior vaginal fornix will provide a more profound cervical block, but for most minor cervical dilations, uterosacral injections cause more pain than they prevent.

Cervical Dilation Technique. If the cervix has not been previously dilated with Laminaria or Dilapan,[22,23] mechanical dilation with Pratt-type dilators (finely tapered and closely graduated) is usually required prior to uterine evacuation. Dilation should not exceed that needed for rapid (less than 5 minutes) uterine aspiration. Ten mm diameter is the maximum needed for gestations under 12 weeks.

Select the smallest dilator likely to easily enter the cervical canal, holding it in the middle like a pencil in order to feel which end is larger. The smaller end is advanced to the internal os with the curve directed posteriorly. When the resistance of the internal os is felt, begin to rotate the dilator (if the fundus is not posteriorly positioned) 180 degrees so that the curve is directed anteriorly as it passes into the uterine cavity. If the curve of the dilator (and all other instruments passed into the uterine cavity) is always directed posteriorly as it enters the external os, perforation of uteri that lie posteriorly will be avoided. Failure to detect a posterior uterus is the most common cause of uterine perforation at the time of first trimester abortion.

If firm resistance is encountered in the canal, the procedure is repeated using a smaller dilator. If resistance is slight to moderate, the tip of the dilator is passed through the internal os into the uterine cavity completing the 180 degrees rotatory motion as it enters the cavity. It is essential to distinguish the rubbery, spring-like resistance of the internal cervical os from the softer, non-specific resistance of cervical stroma in order to avoid developing a false passage with a misdirected dilator.

If the dilators are slippery with mucus and blood, a gauze sponge around the middle of the dilators will prevent slippage. Progressively larger dilators are used, without skipping increments, until adequate dilation is achieved; about 1 mm diameter for every week of gestation. Avoid excessive force to obtain dilation. Pratt dilators are labeled with their circumference in mm; divide by 3 to obtain their diameter, the measurement used for uterine aspiration cannulas.

Uterine Aspiration. All that is needed for rapid, safe uterine evacuation in early pregnancy is a cannula and a source of vacuum. Manufacturers have made both available in several varieties. Rigid, clear plastic cannulas increase in diameter by 1 mm increments from 6 through 14 mm. Flexible plastic cannulas increase from 4 mm through 8 mm in diameter. Rigid cannulas are manufactured in both straight and angulated types. Straight cannulas cause less pain when the cannula is rotated inside the uterine cavity, but curved cannulas provide easier access to the cavity and cornual areas of a retro- or antero-flexed uterus. The choice depends upon the patient's anatomy and the surgeon's preference. Flexible (soft) cannulas are useful for very early gestations with minimal cervical dilation or when anatomic abnormalities, such as cervical myomata and uterine septae or duplications, distort the pathway to the gestational sac.

It is best to select a cannula of the largest size that will easily pass the internal os; too small a cannula will result in loss of intrauterine vacuum and prolong the operation, while too large a cannula will be painful. The cannula is attached to the suction hose handle in such a way that the surgeon is always aware of the direction of the curve, if the cannula had one, in relation to the thumb valve on the handle. The cannula (and any other instrument that enters the uterine cavity) should not be touched; only the portions of those instruments that remain outside the cavity may be handled because "sterile" gloves can become contaminated.

As the cannula passes into the uterine cavity, the vacuum pump is turned on by the surgeon with a foot switch. A negative pressure of 50–70 mm Hg assures rapid and complete evacuation and will not injure the myometrium. The cannula tip is advanced to the uterine fundus where it is rotated at a rate of approximately one revolution per second with the handle of the suction hose. During rotation, the cannula is gradually and gently withdrawn to the external os. Just as its tip exits the cervix, the negative pressure is released with the thumb valve on the handle, not with the pump switch. The cannula is again advanced into the uterine cavity, rotated and withdrawn to the external os. If uterine contents continue to appear in the plastic cannula and the evacuation hose, this procedure is repeated, rotating the cannula first clockwise and then counterclockwise until flow into the cannula and through the hose ceases. At this point the cannula tip is withdrawn from the external os, again taking care to release pressure with the thumb valve on the hose handle just as the tip leaves the external os. This timing of vacuum release is important in order to avoid leaving uterine contents behind or drawing vaginal mucosa into the tip of the suction cannula, a painful experience for the patient.

Sometimes flow through the cannula stops because the placenta or its fragments are too large to pass. Flow can usually be restored simply by releasing pressure with the thumb valve (don't switch off the pump motor) and quickly restoring it by closing the valve. If this technique doesn't work, releasing and restoring vacuum while the cannula is advanced a few cm into the cavity and then quickly withdrawn again in a pumping motion almost always restores flow. Rotation of the cannula during the "pumping" maneuver also helps to fragment the placenta, allowing it to pass through the cannula. If the cannula remains plugged despite these attempts to clear it, simply withdraw the cannula, releasing the vacuum at the external os, but not before, and remove the plug from the end of the cannula with ring forceps.

When all flow of uterine contents and most flow of blood has ceased and when the contraction of the uterus around the cannula makes rotation increasingly difficult, the surgeon can assume that the uterus is evacuated. Completeness of the evacuation should then be evaluated using a malleable, sharp curette, 5–10 mm in breadth. Larger curettes are used in later gestations, but a no. 2 is right for most first trimester abortions. A systematic approach to curettage will help ensure that no area of the uterine cavity is missed. First, place the tip of the curette in the right uterine cornu and withdraw it to the internal os. Repeat this motion with 2 or 3 withdrawals across the anterior uterine fundus and a final one from the left cornu. Turn the curette over and withdraw it 3 or 4 times in succession from left to right, moving across the posterior uterine wall.

During curettage, the empty uterine cavity should provoke a gritty sensation with each stroke of the curette and should feel triangular and symmetrical. Deviations from these findings can indicate retained products of conception, myomata, or uterine anomalies. If curettage reveals a slick area of uterine wall, repeated suctioning in which the cannula's open tip is applied firmly to the abnormal area of the uterus will usually demonstrate retained fetal, or, more likely, placental fragments. When these are suctioned out, the cavity should be re-evaluated with the sharp curette. The sharp curettage is not used to remove uterine contents (the suction cannula does that) but to assess the completeness of evacuation.

The abortion procedure is completed by again inserting the cannula through the cervical canal to the uterine fundus, switching on the vacuum pump and rotating and withdrawing the cannula a final time in order to remove any fragments left behind. At the end of the abortion procedure, the uterus should be firmly contracted around the cannula. Application of vacuum to the uterine cavity should elicit only a small amount of blood and air bubbles, and when the cannula is withdrawn for the final time, only a small trickle of blood should run from the cervical os. The tenaculum is then removed, the cervical lip inspected for bleeding, the blood remaining in the vagina suctioned or sponged away, and the speculum gently withdrawn. The patient's vulva can then be cleaned with remaining chlorhexidine or water, and gently dried.

Postoperative Care. After an abortion under local anesthesia nearly all patients can comfortably walk to a nearby recovery area. They may sit in chairs or lie down. Comfortable reclining chairs are ideal because patients recover more quickly sitting but can lie back if they prefer or if they have a syncopal episode. Vital signs should be taken on the operating table immediately after the procedure, and at least one more time in the recovery room before discharge. In addition, perineal pads should be inspected for bleeding at least once before discharge. Patients should not be discharged until they ambulate independently to the bathroom, take sips of fluids, and show complete recovery from the effects of operative medications. This recovery period generally requires at least 30 minutes, and some patients need to remain longer.

At the time of discharge, patients are again informed of the 3 signs of possible complications: increased (rather than decreased) bleeding, increased pain, and fever. They are instructed to take their temperature for the next 3 mornings and given a thermometer if they do not have one. They are given a telephone number at which they can seek advice and answers to questions at any time during the day or night. An opportunity is given to ask questions about contraception, and patients can begin taking oral contraceptives that night. If the preoperative hematocrit was less than 35, a daily iron supplement for 2 months is indicated. Patients who are still under the influence of preoperative medications should leave in the company of a responsible adult.

Complications of First Trimester Abortion

Excessive Bleeding Immediately After Aspiration

Excessive blood loss occurring promptly after uterine evacuation can result from uterine atony, retained products of conception, uterine perforation, cervical laceration, or the "postabortal syndrome." A pelvic bimanual examination and visualization of the cervix will distinguish among these. Uterine atony, marked by a soft, nontender uterine fundus and a steady trickle of dark blood from the cervix, is initially treated by uterine massage, the intramuscular injection of 0.2 mg ergonovine (Methergine) and repeated uterine massage before discharge. If bleeding persists it may be necessary to repeat this injection and continue oral treatment (ergonovine, 0.2 mg tid for 3 days). If blood loss is great enough to cause tachycardia or hypotension, an intravenous infusion of lactated Ringer's solution should be started. If the response to ergonovine is inadequate, prompt transvaginal, intrauterine injection of carboprost (Hemabate), 200 mg diluted in 10 mL saline, will usually restore uterine tone.

If bleeding is excessive and pelvic examination reveals a slightly tender uterus somewhat larger than expected, the possibility of retained fetal or placental tissue must be considered. Bleeding unresponsive to uterotonic agents also suggests retained tissue. The uterine cavity should then be re-evaluated with the largest sharp curette that will pass through the cervix. If more than 30 minutes have lapsed since the procedure, a second paracervical block and additional parenteral analgesia may be required. If the uterine cavity is asymmetrical or lacks a gritty surface, it should be reaspirated with the largest cannula that will pass the cervix. If nothing can be aspirated, an ultrasonographic evaluation of the uterus should be conducted with the cannula in the uterine cavity. Sonography may reveal unsuspected uterine anomalies, such as an additional uterine horn or a septum, may demonstrate that the cannula is not actually within the uterine cavity, or may localize the retained products. Evacuation can then be carried out under direct ultrasonographic monitoring.

If there are no other explanations for excessive bleeding, a clotting disorder is possible. The diagnosis is made by assessing the clotting capacity of blood in a tube, measuring platelet and fibrinogen levels, as well as prothrombin and partial thromboplastin times. The values of fibrinogen degradation products may also be helpful in following this problem. Patients suspected of having disseminated intravascular coagulation (DIC) should have lost fluid volume rapidly replaced with whole blood, or, lacking that, lactated Ringer's solution, and be transferred to a facility with a blood bank that can provide specific replacement products such as fresh frozen plasma and cryoprecipitate. DIC can occur as an isolated condition or can accompany other complications such as hemorrhage, amniotic fluid embolus, or anesthetic toxicity.

Uterine Perforation

Perforation of the uterus during first trimester abortion occurs from 1 to 2 times per 1,000 operations.[25] Most commonly, perforations occur in the mid fundal area because the surgeon failed to identify a retroverted or retroflexed uterus prior to uterine sounding or cervical dilation. Useful preventive measures are the use of hydrophilic dilators, a bimanual examination immediately before every abortion procedure to determine uterine position, and elimination of uterine sounding.[26,27] If the uterus is not palpable, its location should be determined sonographically, or the direction of the cervical canal should be cautiously determined using a small caliber cervical dilator with its curve directed posteriorly as it traverses the cervical canal. If these measures are taken, many first trimester perforations can be avoided.[9] Uterine perforation rarely results in significant blood loss. The patient's vital signs, hematocrit, and abdominal pain and tenderness will diagnose the rare event of intra-abdominal hemorrhage. Patients who do not have significant blood loss, and for whom uterine evacuation is already completed, should be observed for 2 or 3 hours postoperatively. If their vital signs and hematocrit remain stable and they are without pain, patients can be discharged with cautions to telephone or return should pain or bleeding occur later.

If perforation has occurred and the uterus has not been completely evacuated, evacuation can usually be completed under ultrasonographic guidance by passing a flexible or rigid plastic cannula into the uterine cavity, taking care to avoid the perforation. To improve the image, fill the bladder when using an abdominal sector transducer, or use a small vaginal transducer. When ultrasonography is immediately available, laparoscopy is rarely needed to guide uterine evacuation.

Cervical Laceration

Cervical trauma is a relatively common but rarely serious complication of first trimester abortion, occurring about once per 100 abortions. It is more common when general anesthesia and forceful cervical dilation are employed.[27,28] Bleeding from the tenaculum site is unusual if an atraumatic (Bierer) tenaculum is used. Tenaculum site bleeding can usually be controlled by direct application of a sponge (ring) forceps to the bleeding site; the metal should be applied directly to the bleeding site, and the clamp completely closed over the cervical lip and left in place for 1–2 minutes. Cervical lacerations that continue to bleed can be sutured with O chromic catgut; a single figure of eight usually suffices.

Acute Hematometra

Postabortal hematometra or the "post abortion syndrome" occurs in about one in every 200 abortions and is most common in late first trimester and early second trimester abortions (11–14 weeks).[29] It is easily diagnosed and should be promptly treated. Symptoms include the rapid onset of post abortion pelvic pain, within an hour or two of surgery, without increased vaginal bleeding or changes in vital signs. Pelvic examination reveals a very tender and distended uterus. Treatment is prompt suction evacuation of the accumulated clot and blood, providing immediate relief and followed by intramuscular ergnovine, 0.2 mg, and two days of oral treatment, 0.2 mg tid.

Syncopal Episodes During or After Abortion

Syncopal episodes can be caused by vasovagal reaction, hyperventilation, toxic or allergic reactions to local anesthetics, or shock. Vasovagal reactions are by far the most common cause. The reaction ranges from uneasiness and diaphoresis to severe bradycardia and hypotension. Vasovagal reaction is usually diagnosed by noting bradycardia in response to cervical manipulation or dilation. Lowering the patient's head provides relief. Severe reactions can be treated with subcutaneous or intravenous atropine, 0.6 mg. Since mild vasovagal reactions are a common response to cervical manipulation, we routinely give a prophylactic dose of atropine, 0.4 mg, intravenously with the analgesic agent.

Hyperventilation can be a cause of syncope in abortion patients. It is a response to anxiety and sometimes occurs when patients "over breathe" as a relaxation technique for local anesthesia. It is often accompanied by an inability to breathe comfortably and circumoral paresthesia. Lightheadedness may progress to actual syncope as a result of cerebral vasoconstriction and peripheral vasodilation. It is prevented by helping the anxious patient to breathe deeply but slowly. Recovery is accelerated by re-breathing expired air from a paper bag in order to increase pCO_2.

Reactions to local anesthetics used in the paracervical block have a wide range of manifestations, including syncope. A majority of reactions are toxic and occur because the paracervical block is injected into a highly vascular area. Direct intravenous injection will cause immediate ringing in the patient's ears, occasionally accompanied by paresthesias and lightheadedness. A more profound reaction will lead to dizziness and, finally, syncope. Severe reactions are marked by seizures. Duration of the toxic reaction depends on the rapidity with which the anesthetic agent is cleared from the bloodstream. The amino esters (procaine and chloroprocaine) are rapidly hydrolyzed by plasma cholinesterase. Chloroprocaine is hydrolyzed 3–4 times faster than procaine and has a half-life of only 21 seconds. Amino amide local anesthetics (lidocaine, mepivacaine, bupivacaine) are metabolized at a much slower rate, and some of their metabolites can themselves cause toxic reactions. The elimination half-life of lidocaine, for example, is 1.6 hours. Metabolism occurs primarily in the liver rather than in the blood as for the ester anesthetics. A severe toxic reaction can result in sinus bradycardia, AV block, or even asystole. Severe hypotension, unconsciousness, generalized convulsions, and respiratory arrest can follow.[30] With ester anesthetics, these reactions are self-limited and rarely require treatment. With amide anesthetics, treatment consists of cardiopulmonary resuscitation support. Control of seizures can be achieved with intravenous diazepam, 10 mg.

Inadequate Products of Conception and Ectopic Pregnancy

Failure to identify fetal or placental tissue after first trimester pregnancy termination results from failure to aspirate the uterus, failure to detect products of conception in the aspirated specimen, or ectopic pregnancy. Since ectopic pregnancy is a life-threatening condition, each office or clinic should have a system for managing patients who have inadequate products of conception following uterine aspiration. Our approach is described here.

Counselors, nurses, and physicians should be alert to the possibility of an ectopic pregnancy in patients who report bleeding episodes since their last menstrual period, pelvic pain prior to requesting abortion, or who have risk factors such as a previous ectopic pregnancy, salpingitis, or tubal surgery. The possibility of an ectopic pregnancy should be considered when the physical examination reveals a uterus that seems small for the reported duration of gestation, presence of an adnexal mass, or the presence of unilateral pelvic tenderness. Offices or clinics that perform a high proportion of abortions early in gestation (prior to 8 weeks) have a special responsibility to diagnose ectopic pregnancy because patients with this condition may seek abortion prior to the onset of symptoms that would suggest the diagnosis.

For patients at high risk of ectopic pregnancy, a pelvic examination should be carried out immediately prior to uterine aspiration to assess uterine size, position, and detect adnexal tenderness or masses. If history and physical examination suggest that ectopic pregnancy is a possibility, the uterus should, if possible, be aspirated under sonographic guidance. If the cannula can be identified in the uterine cavity but no gestational sac is seen, ectopic pregnancy should be suspected. Occasionally an adnexal pregnancy will actually be seen, but this cannot be counted on to diagnose ectopic pregnancy.

Following aspiration, all collected tissue should be flushed from the hose and cannula with an isotonic solution for examination. If the aspirate is flushed with water, the villi collapse, making villi difficult to identify, and the opportunity to confirm an intrauterine pregnancy can be lost. In earlier gestations, we have found villi easiest to detect when the washed tissue is placed in a white, translucent plastic container (the kind typically used for pathological specimens) and spread over the bottom making the clear, tubular villi obvious in the light transmitted through the container. Another widely used method is to empty the washed material into a clear flat dish of isotonic solution that can then be set on a horizontally placed light source such as a slide viewer or an x-ray box. Light shining up through the bottom of the container will make easier the distinction between decidual tissue and the products of conception such as the gestational sac, the decidua capsularis, chorionic villi, or the embryo. The additional use of a hands lens is also helpful, especially in very early gestations.

If the surgeon cannot positively identify evidence of intrauterine gestation in the specimen, it should be sent to a pathologist with the diagnosis of "possible ectopic pregnancy" and a request for multiple sections to identify villi. Villi remaining in the uterus after a spontaneous abortion can be difficult to identify without staining because with time they lose their fluid content. Since the pain and bleeding of spontaneous abortion can be hard to distinguish from ectopic pregnancy, the pathologist should be informed that both possibilities are being considered.

If visual examination of the uterine aspirate does not confirm an intrauterine pregnancy, the surgeon must make certain that the uterus is really empty. The best approach is to re-examine the patient in order to detect uterine anomalies, such as a uterus didelphys, and adnexal masses or tenderness that might have been missed at the preoperative evaluation. Uterine aspiration should be repeated using intraoperative sonographic guidance, if available, to ensure that the cannula is correctly placed in the uterine cavity. If the cavity is, in fact, found to be empty, pregnancy should be confirmed with a test for the beta subunit of human chorionic gonadotropin (HCG). A highly sensitive urine test is sufficient. If such a test is positive, and if the patient is at high risk for an ectopic pregnancy from history, signs, or symptoms, treatment is indicated. If the test is positive but there are no risk factors for ectopic pregnancy, spontaneous abortion must be considered, and the HCG levels must be assessed over the following days. If HCG has not decreased or if signs or symptoms of an ectopic pregnancy develop, the patient should be treated laparoscopically or medically with methotrexate, depending on the size of the pregnancy and the clinical situation.

Delayed Complications

Delayed complications of abortion are those occurring several hours to several weeks after the operation. The vast majority of these occur within the first week following the operation, which is why post abortion follow-up should occur within a week of the procedure.

These complications can be classified by the symptoms they produce: bleeding, pain, or continuing symptoms of pregnancy. All 3 kinds of symptoms can be present in some patients (e.g., those with an ectopic pregnancy) while others can present with only a single symptom.

Delayed Bleeding. By far the most common cause of unusually heavy post abortal bleeding is retained products of conception, which follows one of every 200 abortions.[9] Patients with retained products of conception occasionally present several weeks after an abortion, but the great majority report excessive bleeding within one week. Patients may also report uterine contractions, but severe pain or pelvic tenderness suggests that infection is also present. If bleeding has been significant, the cervical os will usually be dilated and clots may be present in the vagina and cervical canal. Treatment is aspiration of the uterus with the largest cannula that will pass the cervix. Cervical dilation to 10 mm is occasionally required. Local anesthesia as described for the abortion procedure usually suffices.

Infection. Uterine tenderness and fever are the most common signs of post abortal endometritis. The risk of post abortion infections is decreased for women who have had previous deliveries and is increased for those with positive chlamydia or gonorrhea cultures.[31] Some studies indicate that prophylactic antibiotics reduce the risk of post abortal infection,[32,33] Most clinicians agree that women at risk of pelvic infection benefit from the use of prophylactic antibiotics prior to therapeutic abortion; others state that women who have not had a previous delivery should receive prophylaxis, while still others believe that all abortion patients would benefit from prophylactic antibiotics.[34,35] Because both gonorrhea and chlamydia, as well as other organisms, can cause post abortion infections, a tetracycline seems the best drug for prophylaxis. Doxycycline, 100 mg an hour before the abortion and 200 mg 30 minutes afterwards, is the most convenient and comprehensive regimen.[36] Tetracycline, 500 mg once before and once after the operation, is also acceptable. Metronidazole, 400 mg an hour before and 4–8 hours afterward, has been tested and is effective treatment for patients with bacterial vaginosis detected at the time of abortion.[37,38]

Patients who present with uterine tenderness, fever, and bleeding require antibiotic treatment as well as uterine reaspiration. The treatment regimen depends on the severity of the infection. Patients who have fevers above 37° (101° F) and signs of peritoneal as well as uterine tenderness require hospitalization and intravenous antibiotics. Outpatient treatment should be reserved for patients whose signs and symptoms are confined to the uterus; doxycycline, 100 mg bid for 10 days, metronidazole, 500 mg bid for 7 days, or amoxicillin and clavulanic acid (Augmentin), 250 mg tid for 7 days, depending on the suspected cause, are all appropriate treatments.

Cervical Stenosis. Patients who experience amenorrhea or hypomenorrhea and cyclic uterine pain after first trimester abortion may have stenosis of the internal os.[39] This condition is more common among women whose abortions are done in the early first trimester with a minimum of cervical dilation and a small diameter, flexible plastic cannula. A possible explanation is that the whistle tip of this type of cannula abrades the internal os and the minimal dilation allows the abraded areas to heal in contact. The result is an inability to pass menstrual effluent and accompanying pain. The condition is easily treated with cervical dilation under paracervical block using Pratt dilators.

Rh Sensitization. Approximately 4% of Rh negative women become sensitized following an induced abortion (a lower proportion in first trimester and a higher proportion in second trimester abortions).[40] Subsequent hemolytic disease of the newborn can be prevented by administering 50 μg of Rh immune globulin to all Rh negative, Du negative women undergoing abortion. A standard dose should be administered for second trimester abortion.

Medical Methods of First Trimester Abortion

Aspiration abortion is safe and effective, but it is not available everywhere, and some women find it difficult to undergo a surgical procedure or to go to a clinic where they may be subject to loss of privacy or harassment. Nonsurgical methods might make abortion available to more women and improve the circumstances under which pregnancies are terminated. Two such methods have undergone clinical testing. The progesterone antagonist mifepristone (RU486) and the antimetabolite methotrexate have both been demonstrated to induce abortion early in pregnancy when combined with a prostaglandin.

France and China were the first countries to approve the marketing of the medical abortifacient mifepristone (now available in Great Britain and Sweden as well), a synthetic relative of the progestational agents in oral contraceptives. Mifepristone acts primarily, but not totally, as an anti-progestational agent.

Both progesterone and RU486 form hormone responsive element-receptor complexes that are similar, but the RU486 complex has a slightly different conformational change (in the hormone binding domain) that prevents full gene activation. The agonistic activity of this progestin antagonist is due to its ability to activate certain, but not all, of the transcription activation functions on the progesterone receptor. The dimethyl (dimethylaminophenyl) side chain at carbon 11 is the principal factor in its antiprogesterone action. There are three major characteristics of its action which are important: a long half-life, high affinity for the progesterone receptor, and active metabolites.

It is likely that abortion with mifepristone is the result of multiple actions. Although mifepristone does not induce labor, it does open and soften the cervix (this may be an action secondary to endogenous prostaglandins). Its major action is its blockade of progesterone receptors in the endometrium. This leads to a disruption of the embryo and the production of prostaglandins. The disruption of the embryo and perhaps a direct action on the trophoblast lead to a decrease in human chorionic gonadotropin (HCG) and a withdrawal of support from the corpus luteum. The success rate is dependent upon the length of pregnancy — the more dependent the pregnancy is upon progesterone from the corpus luteum, the more likely the progesterone antagonist, mifepristone, will result in abortion. The combined mifepristone-prostaglandin analogue method is usually restricted to pregnancies that are not beyond 9 weeks gestation. Other progesterone antagonists have been developed, but only mifepristone has undergone extensive abortion trials. It seems unlikely that mifepristone could have serious adverse effects, and there have been none reported.

A single 600 mg oral dose of mifepristone is followed a day later by the administration of a prostaglandin analogue. Several analogues have been used but the most widely available and best tolerated is misoprostol (Cytotec), 800 mg administered vaginally.[41] The combination allows a reduction in dosage of both agents. When administered in the first 8 weeks of pregnancy, this medical termination results in a success and complication rate similar to that achieved with vacuum curettage.[42] Misoprostol is a stable, orally active synthetic analogue of prostaglandin E_1, available commercially for the treatment of peptic ulcer. By itself it is very ineffective for therapeutic abortion, but combined with mifepristone it provides an effective, simple, inexpensive, completely oral or vaginal method.[43,44]

Mifepristone is most noted for its abortifacient activity and the political controversy surrounding it. However, the combination of its agonistic and antagonistic actions can be exploited for many uses, including contraception, therapy of endometriosis, induction of labor, treatment of Cushing's syndrome, and, potentially, treatment of various cancers.

Lack of progesterone antagonists in the U.S. prompted use of methotrexate as an abortifacient in the same dose used to treat ectopic pregnancy, 50 mg intramuscularly per square meter of body surface area. As with mifepristone, a prostaglandin is added to promote expulsion of the uterine contents, and again vaginal misoprostol is the most useful analogue. The first trials demonstrated that if the prostaglandin was given a week after the injection of methotrexate, this method could be almost as effective as mifepristone.[45] Like mifepristone, efficacy diminishes with advancing gestation beyond 7 weeks (since the last menstrual period).[46–48] Because methotrexate takes longer to act than mifepristone, the prostaglandin is used a week after the initial treatment, and is repeated a day later if expulsion has not occurred. Methotrexate is easily available and inexpensive. It has been used in low doses to treat psoriasis and rheumatoid arthritis, as well as ectopic pregnancy, without adverse effects. It is, however, a known teratogen that can be deadly in high doses, and its use as an abortifacient results in prolonged bleeding and a prolonged time to abortion (up to a month in some cases). Mifepristone is preferable to clinicians who have experience with both methods. There are no direct comparison studies of methotrexate and mifepristone.

Abortion in the Second Trimester

Second trimester abortions can be accomplished surgically or medically. The surgical procedure is termed dilatation and evacuation (D&E). Unlike first trimester abortion, D&E requires extensive cervical dilation, to 1.5–2 cm to allow employment of special forceps (Sopher or Bierer forceps). These forceps can extract uterine contents that are too large for a 14 mm suction cannula. This change from aspiration to D&E occurs at about 14 weeks gestation.

Oral, vaginal, intramuscular, or intra-amniotic administration of prostaglandins, and the intra-amniotic injection of hypertonic saline or urea are the medical methods of second trimester abortion. The combination of mifepristone and misoprostol has been effectively used.[49] They all require the patient to go through labor in a hospital. The D&E procedure is safer and less expensive than medical methods, and it is better tolerated by patients.[50,51] In 1991, 87% of U.S. abortions 16–20 weeks and 80% of those over 20 weeks were by

D&E (however, only 11% of all induced abortions are second trimester abortions).[2]

Preoperative cervical dilatation with hydrophilic dilators (Laminaria or Dilapan) is essential for second trimester abortion.[52] Local rather than general anesthesia also makes second trimester abortion safer.[53,54] Some patients are not good candidates for surgical procedures of any kind under local anesthesia, and others may have special reasons to prefer that an abortion be performed under general anesthesia. Patient requests should be seriously considered, but the clinician also has a responsibility to inform the patient of the risks and benefits of local versus general anesthesia.

The training, experience, and skills of the surgeon are the primary factors that limit the gestational age at which abortion can be safely performed. Most surgeons can assess these factors for themselves and establish a rational limit for gestational age. The attitudes of the staff, including counselors, administrators, and nurses, the availability of emergency support, such as a nearby hospital willing and able to accept the transfer of complicated cases, are also important factors.

Advanced gestational age by itself incurs increased risks for all types of complications. These are multiplied when the duration of pregnancy is discovered, after beginning uterine evacuation, to be beyond the experience and skill of the surgeon or capacity of the equipment. Uterine perforation, infection, bleeding, amniotic fluid embolism, and anesthetic reactions are increased as gestational age increases.[50,55]

Although menstrual history and physical examination are adequate estimators of gestational age for the great majority of patients in early pregnancy, uterine ultrasonography offers a reliable alternative when these are in doubt. For patients whose pregnancies may exceed 16 weeks or be near the limit of a particular surgeon or clinic, or when complicating conditions are suspected such as ectopic pregnancy, uterine malformations, myomata, multiple or other abnormal gestations, fetal demise, or when uterine size and menstrual dates disagree, ultrasonographic measurements should be obtained. Published, generally accepted scales for converting crown-rump length, femur length, and biparietal diameter to menstrual weeks should be consistently applied to images provided by experienced sonographers. These measurements should be photographically documented for the patient's medical record. During D&E operations, real-time sonography helps the surgeon to accurately direct intrauterine forceps and can reduce the risk of uterine perforation, one of the primary hazards of D&E abortion.[56]

References

1. Henshaw SK, Van Vort J, Abortion services in the United States, 1991 and 1992, Fam Plann Perspect 26:100, 1994.

2. Koonin L, Smith J, Ramick M, Abortion surveillance—United States, 1991, MMWR 44(No. SS-2):23, 1995.

3. Henshaw SK, Induced abortions: a world review, 1990, Fam Plann Perspect 22:76, 1990.

4. Lawson H, Frye A, Atrash H, Smith J, Schulman H, Ramick M, Abortion mortality, United States, 1972 through 1987, Am J Obstet Gynecol 171:1365, 1994.

5. Lawson H, Atrash H, Saftlas A, Ectopic pregnancy surveillance, United States, 1970–1986, MMWR 38:11, 1989.

6. Grimes DA, Schulz KF, Cates W Jr, Tyler CW Jr, Local versus general anesthesia: which is safer for performing suction curettage abortions, Am J Obstet Gynecol 135:1030, 1979.

7. Peterson HB, Grimes DA, Cates W Jr, Rubin GL, Comparative risk of death from induced abortion at 12 weeks' gestation performed with local versus general anesthesia, Am J Obstet Gynecol 141:763, 1981.

8. Buehler J, Schulz K, Grimes D, Mogue C, The risk of serious complications from induced abortion: do personal characteristics make a difference? Am J Obstet Gynecol 153:14, 1985.

9. Hakim-Elahi E, Tovell H, Burnhill M, Complications of first trimester abortions: a report of 170,000 cases, Obstet Gynecol 76:129, 1990.

10. Hogue C, Impact of abortion on subsequent fertility, Clin Obstet Gynecol 13:96, 1986.

11. Stubblefield P, Monson R, Schoenbaum, Wolfson CE, Cookson DJ, Ryan KJ, Fertility after induced abortion: a prospective follow-up study, Obstet Gynecol 62:186, 1984.

12. Daling J, Weiss N, Voigt I, Spadoni LR, Soderstrom R, Moore DE, Stadel BV, Tubal infertility in relation to prior induced abortion, Fertil Steril 43:389, 1985.

13. Schoenbaum S, Monson R, Stubblefield P, Darney PD, Ryan KJ, Outcome of the delivery following an induced or spontaneous abortion, Am J Obstet Gynecol 136:19, 1980.

14. Frank PI, McNamee R, Hannaford PC, Kay CR, Hirsch S, The effect of induced abortion on subsequent pregnancy outcome, Br J Obstet Gynecol 98:1015, 1991.

15. Daling J, Chow W, Weiss N, Metch BT, Soderstrom R, Ectopic pregnancy in relation to previous induced abortion, JAMA 253:1005, 1985.

16. **MacKenzie I, Fox A,** A prospective self-controlled study of fertility after second trimester prostaglandin-induced abortion, Am J Obstet Gynecol 158:1137, 1988.

17. **Dagg PKB,** The psychological sequelae of therapeutic abortion — denied and completed, Am J Psychiatry 148:578, 1991.

18. **Newcomb PA, Storer BE, Longnecker MP, Mittendorf R, Greenberg ER, Willett WC,** Pregnancy termination in relation to risk of brest cancer, JAMA 275:283, 1996.

19. **Gammon MD, Bertin JE, Terry MB,** Abortion and the risk of breast cancer. Is there a believable association?, JAMA 275:321, 1996.

20. **Landy U, Lewit S,** Administrative, counseling, and medical practices in National Abortion Federation facilities, Fam Plann Persepct 14:257, 1982.

21. **Landy U,** Abortion counseling — a new component of medical care, Clinics Obstet Gynecol 13:33, 1986.

22. **Darney P, Dorward K,** Cervical dilation before first-trimester elective abortion: a controlled comparison of meteneprost, laminaria and hypan, Obstet Gynecol 70:397, 1987.

23. **Kline S, Meng H, Munsick R,** Cervical dilation from laminaria tents and synthetic osmotic dilators used for 6 hours before abortion, Obstet Gynecol 86:931, 1995.

24. **Wiebe ER,** Comparison of the efficacy of different local anesthetics and techniques of local anesthesia in therapeutic abortions, Am J Obstet Gynecol 167:131, 1992.

25. **Lindell G, Flam F,** Management of uterine perforations in connection with legal abortions, Acta Obstet Gynecol Scand 74:373, 1995.

26. **Grimes D, Schulz K, Cates W Jr,** Prevention of uterine perforation during curettage abortion, JAMA 257:2108, 1983.

27. **Cates W, Schulz K, Grimes D,** The risks associated with teenage abortion, New Engl J Med 379:621, 1983.

28. **Schulz KF, Grimes DA, Cates W Jr,** Measures to prevent cervical injury during suction curettage abortion, Lancet 1:1182, 1983.

29. **Sands RX, Burnhill MS, Hakim-Elahi E,** Post-abortal uterine atony, Obstet Gynecol 43:595, 1974.

30. **Grimes DA, Cates W Jr,** Deaths from paracervical anesthesia used for first trimester abortion, New Engl J Med 295:1397, 1976.

31. **Burkman RT, Tonascia JA, Atienza MF, King TM,** Untreated endocervical gonorrhea and endometritis following elective abortion, Am J Obstet Gynecol 126:648, 1976.

32. **Brewer C,** Prevention of infection after abortion with a supervised single dose of doxycycline, Br Med J 281:780, 1980.

33. Hodgson JE, Major B, Portmann K, Quattlebaum FW, Prophylactic use of tetracycline for first trimester abortions, Obstet Gynecol 45:574, 1975.

34. Park T-X, Flock M, Schulz KF, Grimes DA, Preventing febrile complications of suction curettage abortion, Am J Obstet Gynecol 152:252, 1985.

35. Darj E, Stralin E, Nilsson S, The prophylactic effect of doxycycline on postoperative infection rate after first trimester abortion, Obstet Gynecol 70:755, 1987.

36. Levallois P, Rioux J, Prophylactic antibiotics for suction curettage abortion: results of a clinical controlled trial, Am J Obstet Gynecol 158:100, 1988.

37. Heisterberg L, Petersen K, Metronidazole prophylaxis in elective first trimester abortion, Obstet Gynecol 65:371, 1985.

38. Larsson PG, Platz-Christensen JJ, Thejls H, Forsum U, Pahlson C, Incidence of pelvic inflammatory disease after first trimester legal abortion in women with bacterial vaginosis after treatment with metronidazole: a double-blind, randomized study, Am J Obstet Gynecol 166:100, 1992.

39. Hakim-Elahi E, Postabortal amenorrhea due to cervical stenosis, Obstet Gynecol 48:723, 1976.

40. Grimes D, Ross W, Hutchen R, Rh immunoglobulin utilization after spontaneous and induced abortion, Obstet Gynecol 57:261, 1977.

41. El-Rafaey HJ, Rajasekar D, Abdalla M, Calder L, Templeton A, Induction of abortion with mifepristone (RU 486) and oral or vaginal misoprostol, New Engl J Med 332:983, 1995.

42. Silvestre L, Dubois C, Renault M, Rezvani Y, Baulieu EE, Ulmann A, Voluntary interruption of pregnancy with Mifepristone (RU 486) and a prostaglandin analogue, New Engl J Med 322:645, 1990.

43. Thong KJ, Baird DT, Induction of abortion with mifepristone and misoprostol in early pregnancy, Br J Obstet Gynaecol 99:1004, 1992.

44. Peyron R, Aubeny E, Targosz V, Silvestre L, Renault M, Elkik F, Leclerc P, Ulmann A, Baulieu EE, Early termination of pregnancy with mifepristone (RU 486) and the orally active prostaglandin misoprostol, New Engl J Med 328:1509, 1993.

45. Creinin M, Darney P, Methotrexate and misoprostol for early abortion, Contraception 48:339, 1993.

46. Creinin MD, Vittinghoff E, Methotrexate and misoprostol vs misoprostol alone for early abortion. A randomized controlled trial, JAMA 272:1190, 1994.

47. Creinin MD, Park M, Acceptablility of medical abortion with methotrexate and misoprostol, Contraception 52:41, 1995.

48. Hausknecht RU, Methotrexate and misoprostol to terminate early pregnancy, New Engl J Med 333:538, 1995.

49. El-Rafaey H, Templeton A, Induction of abortion in the second trimester by a combination of misoprostol and mifepristone: a randomized comparison between two misoprostol regimens, Hum Reprod 10:475, 1995.

50. Grimes DA, Schulz KF, Cates W Jr, Tyler CW, Midtrimester abortion by dilation and evacuation, New Engl J Med 296:1141, 1977.

51. Kafrissen M, Schulz K, Grimes D, Cates W Jr, Midtrimester abortion: intra amniotic instillation of hyperosmolar urea and prostaglandin $F_{2\alpha}$ v dilatation and evacuation, JAMA 251:916, 1984.

52. Darney PD, Atkinson E, Hirabayashi K, Uterine perforation during second trimester abortion by cervical dilation and instrumental extraction: a review of 15 cases, Obstet Gynecol 75:441, 1990.

53. Mackay T, Schulz K, Grimes D, Safety of local versus general anesthesia for second trimester dilatation and evacuation abortion, Obstet Gynecol 66:661, 1985.

54. Atrash H, Chelk T, Hogue C, Legal abortion and general anesthesia, Am J Obstet Gynecol 158:420, 1988.

55. Peterson WF, Berry FN, Grace MR, Gulbranson CL, Second trimester abortion by dilatation and evacuation: an analysis of 11,747 cases, Obstet Gynecol 62:185, 1983.

56. Darney PD, Sweet RL, Routine intraoperative ultrasonography for second trimester abortion reduces the incidence of uterine perforation, J Ultrasound Med 8:71, 1989.

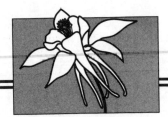

Epilogue

AND SO WE REACH our final paragraph. We do so with optimism. This book documents, within a tick of planet Earth's time, tremendous accomplishments in contraception. These accomplishments reflect initiative, creativity, and dedication. There is reason to believe, as we do, that these human traits will persevere, and we will meet the contraceptive challenges of the future.

Index